a **CORE Curriculum for Diabetes Education**
Fourth Edition

Diabetes Education and Program Management

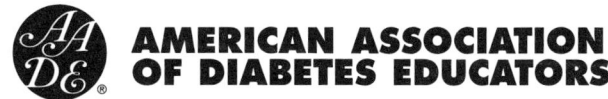

a CORE
Curriculum
for Diabetes
Education
Fourth Edition

Diabetes Education and Program Management

Editor
Marion J. Franz, MS, RD, LD, CDE
Associate Editors
Karmeen Kulkarni, MS, RD, BC-ADM, CDE
William H. Polonsky, PhD, CDE
Peggy Yarborough, MS, RPh, BC-ADM, CDE
Virginia Zamudio, MSN, RN, CDE

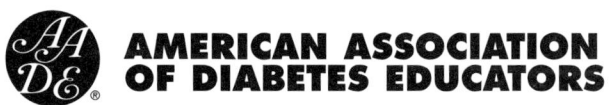

a CORE Curriculum for Diabetes Education, 4th Edition
Diabetes Education and Program Management
Published by the American Association of Diabetes Educators

©2001, American Association of Diabetes Educators, Chicago, Illinois.
ISBN 1-881876-07-1 (Volume Three)
ISBN 1-881876-09-8 (Four-Volume Set)

Library of Congress Control Number: 2001091533

Printed and bound in the United States of America.

All rights reserved. No part of this work covered by copyright herein may be reproduced or copied in any form or by any means—graphic, electronic, or mechanical, including photocopying, recording, or information storage and retrieval systems—without written permission of the publisher.

The information contained in this publication is based on the collective experience of the diabetes educators who assisted in its production. Reasonable steps have been taken to make it as accurate as possible based on published evidence as of March 2001. But the Association cannot warrant the safety or efficacy of any product or procedure described in this publication for application in specific cases. Individuals are advised to consult an appropriate healthcare professional before undertaking any diet or exercise program or taking any medication referred to in this publication. Healthcare professionals must use their own professional judgment, experience, and training in applying the information contained herein. The American Association of Diabetes Educators and its officers, directors, employees, agents, and members assume no liability whatsoever for any personal or other injury, loss, or damages that may result from use of this publication.

a CORE Curriculum for Diabetes Education

Diabetes Education and Program Management

In this Volume:

Table of Contents

Introduction/Acknowledgements vii

Editors ix

Authors x

Reviewers xii

Diabetes Education and Program Management

1 Applied Principles of Teaching and Learning 3

2 Psychosocial Assessment 25

3 Behavior Change 67

4 Cultural Competence in Diabetes Education and Care 99

5 Teaching Persons With Low Literacy Skills 123

6 Psychological Disorders 147

7 Management of Diabetes Education Programs 181

8 Payment for Diabetes Education 225

Index 255

Other Volumes in Core Curriculum, 4th Edition:

Diabetes and Complications

1 Pathophysiology of the Diabetes Disease State
2 Hyperglycemia
3 Chronic Complications of Diabetes: An Overview
4 Diabetic Foot Care and Education
5 Skin and Dental Care
6 Macrovascular Disease
7 Eye Disease and Adaptive Diabetes Education for Visually Impaired Persons
8 Nephropathy
9 Diabetic Neuropathy

Diabetes Management Therapies

1 Medical Nutrition Therapy for Diabetes
2 Exercise
3 Pharmacologic Therapies
4 Monitoring
5 Pattern Management of Blood Glucose
6 Insulin Pump Therapy and Carbohydrate Counting for Pump Therapy: Carbohydrate-to-Insulin Ratios
7 Hypoglycemia
8 Illness and Surgery

Diabetes in the Life Cycle and Research

1 Diabetes During Childhood and Adolescence
2 Pregnancy: Preconception to Postpartum
3 Gestational Diabetes
4 Diabetes in Older Adults
5 Lifestyle for Diabetes Prevention
6 Biological Complementary Therapies in Diabetes
7 The Importance of Research and Outcomes

Introduction/Acknowledgements

It is a very exciting and challenging time for diabetes educators. Exciting because of the many advances that help people with diabetes to better manage their diabetes—new medications, technologies, research that makes lifestyle recommendations easier to understand and apply, the empowerment approach to education—to name just a few. The challenges and frustrations are the difficulties of sharing this information with individuals with diabetes, the lack of opportunities to individualize care, and the lack of time to assist in facilitating behavior changes. Resources—personnel, payment for services, training new educators—are other challenges. Although for years the person with diabetes has been acknowledged as the center of the diabetes team and the person who makes the final decision on what he/she is willing and able to do, often the individual with diabetes is still left out of the decision-making process. The Core Curriculum, 4th Edition cannot solve all the challenges but it can update the educator's knowledge and provide suggestions for skills to assist in facilitating necessary behavior changes for persons with diabetes.

The Core Curriculum was originally planned to help educators prepare for the Certified Diabetes Educator (CDE) exam. This has continued to be a goal for subsequent editions; however, the use and the scope of the Core Curriculum has expanded. It is a key reference for the Advanced Diabetes Management credential exam. Furthermore, the Core Curriculum has evolved into being a diabetes educator's authoritative source of information for diabetes education and management. One of the objectives of this edition is to move this goal one step further ahead. Just as all medicine is moving toward evidence-based practice, this must also be a goal for education. Chapters must have appropriate and adequate references and as a reader you have the right to question statements in the Core Curriculum that do not have adequate documentation. As all of us continue this focus, the Core Curriculum will truly become an evidence-based document.

As with all projects of this magnitude, there are many individuals to whom we are indebted. It begins with the chapter authors who have been willing to share their expertise and provide up-to-date information and management skills for the reader. It continues to the chapter reviewers who provide suggestions to make the chapters stronger. The authors and reviewers are listed in each volume of the Core Curriculum. As an educator, when you see these individuals please extend your thanks to them for the valuable service they have provided. The Associate Editors—Karmeen Kulkarni, William Polonsky, Peggy Yarborough, Virginia Zamudio—have provided valuable assistance in moving the process along efficiently and synthesizing the reviewers' comments to the chapter authors. Dr. Lois Book, RN, Director of Professional Relations, and Kaitrin Hall at the AADE National Office have also provided valuable suggestions for core content and support for the process of writing and editing of the Core Curriculum. We have all been fortunate to work with very competent editorial and publishing professionals. Mary Beach and Jim West at Stenson Bauer Communications have kept the process moving efficiently. Karen Lloyd has provided editorial assistance for the new chapters. Nancy Williams has used her copyreader and editing skills to make sure small details and mistakes were not missed and Michele Montour at Montronics made sure text was accurately typeset. To all these fine professionals, the AADE owes a great deal of gratitude.

But this fourth edition of the Core Curriculum with the new four-volume format would not have been possible without the contributions of previous Core editors. I am proud to join this elite group of educators beginning with Diana Guthrie, Julie Meyer, Kathryn Godley, Virginia Peragallo-Dittko, and continuing to Martha Funnell, editor of the third edition. Each edition has moved the professionalism of the Core forward and, hopefully, we have continued this process. There is still work ahead to make the Core truly evidence-based, and I look forward to future editions.

As authors, reviewers, and editors we have done our best to make this edition of the Core Curriculum a valuable resource for all diabetes educators. We welcome suggestions from you, the reader and professional, who will be using the Core as to how we can continue to make the Core Curriculum better and stronger. But for today, I personally am very proud of this edition. Please use this edition to improve the education and care that you provide for people with diabetes. That ultimately is the final goal, to enrich the lives of persons with diabetes who have been, for all of us, our best educators!

Marion J. Franz, MS, RD, LD, CDE
Editor, Core Curriculum, 4th Edition

Editor

Marion J. Franz, MS, RD, LD, CDE
Nutrition Concepts by Franz, Inc.
Minneapolis, Minnesota

Associate Editors

Karmeen Kulkarni, MS, RD, BC-ADM, CDE
St. Marks Hospital Diabetes Center
Salt Lake City, Utah

William H. Polonsky, PhD, CDE
Department of Psychiatry
University of California
San Diego, California

Peggy Yarborough, MS, RPh, BC-ADM, CDE
Campbell University and Wilson Community Health Center
Wilson, North Carolina

Virginia Zamudio, RN, MSN, CDE
Alamo Diabetes Team
San Antonio, Texas

Authors

Jessie H. Ahroni,
PhD, ARNP, CDE
Veterans Affairs Puget Sound
Health Care System
School of Nursing, University
of Washington
Seattle, Washington

Robert M. Anderson, EdD
Michigan Diabetes Research
and Training Center
University of Michigan
Ann Arbor, Michigan

James D. Anderst, MD
Medical College of Wisconsin
Milwaukee, Wisconsin

Mindy Andrus,
RD, LDN, CDE
East Carolina University
Brody School of Medicine
Greenville, North Carolina

Susan L. Barlow, RD, CDE
Amylin Pharmaceuticals, Inc.
Indianapolis, Indiana

Marla Bernbaum, MD
St. Louis University Health
Sciences Center
Division of Endocrinology
St. Louis, Missouri

Jean Betschart,
MSN, MN, CPNP, CDE
Children's Hospital
of Pittsburgh
Pittsburgh, Pennsylvania

Susan A. Biastre,
RD, LDN, CDE
Women & Infants' Hospital
Providence, Rhode Island

Ann Marie Brooks, RN, CDE
St. Marks Hospital
Diabetes Center
Salt Lake City, Utah

R. Keith Campbell,
RPh, MBA, CDE
Washington State University
Spokane, Washington

Belinda P. Childs, RN, MN,
ARNP, CDE
Mid-America Diabetes
Associates
Wichita, Kansas

Beth Ann Coonrod, PhD,
MPH, RN, CDE
Heritage Valley Health
System
Beaver and Sewickley,
Pennsylvania

Angela D'Antonio, RD
University of South Carolina
Norman J. Arnold School of
Public Health
Columbia, South Carolina

Mayer B. Davidson, MD
Charles R. Drew University
Los Angeles, California

Kristina L. Ernst,
BSN, RN, CDE
Atlanta, Georgia

James A. Fain,
PhD, RN, FAAN
University of Massachusetts
Worcester
Graduate School of Nursing
Worcester, Massachusetts

Eva L. Feldman, MD, PhD
Department of Neurology
University of Michigan
Medical School
Ann Arbor, Michigan

Marion J. Franz,
MS, RD, LD, CDE
Nutrition Concepts
by Franz, Inc.
Minneapolis, Minnesota

Martha Mitchell Funnell,
MS, RN, CDE
Michigan Diabetes Research
and Training Center
University of Michigan
Medical Center
Ann Arbor, Michigan

Patti Geil, MS, RD, CDE
Lexington, Kentucky

Linda Gonder-Frederick, PhD
University of Virginia
Behavioral Medicine Center
Charlottesville, Virginia

Diana W. Guthrie,
RN, ARNP, FAAN, CDE
Professor Emeritus
University of Kansas School
of Medicine
Wichita, Kansas

Richard A. Guthrie,
MD, CDE
Mid-America Diabetes
Associates
Via Christi Regional
Medical Center
University of Kansas School
of Medicine
Wichita, Kansas

Deborah Hinnen,
RN, MN, ARNP,
BC-ADM, CDE
Via Christi Regional
Medical Center
Wichita, Kansas

Carol Homko,
RN, PhD, CDE
Temple University Hospital
Philadelphia, Pennsylvania

Cheryl Hunt,
RN, MSEd, CDE
Health Education
and Resources
Alexandria, Virginia

Donna Jornsay,
BSN, RN, CPNP, CDE
MiniMed
Great Neck, New York

Elaine Boswell King,
MSN, RN, CS, CDE
Vanderbilt Diabetes Research
and Training Center
Nashville, Tennessee

Karmeen Kulkarni,
MS, RD, BC-ADM, CDE
St. Marks Hospital
Diabetes Center
Salt Lake City, Utah

Janie Lipps,
MSN, RN, CS, CDE
Vanderbilt Diabetes Research
and Training Center
Nashville, Tennessee

Nancy Leggett-Frazier,
RN, MSN, CDE
East Carolina University
Brody School of Medicine
Greenville, North Carolina

Elizabeth J. Mayer-Davis,
PhD, RD
University of South Carolina
Norman J. Arnold School of
Public Health
Columbia, South Carolina

Stephania Miller, PhD
Diabetes Research and
Training Center
Vanderbilt University
School of Medicine
Nashville, Tennessee

Catherine A. Mullooly,
MS, RCEP_{SM}, CDE
Joslin Clinic
Boston, Massachusetts

Kathryn Mulcahy,
RN, MSN, CDE
Fairfax Hospital INOVA
Diabetes Center
Fairfax, Virginia

Joseph P. Napora,
PhD, LCSW-C
The Johns Hopkins
University School of Medicine
The Johns Hopkins
Diabetes Center
Baltimore, Maryland

Anne T. Nettles,
RN, MS, CDE
Healthcare Consultant
Minneapolis, Minnesota

Jan Norman, RD, CDE
Washington Department
of Health
Diabetes Control Program
Olympia, Washington

Virginia Peragallo-Dittko,
RN, MA, CDE
Diabetes Education Center
Winthrop-University Hospital
Mineola, New York

Michael A. Pfeifer,
MD, FACE, CDE
East Carolina University
Brody School of Medicine
Greenville, North Carolina

James W. Pichert, PhD
Diabetes Research and
Training Center
Vanderbilt University
Nashville, Tennessee

Robert E. Ratner, MD, CDE
Medstar Research Institute
Washington, DC

Lynne S. Robbins, PhD
University of Washington
Department of
Medical Education
Seattle, Washington

Richard R. Rubin, PhD, CDE
The Johns Hopkins
University School of Medicine
Departments of Medicine
and Pediatrics
Baltimore, Maryland

Stephanie Schwartz,
MPH, RN, CDE
Children With Diabetes .Com
Ann Arbor, Michigan

Laura Shane-McWhorter,
PharmD, BCPS, FASCP, CDE
College of Pharmacy
University of Utah
Salt Lake City, Utah

Tamara Stich,
RN, MSN, CDE
Washington University School
of Medicine
Department of Metabolism
St. Louis, Missouri

Catrine Tudor-Locke, PhD
University of South Carolina
Norman J. Arnold School of
Public Health
Columbia, South Carolina

Frank Vinicor, MD, MPH
Centers for Disease
Control and Prevention
Division of Diabetes
Translation
Atlanta, Georgia

John R. White, Jr.,
RPh, PharmD, PA-C
Washington State University
Spokane, Washington

Peggy C. Yarborough,
RPh, MS, BC-ADM, CDE
Campbell University and
Wilson Community
Health Center
Wilson, North Carolina

Reviewers

Barbara J. Anderson, PhD
Joslin Diabetes Center
Harvard University School
of Medicine
Boston, Massachusetts

Gary M. Arsham, MD, PhD
Arsham Consultants, Inc.
San Francisco, California

Anita K. Austin, RPh, CDE
University of Pittsburgh
Physicians
Pittsburgh, Pennsylvania

David W. Bartels,
PharmD, CDE
University of Illinois at
Chicago College of Pharmacy
Department of Pharmacy
Practice and College of
Medicine at Rockford
Department of Family and
Community Medicine

David S. Bell, MD
University of Alabama
Medical School
Birmingham, Alabama

Kathy J. Berkowitz,
RNC, FNP, CDE
Diabetes Unit, Grady
Health System
Atlanta, Georgia

Liz Blair, ANP, CDE
Joslin Diabetes Center
Boston, Massachusetts

Barbara H. Bodnar,
RN, MS, CDE
West Virginia University
Morgantown, West Virginia

John B. Buse, MD, PhD, CDE
University of North Carolina
Diabetes Care Center
Durham, North Carolina

Denise Charron-Prochownik,
PhD, RN, CPNP
University of Pittsburgh
School of Nursing/
Health Promotion
Pittsburgh, Pennsylvania

Belinda Childs, RN, MN,
ARNP, CDE
Mid-America Diabetes
Associates, PA
Wichita, Kansas

Beth Ann Coonrod,
PhD, MPH, RN, CDE
Heritage Valley Health
System
Beaver and Sewickley,
Pennsylvania

Alicia Correa,
RN, BSN, MBA
Texas Diabetes Institute
San Antonio, Texas

Marjorie Cypress,
MSN, C-ANP, CDE
Lovelace Medical Center
Endocrinology/Diabetes
Department
Albuquerque, New Mexico

Anne Daly,
MS, RD, LD, BC-ADM, CDE
Springfield Diabetes and
Endocrine Center
Springfield, Illinois

Mary Ellinger, RD, CDE
Diabetes Self Care,
Matria Healthcare
Centreville, Virginia

Janine Freeman,
RD, LD, CDE
Diabetes Nutrition Specialist
Atlanta, Georgia

Sandra J. Gillespie,
MMSc, RD, LD, CDE
Diabetes Resource Center
Piedmont Hospital
Atlanta, Georgia

Russell E. Glasgow, PhD
AMC Cancer Research
Center
Denver, Colorado

Kathryn Godley,
MS, RN, CDE
Albany Medical College
Albany, New York

Marilyn R. Graff,
RN, BSN, CDE
MiniMed Professional
Education Department
Sylmar, California

Richard A. Guthrie,
MD, FCAP, CDE
Mid-America Diabetes
Associates, Inc.
Wichita, Kansas

Leo E. Hendricks,
PhD, LICSW, CDE
LHCA's Diabetes Self-
Management Skills
Training Center
Silver Springs, Maryland

Rosetta T. Hendricks,
PhD, RN, CS, FNP, CDE
Veterans Affairs
Medical Center
Washington, DC

Lea Ann Holzmeister,
RD, CDE
Nutrition Consultant
Tempe, Arizona

David Holtzman
Director of
Government Affairs
American Association of
Diabetes Educators
Chicago, Illinois

Bonnie Irvin,
MS, RD, LD, CDE
Iredell Memorial Hospital
Health Care System
Diabetes Center for Learning
Statesville, North Carolina

Timothy J. Ives,
PharmD, MPH
Department of
Family Medicine
University of North Carolina
Chapel Hill, North Carolina

Scott J. Jacober, DO, CDE
Eli Lilly & Co.
Indianapolis, Indiana

Dennis Janisse, CPed
National Pedorthic Services
Milwaukee, Wisconsin

Jane Kadohiro,
DrPH, APRN, CDE
University of Hawaii School
of Nursing and
Dental Hygiene
Honolulu, Hawaii

Ginger Kanzer-Lewis,
RNC, EdM, CDE
GKL Associates
Pomona, New York

Wahida Karmally,
MS, RD, CDE
The Irving Center for Clinical
Research, Columbia
University
New York, New York

Julienne K. Kirk,
PharmD, CDE, BCPS
Department of Family
Medicine
Wake Forest University
School of Medicine
Winston-Salem,
North Carolina

Davida F. Kruger,
MSN, RN, BC-ADM, CDE
Henry Ford Health Systems
Endocrinology/Metabolism
Detroit, Michigan

Andrea J. Lasichak,
MS, RD, CDE
Michigan Diabetes Research
Training Center
University of
Michigan Hospital
Ann Arbor, Michigan

Daniel Lorber,
MD, FACP, CDE
Diabetes Control Foundation
Flushing, New York

Melinda D. Maryniuk,
MEd, RD, FADA, CDE
Joslin Diabetes Center
Boston, Massachusetts

Susan McLaughlin, RD, CDE
On-Site Health &
Wellness, LLC
Omaha, Nebraska

Arlene Monk, RD, LD, CDE
International Diabetes Center
Minneapolis, Minnesota

Arshag D. Mooradian, MD
St. Louis University Medical
Center Division of
Endocrinology
St. Louis, Missouri

Charlotte Reese Nath,
MSN, RN, EdD, CDE
West Virginia University
Department of Family
Medicine
Robert C. Byrd Health
Sciences Center
Morgantown, West Virginia

Jan Nicollerat,
MSN, RN, CS, CDE
Duke University Adult
Diabetes Education Program
Cary, North Carolina

Jan Norman, RD, CD, CDE
Washington State
Department of Health
Olympia, Washington

Belinda O'Connell,
MS, RD, CDE
International Diabetes Center
Minneapolis, Minncsota

Joyce G. Pastors,
RD, MS, CDE
Virginia Center for Diabetes
Professional Education
Charlottesville, Virginia

Teresa L. Pearson,
MS, RN, CDE
Health Partners Center for
Health Promotion
Minneapolis, Minnesota

Suzanne Pecoraro,
RD, MPH, CDE
Diabetes Education Society
Denver, Colorado

Martha Price,
DNSc, ARNP, CDE
Group Health Cooperative
Diabetes Clinical Roadmap
Seattle, Washington

Diane M. Reader, RD, CDE
International Diabetes Center
Minneapolis, Minnesota

Dawn Satterfield,
RNC, MSN, CDE
Centers for Disease Control
and Prevention
Division of Diabetes
Translation
Atlanta, Georgia

J. Terry Saunders, PhD
Virginia Center for Diabetes
Professional Education
Charlottesville, Virginia

Pamela Scarborough,
PT, MS, CDE, CWS
Education 2000 Plus
Dallas, Texas

Gary Scheiner, MS, CDE
Integrated Diabetes Services
Wynnewood, Pennsylvania

Barbara Schreiner,
RN, MN, BC-ADM, CDE
Texas Children's Hospital
Diabetes Care Center
Houston, Texas

Michelle Burdette-Taylor
BT & T Health Education
with a Purpose
San Diego, California

Christine Tobin,
RN, MBA, CDE
Health Care Consultant
Atlanta, Georgia

Elizabeth A. Walker,
RN, DNSc, CDE
Albert Einstein College
of Medicine
Diabetes Research and
Training Center
Bronx, New York

Hope S. Warshaw,
MMSc, RD, CDE
Hope Warshaw Associates
Alexandria, Virginia

Madelyn L. Wheeler,
MS, RD, FADA, CDE
Diabetes Research and
Training Center
Indiana University School
of Medicine
Indianapolis, Indiana

Neil H. White, MD, CDE
Pediatric Endocrinology and
Metabolism
Washington University
St. Louis, Missouri

Ann Sawyer Williams,
MSN, RN, CDE
Cleveland Heights, Ohio

Donald N. Zettervall,
RPH, CDE
The Diabetes Center
Old Saybrook, Connecticut

A Core Curriculum for Diabetes Education
Diabetes Education and Program Management

Applied Principles of Teaching and Learning   1

Robert M. Anderson, EdD
Michigan Diabetes Research and Training Center
University of Michigan
Ann Arbor, Michigan

Introduction
1. Many of the chapters in this core curriculum are concerned with the content of diabetes self-management education programs; that is, they discuss the knowledge and skills to be acquired by persons with diabetes.

2. Diabetes educators need to be knowledgeable about diabetes, but they also need to be skilled teachers to be effective.

3. This chapter is concerned with the educational process relevant to diabetes self-management education and focuses on the program design and educational methods used to help individuals learn about diabetes.

4. How diabetes knowledge and skills are taught can have as much impact on patient outcomes as what is taught.

5. The instructional design of a diabetes self-management education program can affect the patients' acquisition of knowledge and skills, their attitudes about diabetes, their motivation to practice appropriate diabetes self-care, their willingness and ability to change behavior, and their degree of psychosocial adjustment to diabetes.

Objectives
Upon completion of this chapter, the learner will be able to
1. Explain the similarities and differences between the compliance and empowerment approaches to self-management education.
2. Describe 9 issues to consider when designing a diabetes self-management education program.
3. Explain the similarities and differences between formative and summative evaluation.
4. Explain the rationale for employing a multidisciplinary team in diabetes education.
5. List 8 areas to consider when assessing an individual's needs and readiness to learn.
6. Describe 4 characteristics of adult learners.
7. List 10 teaching and learning strategies used in diabetes self-management education.
8. Describe 7 techniques that can be used to enhance learning and decision making.
9. Explain the importance of education follow-up for persons with diabetes.

Approaches to Education
1. The *compliance-based approach*[1-3] to diabetes patient education is intended to improve patient adherence to the treatment recommendations of healthcare professionals.
    A. This approach is based on the assumption that healthcare professionals are diabetes care experts and that patients should, in most cases, comply with their recommendations regarding diabetes self-care.
    B. Patient education is seen as a means of influencing patients to follow treatment recommendations to improve their glucose control and prevent the short- and long-term complications of diabetes.

2 In the *empowerment approach*,[4-8] the primary purpose of diabetes self-management education is to prepare persons with diabetes to make informed decisions about their own diabetes care.
   A This approach assumes that most persons with diabetes are responsible for making important and complex decisions while carrying out the daily treatment of their diabetes.
   B The empowerment approach also assumes that because patients are the ones who experience the consequences of having and treating diabetes, they have both the right and responsibility to be the primary decision makers regarding their own daily diabetes care.

3 Very few educators use one approach all the time to the exclusion of the other approach. Furthermore, educators often adopt a primary approach, which is an amalgam of, or a compromise between, the two approaches.
   A Most educators will use some combination of the 2 approaches based on their own values and understanding of the purposes and methods of patient education as well as the needs of their patients. Thus, instead of the approaches being dichotomous, the approach used is a continuum between the poles of the 2 approaches described above.
   B Patients will have varying needs and tolerance for autonomous decision-making in their diabetes self-care based on a number of factors. For example, a newly diagnosed patient with diabetes may wish to have the majority of decisions made by the healthcare team until he or she becomes more familiar with the cost and benefits of various options in diabetes self-care.

Consideration in the Design of Self-Management Education Programs

1 An education program needs to be designed to fit a particular setting and group of patients. It is important to gear program and educational materials to the disease type, age, education, experience, needs, abilities, and cultural background of participants.

2 Program philosophy is an important consideration because it shapes the design and conduct of the program.[9]
   A The program educators need to agree on whether they believe in the compliance approach, the empowerment approach, or some other educational philosophy that expresses the values and sense of purpose shared among the program educators.
   B A written philosophy statement can be a very useful tool for developing and expressing the program philosophy.[10]
   C The program philosophy provides the context for program goals and objectives and for each patient encounter and educational session.

3 Designing a diabetes self-management education program requires first selecting appropriate goals and objectives and then determining the level(s) of comprehensiveness for the program (ie, deciding what material to include and in what depth).
   A Diabetes self-management education programs need clear and realistic goals. These goals can be somewhat general in nature, such as "The program will prepare

persons with diabetes to make informed choices about their diabetes care goals and methods." Well-written goals will guide the formulation of the program objectives.[11]

- **B** The specific patient behaviors that will contribute to achieving a goal should be expressed as behavioral objectives, such as "Individuals will use their own meters to demonstrate the ability to assess their own blood glucose levels with no errors." Write objectives in terms of observable and measurable behavior that contain a criterion for acceptable performance.[12]
- **C** Diabetes education programs need to offer courses of study with different levels of comprehensiveness. Patients cannot, and should not, learn everything there is to know about diabetes in a single course of study.
  - The basic course should focus on the initial skills that newly diagnosed patients must learn immediately to care for their diabetes.
  - A more comprehensive course in the self-management of diabetes is needed to be available for patients who have had time to adapt to having diabetes.
  - Diabetes education should be available for specific topics such as an overall review, lifestyle flexibility, and special situations (eg, instruction about insulin adjustment when traveling across time zones and the availability of visual aids if visual changes occur).

4 Other important design considerations are issues related to educational format.
- **A** One-to-one teaching and group teaching both have advantages and disadvantages to consider (eg, groups allow patients to share experiences while one-to-one teaching allows the focus of the entire session to be on a single patient).[13,14]
- **B** Other issues to consider are when and where classes will be held and whether classes will be limited to a single type of patient (eg, only those patients with type 1 diabetes).
- **C** Flexibility and adaptability are the keys to developing appropriate educational formats.

5 The design of a self-management education program needs to reflect the philosophy, needs, and values of those groups of people (stakeholders) who have an investment in the program and its outcomes.
- **A** Examples of program stakeholders are persons with diabetes, referring physicians, hospital or clinical administrators, the individual's family, and the program educators.
- **B** A program benefits from having an advisory committee with representatives from each stakeholder group. Diabetes is cared for in the patient's home and community, which makes community representation on the advisory committee appropriate.

6 Availability of resources is an important design consideration.
- **A** The availability of financial resources has a significant impact on the design of the program. The availability of people to teach in the program is an equally important resource.
- **B** Another important consideration is physical resources, such as space, equipment, and education materials.

7 The makeup of the multidisciplinary educational team (eg, nurse, dietitian, physician, psychologist, pharmacist, exercise physiologist) is crucial to the design of a program and should be identified early in the planning process. Team teaching provides the significant benefit of professionals with multidisciplinary expertise, although it also requires investment of time for planning and team meetings.

8 Another important issue is documentation and record keeping.
  A Diabetes education programs need to include a system that allows for documentation of educational assessment, education, and follow-up.
  B Such documentation may be required to meet standards such as the National Standards for Diabetes Self-Management Education Programs[15] and achieve certification or recognition from the American Diabetes Association (ADA).

9 A resource to help in designing diabetes patient education are the ADA National Standards for Diabetes Education Self-Management Programs.[15] These standards address important issues such as needs assessment, program planning and management, communication and coordination, patient access to teaching, content of the educational curriculum, qualifications of the instructors, the importance of follow-up education, patient and program outcomes, evaluation, record keeping, and documentation.[15] (See Chapter 7, Management of Diabetes Education Programs, in Diabetes Education and Program Management, for additional information on designing education programs.)

Evaluation of Program Outcomes

1 *Formative evaluation*,[16-18] also called process evaluation, involves collecting information about how well the program is functioning.
  A This type of evaluation provides information that can be applied almost immediately to change the program and increase its effectiveness.
  B Formative evaluation data often are gathered by having patients complete questionnaires about their level of satisfaction with the course content, physical and social environment, teaching, audiovisual materials, and so on.

2 *Summative evaluation*,[16-18] also called outcome evaluation, involves gathering and analyzing information to determine whether the program achieved the intended outcomes.[19]
  A Summative evaluation domains include knowledge, attitudes, self-care practices, and psychosocial adaptation. Certain metabolic indices such as blood glucose control and weight are sometimes considered outcome measures by education programs.[19]
  B In general, choose to measure outcomes that occur shortly after the end of the program and outcomes that can be attributed to the program with a high degree of confidence.[19] Chapter 7, Management of Diabetes Education Programs, in Diabetes Education and Program Management, discusses in more detail outcome evaluations.

Multidisciplinary Teams in Diabetes Education

1 A coordinated team approach is recommended in diabetes care because of the multidisciplinary nature of the treatment.[20] This approach is particularly appropriate for self-management education where learners must acquire knowledge and skills from a variety of disciplines.

2 Additional benefits of multidisciplinary teams include improved coordination of care and education, multiple reinforcement of the same educational objectives, and consistency of approach to treatment. For example, although a physician may not spend much time teaching, he or she can reinforce the importance of diabetes self-management education and transmit other core messages to the person with diabetes, family members, and significant others, such as the fact that diabetes is a serious disease.[21]

3 A program coordinator should be chosen to plan and coordinate the efforts of the educational team. This person is responsible for scheduling team meetings and preparing the agenda.

4 Team membership is crucial and should include, whenever possible, a nurse, a dietitian, and a physician as core team members. Other team members will vary depending on need and availability but could include a psychologist, social worker, pharmacist, exercise physiologist, or podiatrist.

5 Team meetings can be used for a variety of purposes:
   A To share information gained from individual patient assessments (eg, nursing, nutrition, medical)
   B To develop a plan to respond to the patient's clinical and educational priorities
   C To plan, implement, and evaluate a patient education program
   D To provide for patient referrals and follow-up care and education

Assessing Educational Needs and Readiness to Learn of Persons With Diabetes

1 Teaching and learning are generally divided into 3 domains: knowledge, psychomotor skills, and affective (or attitudinal) learning. Assessment should focus on these 3 domains as well.
   A It is useful to assess individuals' attitudes[22] and health beliefs[23] about diabetes and its care.[24,25] Patients who think they have mild diabetes or are immune from complications are not very likely to be motivated to learn.
   B It is also important to assess individuals' attitudes about participating in the education program. For example, the educator could discuss learning goals by asking questions about what they hope to get out of the education program and their goals related to their daily self-care.[11,16,26]
   C Assess the individual's metabolic goals regarding glucose control, weight, and lipids.[27]
   D Patients' experience with diabetes and/or other health problems can shape their attitudes and affect their readiness to learn and apply diabetes self-care skills. For example, a patient who is admitted to the hospital for gallbladder surgery or a patient who is newly diagnosed with an acute illness is likely to have a diminished readiness to learn about diabetes. Acutely ill patients need to be taught only basic survival skills until they feel well enough to be more active learners.
   E Families can have a significant impact on an individual's attitudes and readiness to learn by providing or withholding support. Patients are more likely to have a positive attitude about learning when family members are supportive and enthusiastic about diabetes education.[28]

2 Current level of self-care is another important area to assess.[27,29] An educator can glean important information about the individual's tolerance for complexity in the regimen and/or which self-care behaviors are most difficult to perform by assessing their current self-care practices.

3 Preferred styles of learning can affect an individual's willingness to participate in the education program and whether they actually learn.

A Some people prefer to read, others like to listen, and still others learn best from discussions.
B Educators can ask how an individual prefers to acquire other types of information not related to diabetes, (eg, newspapers, TV, discussion with friends). This information will provide clues about how to tailor the education to the individual's needs.
C Consider the fact that not everyone wants to be or belongs in a group program; some patients respond better to one-on-one instruction.

4 The psychological status of patients can affect their interest in learning about diabetes. (See Chapter 2, Psychosocial Assessment, in Diabetes Education and Program Management, for additional information on psychological assessment.)
  A Marked denial, depression, and anxiety can interfere with learning, while low-to-moderate anxiety about diabetes can increase readiness to learn.
  B Patients will also display various degrees of alertness and ability to concentrate on educational issues.

5 Severe stress can seriously impair patients' abilities and interests in learning about diabetes.
  A *Stress* is a reaction to factors that force persons to adapt to situations that are perceived on some level as a threat to their well-being.
  B Self-management education (with the possible exception of basic survival skills) should be postponed for patients experiencing severe stress.

6 Assess the individual's social/cultural and religious milieus because of their influence on patients' interest and willingness to learn about and apply specific diabetes self-care recommendations. Tailor diabetes education to the specific cultural needs and perceptions of the participants.[30] (See Chapter 4, Cultural Competence in Diabetes Education and Care, in Diabetes Education and Program Management.)

7 Literacy can be difficult to assess. Years of schooling completed provides only a clue about literacy.
  A Patients' educational and literacy levels can influence how they learn (eg, reading versus listening or viewing illustrations) and the amount of complexity they can tolerate in an education program.
  B Because complexity is part of diabetes self-care, the challenge lies in using this part of the assessment to direct learning and management issues (see Chapter 5, Teaching Persons With Low Literacy Skills, in Diabetes Education and Program Management).

8 An individual's willingness to participate in and benefit from diabetes education is most likely related to their readiness for change.
  A Recent work on smoking cessation and other addictive behaviors has resulted in a stages of change model that now is being applied to diabetes education.[31] (See Chapter 3, Behavior Change, in Diabetes Education and Program Management, for more information on the stages of change model.)
  B The educational process must either create conditions that stimulate the desire for change in an individual and/or capitalize on the readiness to change if it is already present.

C The extent to which patients feel that change is necessary will influence their readiness to participate in an education program.

9 Other assessment areas involve physical factors such as age,[32] mobility, visual acuity, hearing loss, and dexterity. These factors can influence an individual's willingness and ability to learn and apply diabetes self-care skills.

Characteristics of Adult Learners

1 Adults are usually self-directed and must feel a need to learn before they are able to participate fully in the educational process.[33]
   A It is not relevant that the educator feels the patient should learn something if the patient does not also perceive this need.
   B Sometimes, however, the diabetes educator will have to help patients discover what they need to know. For example, if a patient is being started on insulin for the first time, there are certain safety issues that the educator must address. In this case, the educator may have to take a leadership role in pointing out the crucial areas for diabetes education (eg, signs, symptoms, and treatment of hypoglycemia) rather than wait for the patient to discover these educational needs.

2 Adults tend to be problem-oriented learners rather than subject-oriented learners. They usually want to acquire information that will help them solve specific diabetes problems rather than complete a comprehensive study of the subject of diabetes.[33]

3 Adults learn better when their own experience with diabetes is incorporated into diabetes education, including their past experiences and consideration of how these experiences will apply to their learning in the future (eg, Have you dealt with this problem before? What did you do to try and resolve it? What do you think might work this time?).[33]

4 Adults usually prefer to participate actively in the learning process rather than remain passive. Education programs need to provide patients with the opportunity to ask questions, solve problems, share their own experiences, and otherwise be actively engaged in the educational process.[33]

Teaching and Learning Strategies

1 A brief lecture is useful for presenting information. Persons participate in the learning process by listening and taking notes.
   A This kind of instruction provides a very passive learning experience for an individual.
   B This method may be overused[34] because lectures are easier for teachers to plan and control than other more active types of instruction.

2 Discussion is a more participatory and active learning experience than a lecture; it allows patients to acquire information, ask and answer questions, and share feelings and personal experiences.
   A Discussions cannot be planned and controlled as precisely as lectures; therefore, they require the educator to tolerate a certain amount of ambiguity.

B Leading discussions effectively requires certain interpersonal skills on the part of the educator. For example, a discussion leader must know how to gracefully interrupt a nonstop talker so that other members of the group will have a chance to speak.

3 Demonstration is useful for teaching psychomotor or social skills.
  A After a skills demonstration, encourage patients to practice the skills they have seen demonstrated.[34-36]
  B Give patients the opportunity to demonstrate their skills to the educator and receive feedback. Teaching insulin injection and/or home blood glucose monitoring are the classic examples where this teaching sequence is usually employed.

4 Print materials can provide information for individual study, reinforce previously presented information, and serve as a resource for future reference and review.
  A Print materials need to employ readable type (patients with vision loss may need large type) and be written at an appropriate reading level for the learner.
  B Clarity, nontechnical language, and well-designed, purposeful illustrations enhance the effectiveness of printed material (see Chapter 5, Teaching Persons With Low Literacy Skills, in Diabetes Education and Program Management, for more information about choosing and preparing learning materials at reading levels that are appropriate for specific patient populations).
  C Printed materials do not replace interaction with the educator.

5 Audiovisual (AV) aids such as slides, films, videotapes, food models, and overhead transparencies can enhance the presentation of information.[34-36]
  A Varying the presentation by using AV aids can help increase learner concentration and prevent boredom.
  B Learning is reinforced when the same concepts are presented through a variety of formats.
  C Homemade AV materials give the instructor flexibility. They also provide the opportunity for creativity and matching the AVs to the audience.
  D The use of AV media can be very helpful for patients who do not learn well by reading.

6 Role-playing gives patients a chance to practice social skills, explore interpersonal problems (eg, family conflict), discuss alternative solutions, and share feelings in a psychologically safe environment.[37]
  A Role-playing usually works best with a group of learners who are verbal and who know and trust each other and the instructor.
  B Effective role-playing requires an instructor who has good interpersonal skills and has had training and experience in leading small groups.

7 Games can make learning more enjoyable and improve learner participation.
  A Many board games (eg, Trivial Pursuit®) or television game shows (eg, Jeopardy®, Who Wants To Be A Millionaire®) can be adapted for diabetes education. Some games that are appropriate for diabetes education are produced commercially.

8 Computers have been used in diabetes education for the past 10 years. Computerized clinical problems and simulations can provide a useful mechanism for testing and increasing patient knowledge and improving problem-solving skills.[38,39]

9 Patient examples and problem-based case studies provide a psychologically safe and useful way for learners to explore problems related to having diabetes and to discuss solutions. Patient examples can be written to meet the needs of different types of learners and address a variety of learning domains (eg, knowledge, self-care behavior, or attitudes).[40]

10 *Affective exercises*[37] are techniques for helping individuals express, explore, and change feelings and personal values related to having diabetes.
  A Affective exercises can include some of the previously described techniques such as discussion and role-playing, or they can employ activities designed specifically to elicit an affective response.
  B Existing books on values clarification[41] and human relations training[42] provide many techniques that can be adapted for diabetes education.

Techniques That Enhance Learning and Decision-Making

1 Most diabetes educators want their patients to be motivated, involved, responsible, and committed learners.

2 Diabetes education is much more rewarding and enjoyable for both the educator and the participant when the participant is an active and committed learner.

3 The techniques listed can enhance the involvement and learning of most persons.
  A Learning is enhanced when it is related to what the learner already knows. Match what is being taught with the patient's existing frame of reference.[33]
  B Learning is improved when patients have confidence (self-efficacy) in their ability to actually perform the behavior being taught. Continually reinforce the idea that the patient is a person who can master diabetes self-care skills. This process is enhanced when diabetes self-management education is structured as a series of carefully planned, successful experiences.[24,43]
  C Practice and rehearsal increase the retention of knowledge and skills. Patients need to be given opportunities to practice both psychomotor and social skills (eg, asking family members for their support when following a meal plan).[40]
  D Learning is enhanced by feedback. Provide feedback to patients about how well they are acquiring knowledge and skills. Continued learning can be encouraged by making patients aware of their incremental progress.
  E Learning is reinforced and retained when it can be applied immediately and repeatedly. Patients will retain knowledge and skills longer if they have opportunities for frequent application. For example, having patients who might have to use insulin someday attend a class on insulin injection is unlikely to produce any important or lasting learning because the information/skills cannot be used at this time.

F Educators will occasionally need to adjust the pace at which they teach to accommodate variations in an individual's ability to absorb and retain information. Patients do not always learn at a constant rate. Periodic plateaus occur in learning due to the mood, stress level, and health of patients.

G Review and update core diabetes knowledge and skills on a regular basis.

Follow-Up Learning Opportunities

1 Learning needs to be an ongoing activity.

A One of the most serious impediments to effective diabetes education is the notion that diabetes self-management education is a one-time event. Patient's change, their situations change, and their health status changes, so new learning needs arise.

B Patient education also can provide the continuous emotional support and behavioral reinforcement that is necessary for diabetes self-care.

C To be most effective, patient education should be thought of as an ongoing process (similar to medical care) that plays a lifelong role for people with diabetes.[44]

2 Look for opportunities to provide continuing education to your patients.

A These opportunities include interactions with patients that occur during ongoing diabetes care, such as returning to the provider's office or clinic.

B Educators can also offer courses that are promoted as diabetes updates or refresher courses for patients who have already completed basic diabetes education.

C Support groups, periodic health appraisals and screenings, and annual meetings of diabetes professional and patient organizations also provide opportunities for follow-up diabetes education.

Self-Review Questions

1 Explain the similarities and differences between the 2 educational philosophies: the compliance and empowerment approaches.

2 If you were asked to design a self-management education program, what would you do first and why?

3 When designing a self-management education program, whose input would you seek and why?

4 How would you decide what to evaluate in your diabetes education program?

5 Describe characteristics of adult learners that appear to be most relevant for diabetes patient education.

6 Describe the teaching/learning strategies you think are most useful in diabetes self-management education.

7 Describe the teaching/learning strategies you think are least useful in diabetes self-management education.

8 Describe 4 techniques that you believe could enhance the learning of patients.

9 How would you justify the team approach in diabetes education to your supervisors?

10 What could you say to a patient to reinforce the idea that diabetes self-management education needs to be ongoing?

Learning Assessment: Case Study 1

JL is a dietitian who has recently finished her master's degree and a 1-year internship. She has been hired to be a diabetes educator for an 800-bed urban hospital in Texas. For 6 months JL will work with the experienced dietitian who currently is teaching the nutrition component of the diabetes education program. JL is confident that she will know enough about diabetes and nutrition to teach the classes when she takes over in 6 months. However, she is concerned because the current dietitian gives the two 1-hour classes entirely as lectures. JL has been taught that lecturing to patients for 2 hours is not the best educational technique, but she is unsure about what she should substitute for the lectures.

Questions for Discussion

1 JL has 2 hours' worth of material to teach about nutrition and diabetes. Which part of the class should be lecture and which part should be changed to another educational method?
2 How can JL decide which alternative methods to use instead of a lecture?

Discussion

1 JL could begin by following a simple rule of thumb: most adults have an attention span of about 15 to 20 minutes for a lecture. Using this rough guideline she could decide that she wants to use 2 to 3 different teaching/learning activities for each hour of class.

2 Another concept that could help JL choose effective teaching methods is that participants should be able to interact with the information they have learned after 15 to 20 minutes of lecturing. For example, JL could give a 15- to 20-minute presentation about diabetes and nutrition followed by a discussion session among the participants about applying this information in their own lives. This session could be followed by an opportunity to do some problem-solving such as calculating carbohydrate content of favorite foods or practicing how to read nutrition information labels on food.

3 JL's teaching choices should be directed by the following guidelines:
   A Introduce 2 or 3 new methods per hour.
   B Provide an opportunity for patients to participate actively in the learning process.
   C Include activities that will move the patients closer to applying the knowledge in their own lives.
   D Include activities that will give patients the opportunity to share their own experiences and express and meet their own needs to ensure that the education is personally relevant.

Learning Assessment: Case Study 2

MW is a patient with type 2 diabetes who has been using meal planning alone as treatment for the past 5 years. MW's physician has referred him for patient education because his diabetes control has been worsening for the past 18 months and he is being started on oral agents. MW informs you that he doesn't see why he needs diabetes education. He said, "Do they think I'm an idiot, that I can't take a couple of pills without going to an education program? Besides, I feel fine. I don't know why I have to take these pills anyway." The physician is convinced that MW is denying the seriousness of his diabetes and expects you to change his attitude. MW seems resentful that he has been referred to the diabetes patient education program. You are not sure whether he will actually show up for classes.

Question for Discussion

1 What other approaches would you suggest in working with this patient?

Discussion

1 The answer to this question involves judgment, and judgment is always debatable. It is unlikely that you can (or should) persuade MW to value and attend the education program. When trying to persuade people that their point of view is wrong, they are likely to defend that point of view with increasing vigor. It is psychologically threatening to one's self-image to be told that one's point of view is wrong or inappropriate; most people resist such threatening messages.

2 The approach that probably would be most useful with MW would be to ask him a series of questions about his diabetes: how long he has had diabetes, how he feels about having it, his concerns, what he knows about the progression of the disease, and so on. Listen closely and nonjudgmentally to his responses, giving him an opportunity to express and explore his point of view and perceptions. Such exploration may give him a chance to work through some of his thoughts and feelings. It will also help you be perceived as an ally rather than as someone who is judging him.

3 If at the end of such a discussion MW is still unconvinced that he needs to attend the education program, you could acknowledge the validity of his point of view. You should also, however, suggest that he may wish to consider attending at some future time and that you and the program are available to him if and when he should desire to use them.

4 You could suggest as another alternative that MW try at least 1 class or to meet for one-to-one education that will only address his concerns or answer questions.

5 Tell the referring physician that MW is not open to attending a patient education program at this time and that pushing him to do so may in fact increase rather than decrease his resistance to diabetes patient education.

6 If MW feels safe, accepted, and valued by you he is likely to return at some point and participate in the education program.

References

1. Raymond MW. Teaching toward compliance: a patient's perspective. Diabetes Educ. 1984;10:42-44.

2. Resler MM. Teaching strategies that promote adherence. Nurs Clin North Am. 1983;18:799-811.

3. Anderson RM, Funnell MM. Compliance and adherence are dysfunctional concepts in diabetes care. Diabetes Educ. 2000;2:597-604.

4. Anderson RM, Funnell MM, Arnold MS. Using the empowerment approach to help patients change behavior. In: Anderson BJ, Rubin RR, eds. Practical Psychology for Diabetes Clinicians. Alexandria, Va: American Diabetes Association; 1996:163-172.

5. Anderson RM, Funnell MM. From compliance to empowerment. In: The Art of Empowerment: Stories and Strategies for Diabetes Educators. Alexandria, Va: American Diabetes Association; 2000:32-45.

6. Glasgow R, Anderson RM. In diabetes care moving from compliance to adherence is not enough: something entirely different is needed. Diabetes Care. 1999;22:2090-2091.

7. Anderson RM. Patient empowerment and the traditional medical model: a case of irreconcilable differences? Diabetes Care. 1995;18:412-415.

8. Anderson RM, Funnell MM, Butler P, Arnold MS, Fitzgerald JT, Feste CC. Patient empowerment: results of a randomized control trial. Diabetes Care. 1995;18:943-949.

9. Anderson RM, Funnell MM. Vision trumps method. In: The Art of Empowerment: Stories and Strategies for Diabetes Educators. Alexandria, Va: American Diabetes Association; 2000:22-31.

10. Anderson RM, Funnell MM. Theory is the cart, vision is the horse: reflections on research in diabetes patient education. Diabetes Edu. 1999;25(suppl 6):43-51.

11. American Diabetes Association. Diabetes Education Goals. 2nd ed. Arlington, Va; American Diabetes Association; 1995.

12. Mager RF. Preparing Instructional Objectives. Belmont, Calif: Fearon Publishers; 1975.

13. Rabkin SW, Boyko E, Wilson A, Streja DA. A randomized clinical trial comparing behavior modification and individual counseling in the nutritional therapy of non-insulin-independent diabetes mellitus: comparison of the effect on blood sugar, body weight, and serum lipids. Diabetes Care. 1983;6:50-56.

14. Tattersall RB, McCulloch DK, Aveline M. Group therapy in the treatment of diabetes. Diabetes Care. 1985;8:180-188.

15. American Diabetes Association. National standards for diabetes self-management education (standards and review criteria). Diabetes Care. 2001;24(suppl 1):S126-S133.

16. Haire-Joshu D. Systematic evaluation of diabetes self-management programs. In: Haire-Joshu D, ed. Management of Diabetes Mellitus. Perspectives of Care Across the Life Span. 2nd ed. St. Louis: CV Mosby; 1996:553-573.

17. Gronlund NE. Measurement and Evaluation in Teaching. 6th ed. New York: MacMillan Publishing Co; 1990.

18. Mehrens WA, Lehmann IJ. Measurement and Evaluation in Education and Psychology. 3rd ed. New York: Holt, Rinehart, and Winston, Inc; 1984.

19. Glasgow RE. Outcomes of and for diabetes education research. Diabetes Educ. 1999;25(suppl 6):74-88.

20. Anderson RM. The team approach to diabetes: an idea whose time has come. Occup Health Nurs. 1982;30(12):13-14.

21. Anderson RM, Funnell MM. The role of the physician in patient education. Practical Diabetol. 1990;9(3):10-12.

22. Anderson RM, Fitzgerald JT, Funnell MM, Gruppen LD. The third version of the Diabetes Attitude Scale (DAS-3). Diabetes Care. 1998;21:1403-1407.

23. Becker MH, Janz NK. The health belief model applied to understanding diabetes regimen compliance. Diabetes Educ. 1985;11:41-47.

24. Anderson RM, Fitzgerald JT, Funnell MM. The diabetes empowerment scale (DES): a measure of psychosocial self-efficacy. Diabetes Care. 2000;23:739-743.

25. Funnell MM, Merritt JH. Diabetes mellitus and the older adult. In: Haire-Joshu D, ed. Management of Diabetes Mellitus. Perspectives of Care Across the Life Span. 2nd ed. St. Louis: CV Mosby; 1996:755-809.

26. Houston C, Haire-Joshu D. Application of health behavior models to promote behavior change. In: Haire-Joshu D, ed. Management of Diabetes Mellitus. Perspectives of Care Across the Life Span. 2nd ed. St. Louis: CV Mosby; 1996:527-552.

27. Anderson RM, Funnell MM. What do you want? In: The Art of Empowerment: Stories and Strategies for Diabetes Educators. Alexandria, Va: American Diabetes Association; 2000:163-170.

28. Fain JA, D'Eramo-Melkus G. Diabetes mellitus in young and middle adulthood. In: Haire-Joshu D, ed. Management of Diabetes Mellitus. Perspectives of Care Across the Life Span. 2nd ed. St. Louis: CV Mosby; 1996:729-754.

29. Anderson RM, Funnell MM. What is the problem? In: The Art of Empowerment: Stories and Strategies for Diabetes Educators. Alexandria, Va: American Diabetes Association; 2000;145-156.

30. Murphy FG, Satterfield D, Anderson RM, Lyons AE. Diabetes educators as cultural translators. Diabetes Educ. 1993;19:113-16,118.

31. Ruggiero L, Prochaska JO. Introduction: readiness for change: application of the transtheoretical model to diabetes. Diabetes Spectrum. 1993;6:22-24.

32. Grey M, Kanner S, Lacey KO. Characteristics of the learner: children and adolescents. Diabetes Educ. 1999;25(suppl 6):25-33.

33. Walker EA. Characteristics of the adult learner. Diabetes Educ. 1999;25(suppl 6):16-24.

34. Funnell MM, Donnelly MB, Anderson RM, Johnson PD, Oh MS. Perceived effectiveness, cost and availability of patient education methods and materials. Diabetes Educ. 1992;18:139-145.

35. McCulloch DK, Mitchell RD, Ambler J, Tattersall RB. Influence of imaginative teaching of diet on compliance and metabolic control in insulin dependent diabetes. Br Med J. 1983;287:1858-1861.

36. Clement SC, Gay N. A better method for demonstrating the relationship between factors affecting glycemic control. Diabetes Educ. 1992;18:243-246.

37. Anderson RM, Funnell MM. Interactive learning strategies. In: The Art of Empowerment: Stories and Strategies for Diabetes Educators. Alexandria, Va: American Diabetes Association; 2000:188-208.

38. Lewis D. Computer-based patient educators: use by diabetes educators. Diabetes Educ. 1996;22:140-145.

39. Noell J. Changing health-related behaviors: new directions for interactive media. Med Educ Technol. 1994; 4:4-8.

40. Pichert JW, Smeltzer C, Snyder GM, Gregory RP, Smeltzer R, Kinzer CK. Traditional vs anchored instruction for diabetes-related nutritional knowledge, skills, and behavior. Diabetes Educ. 1994;20:45-48.

41. Simon S, Howe L, Kirschenbaum H. Values Clarification. New York: Hart Publishing Co; 1972.

42. Pfeiffer JW, ed. The 1st-28th Annuals: Developing Human Resources. San Diego, Ca: University Associates Inc; 1971-1999.

43 Johnson JA. Self-efficacy theory as a framework for community pharmacy-based diabetes education programs. Diabetes Educ. 1996;22:237-241.

44 McNabb WL, Quinn MT, Rosing L. Weight-loss program for inner-city black women with non-insulin-dependent diabetes mellitus: PATHWAYS. J Am Diet Assn. 1993;93:75-77.

Suggested Readings

Anderson RM, Funnell MM. The Art of Empowerment: Stories and Strategies for Diabetes Educators. Alexandria, Va: American Diabetes Association; 2000.

Anderson RM, Funnell MM, Arnold MS, Barr PA, Edwards GJ, Fitzgerald JT. Accessing the cultural relevance of an education program for urban African Americans with diabetes. Diabetes Educ. 2000;26:280-289.

Association for Supervision in Curriculum Development. Perceiving, Behaving, Becoming: A New Focus for Education. Washington, DC: National Education Association; 1962.

Bonwell C, Eison J. Active learning: creating excitement in the classroom. Washington, DC: ERIC Clearinghouse on Higher Education, George Washington University, School of Education and Human Development, 1991.

Brown SA. Interventions to promote diabetes self-management: state of the science. Diabetes Educ. 1999;25(suppl 6):52-61.

Browne M, Keeley S. Asking the Right Questions: A Guide to Critical Thinking. 3rd ed. Englewood Cliffs, NJ: Prentice Hall, 1990.

Funnell MM, Arnold MS, Barr PA, eds. Life with Diabetes: A Series of Teaching Outlines. Alexandria, Va: American Diabetes Association; 1997.

Funnell MM, Haas LB. National standards for diabetes self-management education programs: a technical review. Diabetes Care. 1995; 18:100-116.

Peyrot M. Behavior change in diabetes education. Diabetes Educ. 1999;25(suppl 6): 62-73.

Vella J. Learning to Listen, Learning to Teach: The Power of Dialogue in Educating Adults. San Francisco: Josey Bass Publishers; 1994.

Walker EA, Wylie-Rosett J, Shamoon H. Health education for diabetes self-management. In: Porte Jr D, Sherwin RS eds. Ellenberg and Rifin's Diabetes Mellitus. 5th ed. Stamford, Ct: Appleton & Lange; 1997.

Westberg J, Hillard J. Fostering Learning in Small Groups: A Practical Guide. New York: Springer Publishing Co; 1996.

Additional Resources
The National Diabetes Education Program (NDEP) is a federally sponsored initiative involving public and private partners whose mission is to improve treatment and outcomes for people with diabetes, to promote early diagnosis, and ultimately to prevent the onset of diabetes. This comprehensive website has extensive information about a wide range of issues related to diabetes for diabetes educators, clinicians, patients, and the public. It also has an extensive set of links to other diabetes websites. The URL is: *http://ndep.nih.gov.* (Accessed November 2000.)

Learning Assessment: Post-Test Questions

Applied Principles of Teaching and Learning

1. The best instructional approach to use in planning a class on self-monitoring of blood glucose for adults with type 2 diabetes would be:
   A Content oriented, primarily didactic in approach
   B Task centered or problem oriented
   C Interactive group discussion
   D Computer simulations

2. The factor that makes the most significant difference when deciding whether to use a lecture method or a group discussion approach to learning is:
   A Relevance of the material to the learner
   B Educator facilitation skills
   C Opportunities to reinforce learning
   D Availability of audiovisual resources

3. DR is planning a diabetes self-management class for the adults at the health maintenance center and trying to decide how much time she should take to present the key concepts for the class. As a diabetes educator, you advise her to allow:
   A 10 minutes and focus on a single topic
   B 15 to 20 minutes with time to ask questions
   C 30 minutes for lecture, 30 minutes for discussion
   D 50 to 60 minutes to adequately cover the subject material

4. JB, a diabetes educator, frequently communicates to the patient the idea that he or she has the ability to perform the skill being taught and provides feedback to that effect to build confidence. This strategy facilitates learning in that it encourages:
   A Self-efficacy
   B Values clarification
   C Knowledge acquisition
   D Problem-solving skills

5. A 65-year-old widower with type 2 diabetes is referred for education regarding weight reduction. Which of the following strategies would be best to try with this person?
   A Develop a calorie-exchange meal plan and explain to the patient
   B Discuss his eating habits, food choices, and meal preparation skills
   C Teach him how to use carbohydrate-counting approach
   D Have him attend lecture on dietary goals for type 2 diabetes

6. What would be the best learning strategy for a college athlete who is starting insulin therapy?
   A Have the person demonstrate how to draw up and administer insulin
   B Discuss insulin administration procedure using printed material
   C Have him or her watch a videotape on insulin administration
   D Enroll him or her in a class on insulin therapy

7. When is the use of role-playing most effective?
   A To help people with diabetes develop rapport with the educator
   B When a high level of trust exists
   C When learners are still in denial
   D When time is limited

8. What level of diabetes education is most appropriate for a person taking insulin who wants to learn how to make medication adjustments?
   A Survival skills
   B Self-management education
   C Behavior change therapy
   D Lifestyle education

9 Which of the following persons with diabetes is most likely to exhibit an increased readiness to learn?
   A An acutely ill patient
   B A patient who thinks he has "a touch of diabetes"
   C A person who exhibits low-to-moderate anxiety about his condition
   D A person dealing with multiple stressors

10 An effective educational program for persons with diabetes:
   A Uses statements of measurable and observable behaviors to achieve goals
   B Presents specific, single-topic sessions on an as-needed basis
   C Emphasizes disease type and needs over cultural background of patient
   D Incorporates the empowerment approach as the only standard for its patient population

See next page for answer key.

Post-Test Answer Key

Applied Principles of Teaching and Learning

1. B
2. A
3. B
4. A
5. B
6. D
7. B
8. B
9. C
10. A

A Core Curriculum for Diabetes Education
Diabetes Education and Program Management

Psychosocial Assessment 2

Richard R. Rubin, PhD, CDE
The Johns Hopkins University School of Medicine
Departments of Medicine and Pediatrics
Baltimore, Maryland

Joseph P. Napora, PhD, LCSW-C
The Johns Hopkins University School of Medicine
The Johns Hopkins Diabetes Center
Baltimore, Maryland

Introduction

1 Diabetes is a demanding disease. Since about 99% of diabetes care is self-care, personal, family, and other resources are critical to the individual's success in day-to-day diabetes management.

2 The first step in helping individuals make informed choices concerning their diabetes is to conduct a comprehensive assessment of their capabilities and resources that includes psychosocial aspects of diabetes.

3 The purpose of incorporating psychosocial assessment is to systematically identify the individual's strengths and vulnerabilities with regard to diabetes self-care.

4 The psychosocial issues involved in such an assessment include 4 categories of determinants: attitudes, beliefs, and intentions; physical and emotional health status; skills; and family and community factors.

5 A thorough assessment needs to be performed when the person with diabetes is seen for the first time, and on a regular basis thereafter. Informal reassessment is done at every visit; and formal reassessment is done as indicated by changes in the individual's life, therapy, or a crisis such as the onset of complications.

6 Once an assessment is done, an individualized education and treatment plan can be developed with the patient. (For more on using information from the psychosocial assessment to facilitate behavior change, see Chapter 3, Behavior Change, in Diabetes Education and Program Management. For more on using information from the psychosocial assessment to help manage psychological disorders, see Chapter 6, Psychological Disorders, in Diabetes Education and Program Management.)

7 Most educators do not have the time to do a complete psychosocial assessment. Consequently, this chapter includes expedient approaches for identifying each critical psychosocial issue for individual patients. In addition, Table 2.1 describes a brief, selective assessment tool. When indicated, more detailed assessment may then be done in areas that seem to be problems for the patient.

Objectives
Upon completion of this chapter, the learner will be able to
1 State the goals of psychosocial assessment for patients with diabetes.
2 Identify psychosocial factors that may affect an individual's capacity for diabetes self-care.
3 Explain the role that each psychosocial factor may play in influencing self-care behavior.
4 Describe practical, effective approaches for assessing relevant psychosocial factors.
5 Select and use tools and techniques for assessing relevant psychosocial factors.

Table 2.1 A Brief, Selective Assessment

When the time required to use a published assessment instrument or to assess the entire protocol in this chapter is prohibitive, the educator can use this practical, time-sensitive initial assessment. All or some of the 7 determinants can be assessed from the table. The remaining determinants (locus-of-control, readiness to change, complications and other health issues, self-management and coping skills, and community factors) can be assessed quickly with questions from the corresponding section of the chapter text.

Health Beliefs

On a scale of 1 (strongly disagree) to 10 (strongly agree), how much do you agree that (1) you'll be healthier in later life if you control your diabetes now and (2) changing your eating habits would help you control your diabetes?

If the responses indicate that the patient may have unfavorable beliefs, refer to Table 2.2 for additional questions that might help to make an accurate assessment.

Self-Efficacy

On a scale of 1 (confidence very low) to 10 (confidence very high), how confident do you feel about your ability (1) to manage your diabetes on a daily basis and (2) to use a blood glucose meter to test your blood glucose level?

If the responses indicate that the patient has low self-efficacy, refer to Table 2.4 for additional questions that might help to make an accurate assessment.

Behavior Intentions

How often do you plan (1) to monitor blood glucose levels and (2) to walk or do other exercise?

For additional behaviors, see Table 2.5.

Stress

Is diabetes stressful for you? What is most stressful about dealing with your diabetes?

Quality of Life

How is diabetes affecting the quality of your life? On a scale of 1 (very unsatisfied) to 10 (very satisfied), are you satisfied with the quality of your life?

Emotional Well-Being

Self-esteem: Having diabetes, how do you feel about yourself?
Depression: How often do you feel sad, tired, low interest in life and things you used to enjoy? *See Table 2.6.*
Anxiety: Do you often feel nervous or on-edge about your diabetes? *See Table 2.7.*
Eating disorder: How often do you eat too much or too little?

Family, Social Support

How much do your family and friends help you to care for your diabetes?

See Table 2.10 for other questions for assessing this dimension of diabetes self-care.

Goals of Psychosocial Assessment

1 Active diabetes self-care is demanding and pervasive.
  A Requires attention every waking moment, 365 days a year.
  B Affects every aspect of a person's life.
  C Frequently involves tasks that are unpleasant, such as finger-sticks, food restrictions, and, for some people, insulin injections.
  D Presents substantial risks.
  - Short-term and long-term complications are prevalent.
  - Efforts to optimize blood glucose levels may increase the likelihood of hypoglycemia without a guarantee of reduced risk of complications.
  - Some factors that affect glycemia and risks for complications are not under the individual's control.

2 The demands and pervasiveness of diabetes self-care may involve various *psychosocial factors* such as health beliefs, behavioral intentions, and stress, factors that may determine diabetes-related behavior.

3 Psychosocial determinants of self-care are assessed to identify barriers to the effective day-to-day management of diabetes.

4 The results of the psychosocial assessment are used to guide educators and the individual with diabetes in creating a plan for diabetes education and treatment.

5 The results of the psychosocial assessment are used by educators to determine when it is appropriate to refer the individual to a mental health specialist.

6 The goals of diabetes education are to reinforce healthy behaviors and to help change unhealthy ones. The *psychosocial assessment* helps identify the individual's strengths and challenges in living with diabetes.

Determinants of Diabetes-Related Behavior

1 Attitudes, beliefs, and intentions determine an individual's ability to make changes. The following identify attitudes, beliefs, and intentions:
  A Health beliefs
  B Locus-of-control
  C Self-efficacy
  D Behavioral intentions
  E Readiness to change

2 Physical and mental health status complications influence self-care behaviors. The following identify physical and mental health status:
  A Emotional well-being
  B Self-esteem
  C Depression
  D Anxiety disorders
  E Eating disorders

F Substance abuse
G Quality of life
H Stress

3 Skills influence level of diabetes self-care and subsequent changes in degree of self-care. The following can be used to evaluate skills:
A Self-management skills
B Coping skills
C Cognitive maturity, functional literacy

4 Family and community factors affect self-care behaviors. The following are family and community factors:
A Family, social support
B Economic
C Cultural, religious
D Factors related to healthcare delivery

Attitudes, Beliefs, and Intentions

Importance of Health Beliefs

1 The control of diabetes requires numerous changes, and the ability to make the necessary adjustments will depend in part on the individual's beliefs and expectations about the outcome.[1] According to the *Health Belief Model*,[2] behavior reflects a patient's subjective interpretation of a situation. In the context of diabetes self-care, the behavior of patients is influenced by 4 perceptions:
A Benefits of self-care
- Persons who feel that active diabetes self-management will yield benefits are more likely to devote themselves to self-care than persons who are pessimistic that self-management will make a difference.
- Recent studies indicate that an individual's belief in the diagnosis and implicit understanding and attitude towards their illness often affects health behaviors such as compliance with medication.[3]

B Cost of self-care
- Financial costs, personal costs such as extra time involved in efforts to actively manage diabetes, and other costs of active management such as increased incidence of hypoglycemia and weight gain all influence self-care behavior. To be open to active self-care, a person must believe that the benefits outweigh the costs.

C Severity of diabetes and its complications
- Perceptions of issues such as impairment, disability, and job loss are relevant. The more severe the perceived consequences of having diabetes, the more likely the individual is to care for his or her diabetes.

D Susceptibility, or how vulnerable the individual feels to the negative consequences of the illness
- People with type 2 diabetes may feel less susceptible if they think they have a "milder" form of diabetes. Conversely, people who have type 1 diabetes, or people who are suffering from complications of diabetes, may feel more susceptible to negative consequences. According to this theory, the more susceptible the person feels, the more likely that person is to practice self-care.

2 Research yields some support for the predictions of the Health Belief Model. In particular, perceived susceptibility and severity seem to predict self-care. However, these relationships may be curvilinear. For example, those experiencing the lowest and highest levels of susceptibility may have the lowest levels of self-care. Those who feel extremely susceptible may not be able to change their behavior because they feel overwhelmed or fatalistic.

Assessing Health Beliefs

1 Health beliefs may be assessed by asking patients to complete a brief questionnaire rating how strongly they agree or disagree with a series of statements that reflect elements of the Health Belief Model as it applies to diabetes and its management, or by incorporating a few questions into the complete educational assessment.

2 Statements that might be included in an assessment of diabetes-related health beliefs are shown in Table 2.2. These statements represent beliefs related to benefit, cost, severity, and susceptibility. Self-care can be facilitated by identifying and discussing beliefs that either support or undermine active self-management. Special attention needs to be given to helping patients recognize the behavioral and health effects of beliefs concerning benefits and costs of diabetes care (see Chapter 3, Behavior Change, in Diabetes Education and Program Management, for more information on this topic).

3 Health beliefs may be expediently assessed by asking the individual how much he or she agrees (on a scale of 1 to 10) with any single statement from the benefit and cost categories of Table 2.2.

Importance of Locus of Control

1 Beliefs concerning who or what controls health-related outcomes also influence self-care behavior. The *Locus-of-Control Theory*[4] suggests three such beliefs (often called orientations): internal orientation, powerful other orientation, and chance orientation.
  A *Internal orientation:* people who have an internal orientation tend to believe that diabetes-related health outcomes are controlled primarily by their own efforts.
  B *Powerful other orientation:* people who have a powerful other orientation tend to believe that outcomes are controlled primarily by other people, generally by healthcare providers, but often by family members or by friends or other acquaintances.
  C *Chance orientation:* people who have a chance orientation believe that outcomes are determined primarily by chance or fate.

2 Research by Peyrot and Rubin[4] supports some important elements of the Locus-of-Control Model.
  A Internal orientation actually consists of two components, autonomy and self-blame (see Table 2.3). Autonomy was associated with a range of positive outcomes including fewer high blood glucose levels and better emotional adjustment. Self-blame was associated with a range of negative outcomes including less frequent SMBG and insulin dose adjustment.

Table 2.2. Statements for Assessing Health Beliefs of People With Diabetes

Benefit	• I'll be healthier in later life if I control my diabetes. • I believe that exercise can help me control my diabetes. • Controlling my blood sugar will help me avoid heart disease. • Changing my eating habits would help me control my diabetes. • Even if I took my medicine as I should, I wouldn't be able to control my diabetes. • I can control my diabetes if I follow my regimen closely. • The better I control my diabetes, the less the risk of complications.
Cost	• It will take a lot of effort to control my diabetes. • I would have to change too many habits to use a meal plan. • Taking my medication interferes with my daily activities. • I'm always hungry when I stick to my meal plan. • It takes a lot of effort to exercise.
Severity	• Diabetes is a serious disease if you don't control it. • Diabetes is the worst thing that could happen to me.
Susceptibility	• My diabetes would be worse day-to-day if I did nothing about it. • I'm more likely to have eye problems if my control is poor. • If my diabetes isn't controlled, I'm likely to die sooner.

  B Powerful other orientation also consists of two components, healthcare provider and nonmedical other (family, friends, acquaintances), each of which was associated with different aspects of self-care. High healthcare provider locus-of-control orientation was associated with less insulin dose adjustment; high nonmedical other locus-of-control orientation was associated with less insulin doses adjustment, fewer late shots, and less binge eating.
  C Chance orientation was associated with a variety of outcomes that reflect a pattern of dysfunction, including more frequent hyperglycemia, less exercise, lower self-esteem, and more depression and anxiety.

3 Self-care can be facilitated by identifying and discussing locus-of-control orientations that support or undermine active self-management. Special attention needs to be devoted to helping individuals recognize the potential effects of a high chance locus-of-control orientation.

Assessing Diabetes Locus of Control

1 Diabetes-specific locus of control can be assessed comprehensively by means of standardized questionnaires.[4,5]

2 The person's beliefs about who or what controls diabetes-related health outcomes can provide critical information concerning approaches that are likely to be meaningful for that individual. Persons with a predominant chance orientation are at special risk for negative outcomes; they need a great deal of support and assistance to shift from this orientation.

3 Locus-of-control orientation can be assessed by asking individuals to complete a brief questionnaire that rates how strongly they agree or disagree with a series of statements that reflect locus-of-control orientation as it applies to diabetes and its management. It can be assessed, also, by incorporating a few questions into the complete educational assessment.

4 The statements in Table 2.3[4] might be included in an assessment of diabetes-related locus-of-control.

5 Diabetes locus-of-control orientation may be expediently assessed by asking patients how much (on a scale of 1 to 10) they agree with any item from each of the categories in Table 2.3.

Table 2.3. Statements for Assessing Locus of Control in People With Diabetes

Internal locus of control—autonomy	• I can avoid complications. • What I do is the main influence on my health. • I am responsible for my health.
Internal locus of control—blame	• When my sugar is high, it's because of something I've done. • When my blood sugar is high it's because I made a mistake. • Complications are the result of carelessness.
Powerful other locus of control—health professional	• Regular doctor's visits avoid problems. • I should call my doctor whenever I feel bad. • I can only do what my doctor tells me. • Health professionals keep me healthy.
Powerful other locus of of control—nonmedical	• My family is the key to controlling my diabetes. • Other people have a big responsibility for my diabetes.
Chance locus of control	• Good health is a matter of good fortune. • If it's meant to be I won't have complications. • My blood sugars will be whatever they will be. • Blood sugars are controlled by accident. • I never know why I'm out of control. • Good control is a matter of luck.

Importance of Self-Efficacy

1 According to *Self-Efficacy Theory*,[6] a patient's sense of self-efficacy or confidence affects self-care behavior. The more confident a patient feels about performing a set of behaviors, the more likely that person is to actually engage in those behaviors.

2 Some studies[7] suggest that people with diabetes who have a high degree of self-efficacy are more active in the care of their diabetes and have better emotional well-being and glycemic control than people who have a low degree of self-efficacy.

3 In a long-term study, patients who were taught to moderate insulin dosages as needed (in contrast to conventional treatment based on scheduled, rigid food intake and insulin delivery) felt increasingly free from being under the control of physician and treatment-related restrictions, which, along with higher perceived self-efficacy, contributed to a feeling of empowerment. The resultant feeling of empowerment was associated with satisfaction and significant improvement of glycemic control.[8]

Assessing Self-Efficacy

1 The *Diabetes Empowerment Scale* (DES), a 28-item questionnaire, was designed to measure diabetes-related psychosocial self-efficacy. Knowing how patients perceive their ability to perform diabetes self-care behaviors helps the educator to identify specific aspects of self-management that might need special attention.[9]

2 A 30-item questionnaire,[10] originally developed for use with adolescents, is another effective way to measure a patient's perceptions of diabetes self-efficacy, the confidence a person feels about performing diabetes self-care behaviors.

3 Diabetes self-efficacy can be assessed by asking individuals to complete a brief questionnaire rating how strongly they agree or disagree with a series of statements that reflect how confident they feel about managing a variety of daily diabetes-related activities or by incorporating a few questions into the complete educational assessment.

4 The statements in Table 2.4 might be included in an assessment of diabetes-related self-efficacy. This questionnaire, based on the work of Grossman and associates,[11] has been used by Rubin and Peyrot in their ongoing research.[6,12,13] Respondents are asked how sure they are that they can do what is stated.

5 Diabetes self-efficacy may be expediently assessed by asking patients how confident they feel (on a scale of 1 to 10) about their ability to manage their diabetes on a daily basis.

Importance of Behavioral Intentions

1 *Behavioral intentions* (in addition to health beliefs, locus-of-control orientation, and self-efficacy) may predict actual self-care behavior.

2 Work by Peyrot and Rubin[13] suggests that a person's intention to make changes in diabetes self-care behavior powerfully predicts actual behavior change 6 and 12 months later. This relationship is stronger for self-regulation behaviors such as SMBG and insulin adjustment than it is for lifestyle behaviors such as food/eating habits and exercise.

Table 2.4. Statements for Assessing Self-Efficacy of People With Diabetes[6]

I feel sure I can:
1. Take insulin or other medication
2. Figure out meals and snacks at home
3. Figure out foods to eat when away from home
4. Keep track of blood sugar levels
5. Test for ketones
6. Adjust insulin timing or dosage for a lot of extra exercise
7. Figure out how much to eat before activities
8. Figure out how much insulin to take when sick
9. Prevent low blood sugar reactions
10. Talk to my doctor and get the things I need
11. Sleep away from home in a place where no one knows I have diabetes
12. Keep myself free of high blood sugars
13. Avoid having ketones
14. Change my doctor if I don't like him/her
15. Stop a reaction when I'm having one
16. Ask for help when I'm sick
17. Tell a friend or people at work that I have diabetes
18. Confront my doctor if I feel he/she is not being fair
19. Prevent blindness and other complications from my diabetes
20. Get as much attention from people when my diabetes is under control as I get when it isn't
21. Regularly wear a medical alert tag or bracelet that says I have diabetes
22. Sneak food without anyone but me knowing
23. Follow my doctor's orders for taking care of my diabetes
24. Run my life well despite having diabetes

Assessing Behavioral Intentions

1. Peyrot and Rubin[14] developed an approach for assessing self-care behavioral intentions in people with diabetes. A questionnaire was used to measure self-reported, self-care behavior of patients entering a 5-day intensive outpatient diabetes education program. At the end of the program participants were asked to complete a questionnaire to determine what they intended to do regarding each of the same self-care behaviors. Six months later, participants completed a third questionnaire identical to the preprogram instrument, which assessed actual self-care behavior.

2. The specific behaviors that might be included in an assessment of diabetes-related self-care behaviors and intentions are shown in Table 2.5. Respondents are asked how often they do (or intend to do) what is stated.

3. The results of an assessment of behavioral intentions can be formalized in a *behavioral contract* with the patient that can be used as a guide and reminder for ongoing

self-care. At the next visit to the educator, actual behavior can be compared with earlier behavioral intentions, allowing the patient to adjust intentions and plan for future changes. (For more on contracting as a means to facilitate behavior change, see Chapter 3, Behavior Change, in Diabetes Education and Program Management.)

Table 2.5. Specific Behaviors for Assessing Diabetes Self-Care Behaviors and Intentions

How often do you plan to:
1. Monitor blood glucose levels
2. Adjust insulin doses
3. Take medications on time
4. Use your meal plan
5. Walk or do other exercise

Importance of Readiness to Change

1. The *transtheoretical model of behavioral change*[15] postulates that the cessation of high-risk behaviors such as smoking and the implementation of health-enhancing behaviors such as exercise involve progression through 5 stages of change:
   A. *Precontemplation*—not thinking about change
   B. *Contemplation*—considering change in the foreseeable future
   C. *Preparation*—seriously considering change in the near future
   D. *Action*—in the process of behavior change
   E. *Maintenance*—continued change for an extended period

2. Progression through the stages may not be linear as many individuals are likely to relapse and recycle through earlier stages.

3. In a study of smokers with diabetes, the findings attest to the importance of assessing stage of change and providing stage-matched interventions.[16]

4. Although the transtheoretical model has not been studied adequately across other health-enhancing behaviors, treatment interventions are likely to be more effective when they are consistent with the person's stage of readiness to change (see Chapter 3, Behavior Change, in Diabetes Education and Program Management).

Assessing Readiness to Change

1. Assess the patient's stage of change for each diabetes-related health behavior (eg, SMBG, insulin use, meal planning) as it will likely vary for different behaviors.

2. Readiness to change any specific diabetes-related behavior may be assessed by asking the patient whether he or she is already engaged in that behavior, and if so, for more than 6 months (maintenance stage) or less than 6 months (action stage). If the patient

is not engaged in the behavior, is he or she planning to do so in the next month (preparation stage), the next 6 months (contemplation stage), or not at all (precontemplation stage).

3 Approaches that facilitate or maintain each behavioral objective will also need to vary, and the results of the readiness to change assessment may be used to guide subsequent educational interventions (see Chapter 3, Behavior Change, in Diabetes Education and Program Management, for more information).

Physical and Emotional Health Status

Importance of Physical Health Status

1 A patient's health status influences self-care behavior. Acute and chronic complications of diabetes may either hamper or facilitate behavior change in the direction of active self-care.

2 Acute complications may adversely affect self-care behavior. For example, hypoglycemic episodes may discourage efforts to achieve tight control; hyperglycemia may lead to exhaustion which, in turn, may sap energy required for self-care.

3 Acute complications may also encourage self-care. For example, blurry vision caused by hyperglycemia may be so frightening that the patient is motivated to more actively manage his or her diabetes.

4 Chronic complications can also have an adverse effect on self-care. For example, neuropathy or cardiovascular complications may interfere with exercise, and poor vision may interfere with the patient's ability to self-monitor blood glucose levels.

5 Chronic complications may also encourage better self-care. Patients often report that they were "scared straight" by the onset of complications.

6 Similarly, other acute or chronic illnesses that coincide with diabetes may hamper or facilitate change in the direction of self-care.

Assessing Physical Health Status

1 A complete history of the patient's health status, including acute and chronic complications of diabetes and other health issues and problems, is essential for effective educational or treatment planning.

2 These issues may critically influence a patient's ability and motivation for self-care.

Importance of Emotional Well-Being

1 The demands of diabetes are formidable, including pervasive limitation of food intake; blood testing; loss of spontaneity; the threat, discomfort, and danger of hypoglycemia; and the threat, discomfort, and danger of complications.

2 Coping with these demands requires being attentive to details, applying a variety of self-care and coping skills, tolerating frequent frustration, and being reasonably stable emotionally.

3 The need for continual adjustment to the disease can cause a range of negative emotions, including anger, guilt, depression, and anxiety; however, a causal relationship should not be presumed, as a negative effect can be caused by factors other than diabetes.

4 Each negative emotion or any combination can compromise diabetes self-care and metabolic control.

5 Emotional well-being is positively correlated with patient self-care behavior and with glycemic control in type 2 diabetes.[17] The causal relationships between emotional status and self-care are probably reciprocal (ie, high levels of emotional well-being tend to facilitate self-care and high levels of self-care tend to facilitate emotional well-being).

Assessing Emotional Well-Being

1 Self-esteem is positively related to self-care; depression and anxiety are negatively related to self-care.[4,8]

  A Scales that take only a few minutes to administer and score have been developed for measuring self-esteem and stability of self.[18] *Stability of self* measures the consistency of the respondent's self-concept in the face of potentially challenging evidence.

2 Major depression affects approximately 1 of every 5 patients with diabetes and severely impairs quality of life and all aspects of functioning, including sleep patterns, sexual functioning, self-care behavior, and metabolic control.[19,20] Depression in patients with diabetes has been associated also with significant physical decline.[21]

  A A large-scale survey of office-based encounters between physicians and diabetes patients indicated that a significant proportion of depressed patients are not diagnosed for the disorder.[21]

  B Several standardized tests are available to help the healthcare provider screen for common psychiatric disorders that can have a significant impact on the management of diabetes.

  - One of the most frequently used measures is the *SF-36 scale*.[22] Patients can complete the SF-36 in less than 10 minutes, and the measure can be scored by hand.
  - Several easy-to-administer and score instruments for measuring depression are readily available, including the *Center for Epidemiological Studies Depression Scale* (CES-D)[23] and the *Zung Depression Scale* (ZDS).[24]
  - The *Hospital Anxiety and Depression Scale* (HADS) is a short questionnaire to measure psychological symptoms in a clinic setting.[25]

  C The educator can screen individuals for depression by asking a series of simple questions concerning symptoms. A person who has 5 or more specific symptoms for a period of at least 2 weeks may be having a major depressive episode. A person with 2 or more symptoms for at least 2 years is probably suffering from a dysthymic disorder. The symptoms of clinical depression are listed in Table 2.6. Ask patients if they have each symptom; if yes, ask for how long and how often.

- **D** Because some of the symptoms of clinical depression (specifically items 2 through 6 in Table 2.6) are similar or identical to symptoms of hyperglycemia, it may be difficult to ascertain whether a patient with these symptoms is depressed, hyperglycemic, or both. Thus, it is important to pay close attention to the other symptoms listed in the table when a possibly depressed patient is chronically hyperglycemic.
- **E** While most educators are not mental health professionals, an understanding of current treatment options may be useful. Approaches to treating depressed patients who have diabetes are addressed in Chapter 6, Psychological Disorders, in Diabetes Education and Program Management.

Table 2.6. Symptoms of Clinical Depression

1. Depressed mood (feeling sad or empty) most of the day, nearly every day
2. Significant weight loss when not dieting or weight gain (eg, a change of more than 5% of body weight in a month), or a decrease or increase in appetite nearly every day
3. Trouble sleeping or sleeping too much nearly every day
4. Feeling very agitated or physically sluggish nearly every day
5. Fatigue or loss of energy nearly every day
6. Markedly diminished interest or pleasure in all or almost all activities most of day, nearly every day
7. Feeling worthless or excessively or inappropriately guilty nearly every day
8. Diminished ability to think or concentrate, or indecisiveness, nearly every day
9. Recurrent thoughts of death (not just fear of dying), recurrent thoughts of suicide, a suicide attempt or a specific plan to commit suicide

3. Clinical anxiety disorder is another problem common among people with diabetes.[20] In a study of adults with either type 1 or type 2 diabetes in a clinic setting, 28% of participants reported moderate to severe levels of depression or anxiety or both.[25] An anxiety disorder often interferes with a person's ability to effectively manage diabetes and with other aspects of life as well.[26]
   - **A** An educator can screen patients for anxiety by asking a series of simple questions concerning symptoms. A person that has been seriously anxious for at least 6 months about a number of events and activities and during that period has had 3 or more specific symptoms for more days than not is probably suffering from a *clinical anxiety disorder*. The symptoms of clinical anxiety disorder are listed on Table 2.7.
   - **B** Some of the symptoms of clinical anxiety disorder (eg, sleep disturbance, fatigue, irritability) overlap with those of clinical depression.
   - **C** The *Hospital Anxiety and Depression Scale* (HADS) is a short questionnaire for measuring psychological symptoms in a clinic setting.[25]

Table 2.7. Symptoms of Clinical Anxiety Disorder

1. Restlessness or feeling keyed-up or on-edge
2. Being easily fatigued
3. Difficulty concentrating or mind going blank
4. Irritability
5. Muscle tension
6. Sleep disturbance (difficulty falling or staying asleep or restless, unsatisfying sleep)

    D The fear of hypoglycemia can lead to its avoidance, which can lead to deterioration in diabetes control.[27]

    E Injection-related anxiety may influence compliance, glycemic control, and quality of life in patients with insulin-treated diabetes.[28] In addition to screening for injection-related anxiety, the *Diabetes Fear of Injecting and Self-Testing Questionnaire* (D-FISQ) correlates with fear of hypoglycemia, trait anxiety, and fear of illness or death.[29]

    F Approaches to treating patients who have diabetes and suffer from anxiety disorder are addressed in Chapter 6, Psychological Disorders, in Diabetes Education and Program Management.

4 The problem of eating disorders in people with diabetes has received increased attention in the past few years. There are two types of *eating disorders*.

    A *Anorexia nervosa* is characterized by a severe, self-imposed restriction in caloric intake, often combined with extreme levels of exercise.

    B *Bulimia nervosa* is characterized by binge eating followed by purging, usually in the form of vomiting or the use of diuretic medications or laxatives. The diagnostic criteria for bulimia nervosa includes the omission or reduction of insulin doses in order to reduce the metabolism of food consumed during eating binges.[30]

    C Either type of eating disorder enormously complicates diabetes management, often leading to acute emergencies and contributing to chronic complications.

    D *Subclinical eating disorders* (ie, disordered eating that does not meet the criteria for either anorexia or bulimia) are common in persons with type 1 and type 2 diabetes and can seriously compromise metabolic control and long-term health.

    E Although some young men suffer from clinical eating disorders, anorexia and bulimia are about 10 times more common among young women, probably because of the far more intense pressure that American society places on young women to be thin. Specific aspects of diabetes and its management (eg, weight gain associated with initiation of insulin treatment, food restraint, and food preoccupation) may trigger the body dissatisfaction and drive for thinness that accompany eating disturbances.[31]

    F Insulin manipulation is an especially troubling manifestation of eating-disordered behavior that is unique to people with diabetes. Researchers estimate that between one third and one half of all young women with diabetes frequently take less insulin than required for blood glucose control in order to control their weight.[32] Severe insulin omission in binge-eating, type 1 females has been associated with poor metabolic control.[33]

G The healthcare provider can screen patients for clinical and subclinical eating disorders by asking a series of simple questions concerning symptoms. Keep in mind that it may be difficult for an individual to acknowledge an eating disorder, especially anorexia or bulimia. Sometimes it may also be difficult to distinguish between a normal (and even) positive focus on food and body image, which are part of living with diabetes, and the abnormal concerns and behavior that reflect an eating disorder. The educator can ask the patient if he or she has any of the signs and symptoms in Table 2.8. A person who has any of these signs and symptoms is probably suffering from a clinical eating disorder.

H Approaches for treating patients who have diabetes and suffer from clinical or subclinical eating disorders are addressed in Chapter 6, Psychological Disorders, in Diabetes Education and Program Management.

Table 2.8. Signs and Symptoms of Clinical Eating Disorders

1 Weighs less than 85% of normal weight for height, body frame, and age
2 Has intense fear of gaining weight or becoming fat, even though underweight
3 Sees self as fat when others say too thin
4 Exercises far more than is necessary to stay fit
5 Misses at least 3 consecutive menstrual cycles
6 Denies the seriousness of low body weight
7 Binge eats (eats very large amounts of food at a single sitting) at least twice a week for 3 months
8 Feels unable to stop eating or control what or how much is eaten
9 Omitting or reducing insulin doses

Importance of Substance Abuse

1 Substance abuse, in the form of smoking, excessive consumption of alcohol, or abuse of prescription or so-called recreational drugs, can cause serious problems for diabetes self-care and metabolic control. These types of abuses may also dramatically increase the risk for developing long-term complications of diabetes.

A Excessive intake of alcohol or other substances can impair self-care and metabolic control in various ways, including excessive caloric intake, poor nutrition, and inability to think clearly and make sound diabetes-related decisions.

B Diabetes increases the risk of heart attack or stroke, and smoking may increase the risk substantially.

C The diabetes healthcare team needs to vigorously support patients' efforts to stop excessive alcohol intake, drug abuse, and smoking.

Assessing Substance Abuse

1 Because of the serious effects of excessive alcohol intake, inappropriate drug use, and smoking, detection and assessment of these behaviors may be critical both to the patient's ability to manage diabetes and to his general well-being.

A Symptoms of excessive alcohol intake may appear similar to ketoacidosis, including fruity-smelling breath, flushed face, irritability, staggering gait, drowsiness, and coma.
  B Excessive alcohol intake may also trigger or mimic hypoglycemia.
  C Ask patients directly about their alcohol consumption, including questions about how much alcohol is consumed each week, how much is the most consumed in 1 day over the past 3 months, and how much it takes to make the person intoxicated.

2 Like alcohol abuse or dependence, the uncontrolled use of drugs can seriously diminish the user's ability to maintain a healthy regimen of diabetes management.
  A Signs of drug abuse vary as widely as a function of the substance abused.
  B Some typical signs of *drug abuse* include bloodshot eyes, constricted or dilated pupils, confusion, inappropriate behavior with emotional mood swings, anorexia or overeating, dramatically pressured or slowed speech, needle marks, and poor physical condition.
  C *Stimulants* such as amphetamines and cocaine and depressants such as barbiturates and heroin affect memory and appetite and, in turn, diabetes self-care and metabolic control.
  D *Hallucinogens* such as lysergic acid diethylamide (LSD), phencyclidine (PCP), and marijuana can increase appetite leading to extra caloric intake and, often, higher blood glucose levels.
  E Ask patients who may be abusing drugs directly about their use even though most people will be wary about revealing that they are engaged in this activity.

3 Because smoking is a risk factor for many disease states, all of which are complicated by diabetes, smoking behavior is important to assess.
  A Ask patients directly about whether and how much they smoke and about their use of smokeless tobacco products.
  B Ask patients who smoke if they are interested in information on or help with smoking cessation and provide any requested resources.

Importance of Quality of Life (QOL)

1 Snoek[34] noted that although there is no consensus on the definition of *quality of life*, it is generally agreed that QOL encompasses aspects of psychosocial and physical well-being and should reflect the patient's subjective evaluation of well-being.

2 There is general agreement, too, that improving QOL is the primary goal of diabetes-care.[35]

3 Factors associated with a significant decrease in diabetes-related quality of life include dependence upon insulin, depression, diabetic retinopathy, and the presence of co-morbidities in general.[36]

Assessing Quality of Life

1 *Health-related quality of life* (HRQL) refers to an individual's subjective perception of well-being as it relates to health status.

2 HRQL assessment is multidimensional and typically includes several domains: physical functioning, social functioning, pain, emotional well-being, and satisfaction with treatment.

3 Approaches to assessing HRQL include generic, situation-specific, and illness-specific measures.
   A Some popular generic measures of HRQL are the *Medical Outcomes Survey (SF-36)*,[22] the *Quality of Well-Being Instrument*,[37] and the *Sickness Impact Profile*.[38]
   B Illness-specific measures focus on specific problems posed by an individual illness. A *diabetes-specific quality-of-life* assessment may evaluate the impact of experiences such as hypoglycemia, insulin injections, blood glucose monitoring, and dietary restrictions. Some of these instruments include items or subscales concerning the impact of diabetes on physical, psychological, and social functioning.[39]
   C The *Diabetes Quality of Life Measure* (DQOL) is a widely used diabetes-specific assessment of quality of life.[40] The DQOL was originally developed by the Diabetes Control and Complications Trial (DCCT) Research Group to evaluate the relative burden of different diabetes treatment approaches.
   D The DQOL consists of 46 items and assesses quality of life in 4 areas: satisfaction with treatment, impact of treatment, worry about the future effects of diabetes, and worry about social and vocational issues.
   • There is a modified version of this instrument for youths.[41]
   E Another measure that may be useful for assessing HRQL in people with diabetes is the 8-item *Diabetes Treatment Satisfaction Questionnaire*.[42]
   F Some more recent measures include the 64-item *Diabetes-Specific Quality of Life Scale* (DSQOLS),[43] the 57-item *Diabetes Quality of Life Clinical Trial Questionnaire—Revised* (DQLCTQ-R),[44] and the 15-item *Audit of Diabetes-Dependent Quality of Life* (ADDQoL).[45]

4 Illness-specific measures and situation-specific questions are probably the most effective way of assessing HRQL in people with diabetes.[34]

5 The presence of potential problems with diabetes-related quality of life may be expediently identified by asking the patient, "How is diabetes affecting your quality of life?"

Importance of Stress

1 Stress—acute or chronic—may impair a patient's ability for self-care and diabetes control.[46-48]
   A *Stress* is a physical and emotional reaction to a situation that is perceived both as a threat to one's well being and as unmanageable. A *stressor* is a condition or situation that causes stress.
   B There are several potential stressors common to diabetes, including being diagnosed with diabetes, having type 2 diabetes and having to start on insulin, complications, the anticipation of complications, the risk of hypoglycemia, and being pushed by others about self-care behavior.
   C The identification and containment of stressors should be a part of a patient's overall treatment program.

Assessing Stress

1 The 45-item *Questionnaire on Stress in Patients with Diabetes—Revised* (QSD-R)[49] and the 20-item *Problem Areas in Diabetes Scale* (PAID)[50] can be used to assess aspects of stress for patients with the disease.

2 Stressors often can be expediently assessed by asking patients directly about the stress in their lives. In one study, perceived stress was measured by asking subjects to rate 2 items on a scale of 1 (almost never) to 5 (almost always): (a) I have a lot of stress in my life, and (b) How often are you stressed more than you want to be.[51] A rating of 3 to 5 on either item would indicate that the individual's stress level should be assessed in more detail.

A Asking the person what is troublesome about dealing with diabetes may reveal a chronic stressor. When a possible stressor is identified, obtaining information about the symptoms the patient associates with the problem will help to assess the seriousness of the situation.

B Look for significant changes in functioning and in quality of life as an indication that a stressor is involved. If a patient said that he had been in good control until some point in time when his blood sugar levels went wild, ask if any significant events had occurred around the time that his control faltered.

C The individual may not be able to make an association between a stressful experience and a change in level of functioning, so it may be expedient to simply ask if there has been a problem, an illness, accident, or any other event that had an emotional impact on the person.

3 Chronic stress in response to an identifiable stressor and causing significant functional impairment may meet the criteria for the diagnosis of an Adjustment Disorder (see Chapter 6, Psychological Disorders, in Diabetes Education and Program Management).

4 The stress of diabetes may be reduced with coping skills training.

Skills

Importance of Self-Management Skills

1 Self-management skills (along with other psychosocial factors such as health beliefs and self-efficacy) may influence the current level of diabetes self-care and subsequent changes in degree of self-care.

2 *Skill* may be defined as knowledge in action because it is achieved through the acquisition of knowledge and through guided practice.

3 The foundation of *self-management skill* is the ability to solve problems by coordinating activities and using information and experience to make decisions. Self-management skill also involves the ability to coordinate a variety of specific tasks to promote physical well-being and quality of life (eg, coordinating the amount and timing of food, medication, and exercise when on vacation or sick-day management); the ability to effectively utilize family, social, and professional support; and the ability to set and pursue goals.

4 Some authors and researchers do not make a distinction between self-care and self-management, using these terms synonymously.

Assessing Self-Management Skills

1 An individual's ability to implement self-management behaviors, which can seriously affect the level of self-care, also informs the planning of individualized treatment or education.

2 The level of problem-solving skills seems to be a powerful predictor of health outcomes. Problem-solving skills can be assessed by observing the patient in the process of solving a diabetes-related problem.

3 The person's ability to coordinate activities to maintain physical well-being and quality of life, as well as other aspects of self-management, can be assessed by asking patients how they deal with potentially problematic diabetes-related situations. Example: "As a single, working mother with two young children, how do you manage your diabetes in the mornings, which must get pretty hectic at times?"

4 The development of self-management skills is addressed in Chapter 3, Behavior Change, in Diabetes Education and Program Management.

Importance of Coping Skills

1 *Diabetes coping skills* are behaviors that eliminate or modify the stressors common to diabetes (eg, rigid regimen, fear of complications), stressors that might cause emotional distress and impair self-care.

2 Research has shown that coping may be associated with better self-care[6] and with certain metabolic (eg, glycosylated hemoglobin and body weight) and psychosocial outcomes (eg, depression and quality of life).[52-54]

3 Improved coping skills can lead to improved metabolic control indirectly, by facilitating self-care, and directly, by reducing the acute effects of stress on glycemia.[55]

4 Self-care behavior can be affected by the patient's skill in coping with the emotional stresses of day-to-day life with diabetes. Clinical experience reveals that the major barriers to self-care are often emotional (eg, frustration and feeling overwhelmed).

Assessing Coping Skills

1 Coping style can be evaluated using a variety of structured instruments.[52,56]

2 *Kovacs' Issues in Coping With Diabetes Scales for Children and Parents*[57] is a reliable and valid instrument for measuring coping with diabetes.

3 In one study, a "coping styles" questionnaire that distinguished between emotional and self-control styles of coping was used to study stress, coping, and regimen adherence as determinants of metabolic control.[58]

4 The *Ways of Coping Checklist*[59] and the *Adolescent Coping Orientation for Problem Experiences Scale*[60] also assess coping among people with diabetes.

5 Coping skills may be expediently assessed by asking patients how they would respond to typical day-to-day diabetes-related problems and other difficult situations.

6 Examples of specific questions to include are "Is your diabetes and its care causing you stress? If so, how?" "What are you currently doing to try to cope with the stress? What could help you cope better?" "Have you ever been able to cope successfully with a stressful situation before; if so, how did you do it?" "Have you been successful in coping with stress in the past? If so, what did you do at the time?"

7 Weissberg-Benchell and Pichert[61] identified guidelines for assessing coping skills via the interview process:
  A The best questions are nonjudgmental.
  B Do not ask questions that can be answered "Yes" or "No." Ask open-ended questions.
  C Helpful questions reveal new information about the patient.
  D Helpful questions encourage patients to think about diabetes differently.
  E You seldom have time for complete questioning so prioritizing is essential.

8 Specific skills for helping patients to cope with diabetes-related problems and stressors are presented in Chapter 3, Behavior Change, in Diabetes Education and Program Management.

Importance of Cognitive Maturity, Functional Literacy

1 Self-care behavior reflects the level of cognitive maturity a person has achieved.
  A Recent studies indicate that school-age children make more mistakes with more responsibility for their diabetes management, mistakes that lead to poorer metabolic control than when their parents are involved. Studies in children with diabetes, ages 6 to 12, have shown that parental involvement is related to better diabetes control.[62]
  B Some young people (up to age 15) are not cognitively ready to assume responsibility for independent self-care.[63]
  C To be considered *cognitively mature*, a young person must be able to reason about abstract concepts that are inherent in diabetes management (eg, balancing multiple unknowns and making causal connections between events that are not temporally connected in experience).
  D Parents, motivated by frustration or the advice of health professionals, often withdraw from responsibility for their child's diabetes care. When young children are not ready to assume the responsibility divested by their parents, gaps in care may develop.[64] These gaps can go unrecognized and lead to critical health-related difficulties.
  E Some adults may also be cognitively immature or have other learning difficulties that pose problems for independent diabetes self-care (see Chapter 5, Teaching Patients With Low Literacy Skills, in Diabetes Education and Program Management, for more information about this issue).

F The lack of cognitive maturity may lead to poor metabolic control with the demands of a complex treatment regimen.[65]

Assessing Cognitive Maturity, Functional Literacy

1 Cognitive immaturity may preclude children and young adolescents from assuming substantial responsibility for their self-care. Although the educator may choose not to assess cognitive maturity directly, this issue should be considered when working with young patients (see Chapter 1, Diabetes During Childhood and Adolescence, in Diabetes in the Life Cycle and Research, for more information about these issues).

2 Assessing the literacy skills of patients (including functional and health literacy) presents a challenge to many educators. *Health literacy* is defined by the National Library of Medicine as the degree to which people can obtain, process, and understand basic health information and services they need to make appropriate health decisions.[66] (See Chapter 5, Teaching Patients With Low Literacy Skills, in Diabetes Education and Program Management, for information about assessment and education of persons with low literacy skills).

Family and Community Factors

Importance of Family, Social Support

1 Self-care behavior may be powerfully affected by amount and type of social support provided by family, friends, and others and even by the healthcare provider.[67] Much of diabetes self-care takes place in a social context, so assessing and understanding social influences is often critical to facilitating effective self-care. The major social influences on diabetes in patients throughout the life span is shown in Table 2.9.

Table 2.9. Major Social Influences on Diabetes Self-Care Through the Life Span

Patient	Major Influence
Children	Parents
Adolescents	Peers
Adults	Spouses, other family members, friends, coworkers

2 Social support may help individuals mobilize positive coping strategies for dealing with the demands of daily life with diabetes, or it may help by buffering the effects of stress on these individuals.

3 Individuals are often more able to engage in self-care when their social networks provide practical and emotional support for diabetes self-management efforts.[68]

4 Individuals whose social networks are nonsupportive, either practically or emotionally, are often less motivated to take care of their diabetes.

Assessing Family, Social Support

1 To clarify the strengths and weaknesses of an individual's social support network, the educator may ask all or some of the questions in Table 2.10 to determine the following information:

A What practical and emotional help patients receive from those around them
B What barriers to self-care other people represent
C What changes the patient wants in the area of support

Table 2.10. Critical Questions for Assessing Social Support Available to People With Diabetes

1 Who helps you in your effort to manage your diabetes?
2 What does he/she/they do that you find helpful? Please be as specific as possible.
3 Would you say this support is more practical or emotional?
4 Does anyone provide you with practical/emotional support (whichever was not mentioned in response to prior question) for managing your diabetes? If someone does, tell me about it, being as specific as possible.
5 Does anyone important to you make it harder to manage your diabetes? If so, who is this person? What does this person do that makes it harder for you to manage your diabetes? Please be as specific as possible.
6 What would you like in the way of support for day-to-day diabetes management that you are not getting now?
7 What one thing could you do to make it more likely you will get the support you want? Anything else?
8 What can I do to help you get the support you want? (Suggest options such as joint meeting with family, materials for family to read, educational or support group programs to attend, etc.)

2 The support of family members can encourage and reinforce self-care, just as the lack of support can have a negative effect. For example, whether a family member views aspects of a diabetes regimen as a cooperative endeavor or an imposition may affect the behavior of the one with diabetes. Consequently, attention should be given to how family members react to the needs of the individual with diabetes.[69]

3 The educator may find it useful to involve important members of the individual's social network in assessment, education, and treatment plans. Some comprehensive education programs use this approach as do many support groups (see Chapter 3, Behavior Change, in Diabetes Education and Program Management, for more information on these and other interventions).

Importance of Economic Factors

1 Paying for essential health services is a problem for many people who have diabetes, even for those with medical insurance coverage. Out-of-pocket medical expenses for people with diabetes are three times greater than for people who do not have diabetes. In addition, there are patients who are not able to pay for basic necessities such as food and shelter. Effective self-care and good health are hard to attain for those who lack the resources to pay for food, housing, and basic medical care.

Assessing Economic Factors

1 Because financial resources are required to pay for food, shelter, and medical care, diabetes educators should ask patients directly about any concerns they have in this area.

2 People with diabetes may have difficulty getting and keeping health insurance, and The Health Insurance Portability and Accountability Act of 1996 will help in this endeavor.[69]

3 Become familiar with community resources that may be available to help patients who cannot pay for basic necessities.
  A Medical assistance may be available through Medicaid or Medicare.[69]
  B Some organizations such as the American Diabetes Association (ADA), the Juvenile Diabetes Research Foundation International (JDRF), and the American Association of Diabetes Educators (AADE) offer information about services for those with limited financial resources. In addition, Lions Club International offers assistance to those with visual impairment.
  C Community food banks have appropriate choices of foods for people with diabetes and may assist in providing staples on a monthly basis.
  D State vocational rehabilitation agencies may provide vocational counseling, job placement, and financial assistance for job training and education.
  E The Salvation Army and the American Red Cross often can help with emergency financial assistance.
  F State social service agencies may assist in obtaining essential staples.

Importance of Cultural and Religious Influences

1 Cultural influences on diabetes care must be recognized as well. We all are influenced by our cultural background and religious beliefs. Not taking a patient's cultural beliefs and behaviors into account may result in patient distrust, dissatisfaction, and treatment failure.
  A Some cultural values (eg, the view that being overweight is desirable or that having diabetes may be seen as a sign of imperfection or contamination) and practices (eg, considering it impolite to refuse food that is offered when visiting another person's home or eating a starch-ladened diet) may be inconsistent with standard approaches to diabetes self-management. In addition, these practices may lead to increased incidence of obesity, which may increase susceptibility to type 2 diabetes.[70]
  B Some religious beliefs and practices (eg, fasting or "divine healing") may be contrary to conventional diabetes self-management.

C On the other hand, some cultural and religious beliefs and practices can be sources of support in coping (see Chapter 4, Cultural Competence in Diabetes Education and Care, in Diabetes Education and Program Management, for more information about these issues).

Assessing Cultural and Religious Influences

1 Recognizing, assessing, respecting, and working with cultural and religious influences can be a challenge for many educators. The challenge diminishes in proportion to the educator's familiarity with relevant cultural and religious influences.

2 When the educator perceives a conflict concerning religious or cultural backgrounds, it would be expedient to ask an open-ended question such as, "Is there anything about your background or upbringing that makes this aspect of diabetes care a problem?"

3 To communicate effectively with some patients, the educator may need to work with an appropriate interpreter.

Factors Related to Healthcare Delivery

1 Certain factors related to healthcare delivery may affect the patient's ability to achieve and maintain effective self-care.
  - **A** Minority cultures prefer (or may need) to be spoken to in their native language, which may not be available in any given treatment facility.[71]
  - **B** Although studies have shown that comprehensive diabetes management can reduce complications and fatalities, a recent study concluded that primary care is doing poorly with regard to helping people with diabetes to help themselves.[72]
  - **C** Practitioners' perspectives tend to be rooted in a clinical context, emphasizing technical considerations, whereas patients' perspectives exist within a life-world context based on practical and experiential considerations.[73]
  - **D** Although educational and behavioral interventions such as training in self-management and coping skills has contributed substantially to diabetes care and health care in general, these services are often denied or limited by health insurance and health care systems.[74]

Assessing Factors Related to Healthcare Delivery

1 Behavioral scientists and practitioners need to educate other care providers and insurance carriers about the positive effects of behavioral changes on metabolic control and quality of life.[74]

2 Applying practical behavioral interventions (eg, stress management skills training) and utilizing behavioral measures as outcomes in research and treatment centers will advance the recognition and appreciation of the role of behavior change in self-care.

3 Ask patients if they have been denied treatment or education services by their insurance carrier.

Key Educational Considerations

1 Helping individuals make informed decisions and appropriate behavior changes concerning their diabetes is a primary responsibility of diabetes educators. The first step in addressing this responsibility is to conduct a thorough assessment, including an assessment of psychosocial factors that may influence a person's capacity for self-care and metabolic control. In planning and conducting psychosocial assessments, apply the following key considerations.

   A Psychosocial factors powerfully influence not only a person's overall capacity for self-care, but also the unique details of that person's approach to day-to-day management.

   B Assess each determinant of diabetes-related behavior: health beliefs and attitudes; locus of control; self-efficacy; self-management; stress; coping skills; quality of life and emotional well-being; health status; family and social support; contextual factors such as barriers to learning, economic considerations, religious and cultural influences; and readiness to change.

   C Assess psychosocial influences on self-care during the first meeting with a patient and on a regular basis thereafter.

2 Psychosocial assessment is useful for both the educator and the patient because it establishes at the outset that education and care are cooperative endeavors based on the nature and uniqueness of the individual patient.

3 Each potential psychosocial influence on behavior may be assessed using either published instruments, items from published instruments, or open-ended questions.

4 This chapter identified specific questions in each psychosocial domain which may be used to expediently screen for possible problems in that domain. If such problems are identified, the educator may choose to do a fuller assessment of that domain.

5 In some cases, psychosocial assessment will reveal problems that can only be resolved using skills outside of the educator's area of expertise. Developing a network of specialists, including mental health professionals, social workers, and others, to provide expert evaluation, treatment, and case management services on an as-needed basis can greatly facilitate patient access to such services. An important role for the educator in this network is to provide information about diabetes to these professionals.

Self-Review Questions

1 Define the educator's goals in doing a psychosocial assessment.
2 Describe how health beliefs and attitudes influence a person's self-care behavior.
3 List simple, practical instruments or questions you can use to assess various aspects of a person's diabetes-related health beliefs and attitudes.
4 Define behavioral intentions and why they are important to assess.
5 When assessing overall quality of life in a person with diabetes, should you use a diabetes-specific measure? Why?
6 List the 3 clinical psychological disorders that seem to be more common among people with diabetes.

7 Describe how social support influences a person's day-to-day diabetes self-care.

8 List questions you could ask a person with diabetes to assess available social support.

9 Why is it important to assess the patient's level of stress, and how can it be done expeditiously?

10 State why it is important to assess readiness to change.

11 List contextual influences to assess in patients with diabetes.

12 Define self-efficacy and why it is important to assess.

13 Differentiate self-management and coping skills.

14 Identify the 3 beliefs or orientations defined in Locus of Control Theory and evaluate each one in terms of diabetes self-care behavior.

Learning Assessment: Case Study 1

LB is a 44-year-old African-American female who was diagnosed with type 2 diabetes 2 years ago. She lives in the home she shared with her husband before they divorced 6 years ago. Two of her 4 adult children and 1 of her grandchildren also live with her. LB's glucose readings are generally very high, and she has problems with many aspects of diabetes self-care, especially SMBG (which she does only a few times a week), meal planning, and exercise (which she does rarely). LB is already reporting some symptoms of neuropathy, and her most recent lab work revealed albumin in her urine. Insulin treatment has been recommended to LB, but she is very upset at the prospect of taking shots. When questioned, she responds, "I just can't take it! I'm already stretched to the limit. I have lots of stress at home, I'm the only one bringing in any money, and I feel rotten all the time. No way could I deal with insulin on top of all that. Everyone else in my family died young from diabetes and I guess the same thing will happen to me."

Questions for Discussion

1 What psychosocial factors might be contributing to LB's resistance to initiating insulin therapy?

2 Which of these factors would you assess first?

3 What questions would you ask to assess these issues?

4 Because LB is experiencing a lot of stress, what determinant of diabetes-related behavior might you want to assess thoroughly?

Discussion

1 LB's presentation suggests that she is feeling overwhelmed by a variety of psychosocial issues. Her family situation seems to make her life and her diabetes management more difficult rather than easier.

2 LB's diabetes-related beliefs and attitudes, based in part on the experience of other family members who had diabetes, reinforce her pessimism concerning the possibility of living well with diabetes.

  A There is a high prevalence of type 2 diabetes among African Americans; and the incidence of complications from diabetes, such as amputations and mortality, are higher for African Americans than white Americans.

B LB should be informed of the advances in medical resources and treatment modalities that probably were not available to some members of her family and, thus, put them at greater risk of complications and early death than she would be with better control.

3 LB may be depressed, her quality of life is clearly poor, her economic situation appears to be precarious, and her coping skills are not adequate for helping her take effective control of her diabetes in the face of other pressures.

4 The diabetes educator must protect herself from feeling as overwhelmed as LB feels. This may be difficult given the severity of LB's problems, and the educator may benefit from seeking the support of colleagues.[75]

5 Under these circumstances a step-by-step approach is essential. A useful first step might be to simply acknowledge the frustration and pessimism LB so obviously feels.

6 Next, the educator could clarify the fact that change may be slow, but it is possible beginning with LB and the educator working together to identify LB's most pressing problem.
   A Prioritizing in this way may help both LB and the educator feel less overwhelmed and help them focus on problem-solving.
   B Keep in mind that this approach has the best chance of success if the priorities are set by LB herself.

7 If this approach works, LB will feel more confident in her working relationship with the educator and in her own ability to deal with her diabetes-related difficulties.

8 If LB is unable to engage in setting priorities, it is probably because she is feeling overwhelmed by stress, including the non-diabetes-related stress in her life.
   A It might be immediately beneficial to teach LB coping skills such as identifying and utilizing available resources.
   B Consider referring LB to a social worker or other mental health professional. The services of these specialists may improve LB's capacity to work with the educator and make informed choices for her life with diabetes.

Learning Assessment: Case Study 2

ZM is a 62-year-old man who was diagnosed with type 2 diabetes at the age of 41 years. He takes insulin by injection 3 times a day, performs SMBG 4 times a day, and walks 5 times a week for at least 30 minutes. Despite ZM's efforts in these aspects of his diabetes self-care, he has hypertension and hyperlipidemia, neither of which is well controlled. ZM has also been steadily gaining weight the last 4 to 5 years and now weighs 35 lbs more than he did 5 years ago. His wife always comes to clinic visits with him.

When ZM is asked about his situation, he says, "I know I have a problem. I live to eat. That's a major source of stress between my wife and me. On the one hand she's often hassling me to eat healthier, but on the other hand, she keeps bringing the cake and candy and ice cream into the house and stuffing her face with it. Now that I think about it, we hassle about a lot of things, especially when it comes to my diabetes. She's the reason I take my shots and test my blood and walk as regularly as I do. She's always reminding me and even nagging me if she has to. She is so into my diabetes it's almost like it's her disease and not mine. Now don't get me wrong, there are times I really appreciate the help. But other times it drives me crazy. The latest thing between us is smoking. She quit 6 months ago and now she's trying to get me to do the same."

Questions for Discussion

1 What 3 psychosocial factors need to be addressed by ZM and the educator?
2 How important is ZM's wife to his self-care? What questions might you ask to help ZM identify what he wants from his wife in terms of diabetes care?
3 What strategies might you use to include ZM's wife in the assessment and educational process?

Discussion

1 ZM's presentation suggests 3 psychosocial issues that need to be addressed.
   A Most obvious among these issues is how ZM and his wife interact concerning his diabetes care.
   B A second related issue is ZM's attitudes about his diabetes and its management.
   C Finally, given ZM's medical history, his smoking is also a concern.

2 It appears that ZM's wife both helps and hinders his diabetes management efforts. It also seems that ZM is ambivalent about his wife's involvement, sometimes welcoming it and other times not.
   A The educator might ask ZM and his wife to say as specifically as possible what determines whether her involvement is helpful. Questions like "When is it helpful? When is it not? What makes the difference? How do you know when it is helpful? What happens when it is not helpful?" may be useful in identifying the determinants of true helpfulnesss in their relationship.
   B Based on this information, the educator might ask ZM if it would be helpful for him and his wife to draft a "contract" specifying when and in what ways she will participate in his diabetes care.

3 The educator might also discuss with the couple the difference between support and pushing. Support is almost always helpful; pushing is generally not.
   A Support is helping someone do what he says he wants to do.
   B Pushing is trying to get someone to do what you believe he should do.

4 That ZM attributed essential self-care behaviors to his wife, the educator might explore several determinants of diabetes-related behavior, including health beliefs, locus of control, and readiness to change.

5 Assess ZM's readiness to stop smoking and offer appropriate resources, including support from his wife.

6 Many of the psychosocial issues depicted in this case study are likely to be seen in relations between children with diabetes and their parents: conflicting perceptions of support and pushing, readiness to change, health beliefs, locus of control.

Learning Assessment: Case Study 3

TJ is a 15-year-old boy who has had type 1 diabetes for 8 years. Although his physician has recommended that he should take 3 injections of insulin each day and perform SMBG 4 times daily, TJ rarely meets these criteria. He also has difficulty following a diabetes-oriented meal plan. TJ says that all of these demands interfere with the activities that are important to him. His A1C is consistently between 10% to 11%, and he has had several incidents of ketoacidosis.

TJ is physically active; he is playing junior varsity basketball and baseball for his high school. His brother is a senior at the same school and a star athlete. His brother tries to bully TJ into taking better care of himself. When TJ has an incident of ketoacidosis, his brother calls him a wimp and accuses him of misbehaving to get attention. Sometimes, his older brother tries to scare TJ into better diabetes care by telling him that horrible things are going to happen in the future if he does not change his behavior. His parents (frustrated by their inability to affect a change in TJ's attitude and frightened by the results of his behavior) do not try to stop the bullying, perhaps hoping that their older son's approach might work when all else has failed.

TJ's friends are dating and his attempts at dating have been distressing for him. On the few dates he has had, he chose not to tell his dates that he had diabetes because he believed he would have been turned down if they knew it. To prevent the possibility of an episode of hypoglycemia, he took less insulin and increased the intake of carbohydrates, which resulted in excessively high blood sugar levels. Feeling poorly, his behavior did not win his date's favor, leaving him feeling both physically and emotionally distressed.

Questions for Discussion

1 Which psychosocial determinants of diabetes-related behavior are of concern here?
2 The situation is complex, and the risk might be that everyone (including the educator) is overwhelmed by the weight of so many problems. Would it be beneficial to focus on 1 or a few determinants; if so, which one(s)?
3 Might you conclude that TJ is in the "precontemplation" state of readiness to change and forego any further assessment of his situation?
4 What psychosocial factors need to be assessed with regard to TJ's brother's behavior?
5 It appears that TJ's parents are suffering from burnout. Would you try to involve them in their son's education and treatment plan? How would you assess this problem?
6 Which psychosocial issues need to be addressed to help TJ to date with a reasonable degree of comfort and confidence?

Discussion

1 TJ's diabetes-related self-care behavior is inadequate as reflected by poor metabolic control and incidents of ketoacidosis.

2 TJ's situation is complex, which is common for adolescents with diabetes.

3 While some determinants are obvious and others less so, many of the determinants of diabetes-related behavior need to be considered.
- **A** Two aspects of health beliefs may be contributing to TJ's struggle with diabetes: susceptibility and severity. At his young age, he may neither feel susceptible to the negative consequences of poor control nor appreciate the seriousness of diabetes and its complications.
- **B** TJ's concern about becoming hypoglycemic on a date may indicate a lack of self-efficacy, a lack of confidence in his ability to maintain metabolic control in a social setting.
- **C** It appears that TJ does not intend to make the behavior changes necessary to follow the regimen prescribed by his physician in spite of the consequences, including incidents of ketoacidosis.
- **D** TJ's distress about dating may be a consequence of inadequate self-management skills. He may not be capable of coordinating the various activities of dating with the tasks of self-care.
- **E** There are several aspects of TJ's situation that may be stressful. The relationship with his brother is very conflicted, and there are signs that the relationship with his parents has been contentious. Since stress may be impairing diabetes self-care, the assessment of TJ's coping skills is warranted.
- **F** Healthy family support would likely help TJ to make some essential diabetes-related behavior changes. The very aggressive style of TJ's brother and the passive approach of his parents concerning his diabetes need to be addressed. Some ways to develop family support include involving the family in the education program, relieving some of their anxieties about diabetes, and helping them to "contract" for when and how they will participate in TJ's diabetes care.
- **G** TJ appears to be in the precontemplation stage of readiness; he is not thinking about changing his diabetes-related behavior. The problem may be what the transtheoretical model of change refers to as "decisional balance," which involves weighing the pros and cons of changing a particular behavior.[71] For TJ, the benefits of diabetes self-care behavior are negligible as compared to the disadvantages of giving up activities that he values highly. Consider helping him to integrate diabetes-related and unrelated activities so that the latter is enhanced. The educator might begin to address this matter with an assessment of TJ's health beliefs.

4 Empowering TJ for better metabolic control might begin with assessing his level of self-efficacy. If he was more confident of his ability to manage the diabetes over a range of circumstances, he might be more motivated to make some essential changes.

References

1. Rapley P, Fruin DJ. Self-efficacy in chronic illness: the juxtaposition of general and regimen-specific efficacy. Int J Nurs Pract. 1999;4:209-215.

2. Becker MH, Janz NK. The health belief model applied to understanding diabetes regimen compliance. Diabetes Educ. 1985;11:41-47.

3. Cooper AF. Whose illness is it anyway? Why patient perceptions matter. Int J Clin Pract. 1998;52:551-556.

4. Peyrot M, Rubin RR. Structure and correlates of diabetes-specific locus of control. Diabetes Care. 1994;17:994-1001.

5. Ferraro LA, Price JH, Desmond SM, Roberts SM. Development of a diabetes locus of control scale. Psychol Rep. 1987;61:763-770.

6. Rubin RR, Peyrot M, Saudek CD. The effect of a diabetes education program incorporating coping skills training on emotional well-being and diabetes self-efficacy. Diabetes Educ. 1993;19:210-214.

7. Bandura A. Social Foundations of Thought and Action: A Social Cognitive Theory. Englewood Cliffs, NJ: Prentice-Hall; 1986.

8. Rubin RR, Peyrot M. Psychosocial problems and interventions in diabetes: a review of the literature. Diabetes Care. 1992;15: 1640-1657.

9. Howorka K, Pumpria J, Wagner-Nosiska D, Grillmayr H, Schlusche C, Schabmann A. Empowering diabetes out-patients with structured education: short-term and long-term effects of functional insulin treatment on perceived control over diabetes. J Psychosom Res. 2000;48:37-44.

10. Anderson RM, Funnell MM, Fitzgerald JT, Marrero DG. The diabetes empowerment scale: a measure of psychosocial self-efficacy. Diabetes Care. 2000;23:739-743.

11. Grossman HY, Brink S, Hauser S. Self-efficacy in adolescent girls and boys with insulin-dependent diabetes mellitus. Diabetes Care. 1987;10:324-329.

12. Rubin RR, Peyrot M, Saudek CD. Effect of diabetes education on self-care, metabolic control, and emotional well-being. Diabetes Care. 1989;12:673-679.

13. Rubin RR, Peyrot M, Saudek CD. Differential effect of diabetes education on self-regulation and life-style behaviors. Diabetes Care. 1991;14:335-338.

14. Peyrot M, Rubin RR. The effect of self-efficacy and behavioral intentions on self-care improvement following diabetes education. Diabetes. 1995;44(suppl 1):96A.

15. Ruggiero L, Prochaska JO, eds. From research to practice: readiness for change. Diabetes Spectrum. 1993;6:21-60.

16. Ruggiero L, Rossi JS, Prochaska JO, et al. Smoking and diabetes: readiness for change and provider advice. Addict. Behav. 1999;24:573-578.

17. Van der Does FE, De Neeling JN, Snoek FJ, et al. Symptoms and well-being in relation to glycemic control in type II diabetes. Diabetes Care. 1996;19:204-210.

18. Rosenberg M. Conceiving the Self. New York: Basic; 1979.

19. Gavard JA, Lustman PJ, Clouse RE. Prevalence of depression in adults with diabetes: an epidemiological evaluation. Diabetes Care. 1993;16:1167-1178.

20. Peyrot M, Rubin RR. Levels and risks of depression and anxiety symptomatology among diabetic adults. Diabetes Care. 1997;20:585-590.

21. Sclar DA, Robison LM, Skaer TL, Galin RS. Depression in diabetes mellitus: a national survey of office-based encounters, 1990-1995. Diabetes Educ. 1999;25:331-340.

22. Ware JE Jr, Shelbourne CD. The MOS 36-item short-form health survey (SF-36). I: conceptual framework and item selection. Med Care. 1992;30:473-483.

23. Radloff LS. The CES-D scale: a self-report depression scale for research in the general population. Applied Psychological Measurement. 1977;1:385-400.

24. Zung WWK. A self-rating depression scale. Arch. Gen. Psychiatry. 1965;12:63-70.

25. Lloyd CE, Dyer PH, Barnett AH. Prevalence of symptoms of depression and anxiety in a diabetes clinic population. Diabet Med. 2000;17:198-202.

26. Kohen D, Burgess AP, Catalan J, Lant A. The role of anxiety and depression in quality of life and symptom reporting in people with diabetes mellitus. Qual Life Res. 1998;7:197-204.

27. Green L, Feher M, Catalan J. Fears and phobias in people with diabetes. Diabetes Metab Res Rev. 2000;4:287-293.

28. Zambanini A, Newson RB, Maisey M, Feher M. Injection related anxiety in insulin-treated diabetes. Diabetes Res Clin Pract. 1999;46:239-246.

29. Mollema ED, Snoek FJ, Pouwer F, Heine RJ, van der Ploeg HM. Diabetes fear of injecting and self-testing questionnaire: a psychometric evaluation. Diabetes Care. 2000;23:765-769.

30. Diagnostic and Statistical Manual of Mental Disorders, 4th ed. Washington: American Psychiatric Association; 1994.

31. Daneman D, Olmsted M, Rydall A, Maharaj S, Rodin G. Eating disorders in young women with type 1 diabetes. Prevalence, problems and prevention. Horm Res. 1998;50(suppl 1):79-86.

32. Rydall AC, Rodin GM, Olmsted MP, et al. Disordered eating behavior and micro-vascular complications in young women with insulin-dependent diabetes mellitus. N Engl J Med. 1997;336:1849-1854.

33. Takii M, Komaki G, Uchigata Y, Maeda M, Omori Y, Kubo C. Differences between bulimia nervosa and binge-eating disorder in females with type 1 diabetes: the important role of insulin omission. J Psychosom Res. 1999;47:221-231.

34. Snoek FJ. Quality of life: a closer look at measuring patient's well-being. Diabetes Spectrum. 2000;13:24-28.

35. Rubin RR, Peyrot M. Quality of life and diabetes. Diabetes Metab Res Rev. 1999;15:205-218.

36. Brown GC, Brown MM, Sharma S, Brown H, Gozum M, Denton P. Quality of life associated with diabetes mellitus in an adult population. J Diabetes Complications. 2000;14:18-24.

37. Bush JM, Kaplan RM. Health-related quality of life measurement. Health Psychol. 1982;1:61-80.

38. Bergner M, Bobbitt RA, Carter WB, et al. The sickness impact profile: development and revision of a health status measure. Med Care. 1981;19:787-805.

39. Polonsky WH. Understanding and assessing diabetes-specific quality of life. Diabetes Spectrum. 2000;13:36-41.

40. Jacobson A. Quality of life in patients with diabetes mellitus. Semin Clin Neuropsychiatry. 1997;2:82-93.

41. Ingersoll G, Marrero D. A modified quality-of-life measure for youths: psychometric properties. Diabetes Educ. 1991;17:114-118.

42. Bradley C, Lewis KS. Measures of psychological well-being and treatment satisfaction developed from the responses of people with tablet-treated diabetes. Diabetic Med. 1990;7:445-451.

43. Bott U, Muhlhauser I, Overman H, Berger M. Validation of a diabetes-specific quality-of-life scale for patients with type 1 diabetes. Diabetes Care. 1998;21:757-769.

44. Shen W, Kotsanos JG, Huster WJ, Mathias SD, Andrejasich CM, Patrick DL. Development and validation of the Diabetes Quality of Life Clinical Trial Questionnaire. Med Care. 1999;37:AS45-66.

45. Bradley C, Todd C, Gorton T, Symonds E, Martin A, Plowright R. The development of an individualized questionnaire measure of perceived impact of diabetes on quality of life: the ADDQoL. Quality Life Research. 1999;8:79-91.

46. Lloyd CE, Dyer PH, Lancashire RJ, Harris T, Daniels JE, Barnett AH. Association between stress and glycemic control in adults with type 1 (insulin-dependent) diabetes. Diabetes Care. 1999;22:1278-1283.

47. Peyrot M, McMurry JF, Kruger DF. A biopsychosocial model of glycemic control in diabetes: stress, coping and regimen adherence. J Health Soc Behav. 1999;40:141-158.

48. MacLean D, Lo R. The non-insulin-dependent diabetic: success and failure in compliance. Aust J Adv Nurs. 1998;15:33-42.

49. Herschbach P, Duran G, Waadt S, Zettler A, Amm C, Marten-Mittag B. Psychometric properties of the Questionnaire on Stress in Patients with Diabetes—Revised (QSD-R). Health Psychol. 1997;16:171-174.

50. Polonsky W, Anderson BJ, Lohrer PA, et al. Assessment of diabetes-related distress. Diabetes Care. 1995;18:754-760.

51. Barnfather JS, Ronis DL. Test of a model of psychosocial resources, stress, and health among undereducated adults. Res Nurs Health. 2000;23:55-66.

52. Grey M. Coping with diabetes. Diabetes Spectrum. 2000;13:167-169.

53. Lloyd CE, Dyer PH, Lancashire RJ, Harris T, Daniels JE, Barnett AH. Association between stress and glycemic control in adults with type 1 (insulin dependent) diabetes. Diabetes Care. 1999;8:1278-1283.

54. Bell RA, Summerson JH, Spangler JG, Konen JC. Body fat, fat distribution, and psychosocial factors among patients with type 2 diabetes mellitus. Behavioral Medicine. 1998;24:138-143.

55. Bradley C, Lewis KS, Jennings AM, Ward, JD. Scales to measure perceived control developed specifically for people with tablet-treated diabetes. Diabetic Med. 1990;7:685-694.

56. Kurtz SMS. Adherence to diabetes regimens: empirical status and clinical applications. Diabetes Educ. 1990;16:50-59.

57. Kovacs M, Brent D, Feinberg TF, Paulauskas S, Reid J. Children's self-reports of psychologic adjustment and coping strategies during the first year of insulin-dependent diabetes mellitus. Diabetes Care. 1986;9:472-479.

58. Peyrot M, McMurry JF Jr, Kruger DF. A biopsychosocial model of glycemic control in diabetes: stress, coping, and regimen adherence. J Health Soc Behav. 1999;40:141-158.

59. Lazarus RS, Folkman S. Coping and adaptation. In: The Handbook of Behavioral Medicine. New York: Guilford; 1984.

60. Patterson JM, McCubbin HI. A-COPE adolescent coping orientation for problem experiences. In: Family Assessment Resiliency, Coping, and Adaptation. Madison, Wis; 1995.

61. Weissberg-Benchell J, Pichert JW. Counseling techniques for clinicians and educators. Diabetes Spectrum. 1999;12:103-107.

62. Anderson B, Laffel LM. Diabetes self-care tasks: what can a kid do? Diabetes Interview. 2000;9:57.

63. Ingersoll GM, Orr DP, Herrold AJ, Golden MP. Cognitive maturity and self-management among adolescents with insulin-dependent diabetes mellitus. J Pediatr. 1986;108:620-623.

64. Brackenridge BP, Rubin RR. Sweet Kids: How to Balance Diabetes Control and Good Nutrition with Family Peace. Alexandria, Va: American Diabetes Association; 1996.

65. Timms N, Lowes L. Autonomy or noncompliance in adolescent diabetes? Br J Nurs. 1999;8:794-800.

66. Health literacy: report of the Council on Scientific Affairs: Ad Hoc Committee on Health Literacy for the Council on Scientific Affairs, American Medical Association. JAMA. 1999;281:552-557.

67. Peyrot M, McMurry JF Jr. Psychosocial factors in diabetes control: adjustment of insulin-dependent adults. Psychosom. Med 1985;47:542-557.

68. Lo R. Correlates of expected success at adherence to health regimen of people with IDDM. J Adv Nurs. 1999;30:418-424.

69. Guffey L, ed. American Diabetes Association Complete Guide to Diabetes, 2nd ed. Alexandria, Va; American Diabetes Association; 1999.

70. Haffner SM. Epidemiology of type 2 diabetes: risk factors. Diabetes Care. 1998;21:(suppl 3):C3-C6.

71. Brown SA. Diabetes interventions for minority populations: "We're really not that different, you and I." Diabetes Spectrum. 1998;11:145-149.

72. Glasgow RE, Strycker LA. Preventive care practices for diabetes management in two primary care samples. Am J Preven Med. 2000;19:9-14.

73. Hunt LM, Arar NH, Larme AC. Contrasting patient and practitioner perspectives in type 2 diabetes management. West J Nurs Res. 1998;20:656-676.

74. Glasgow RE, Fisher EB, Anderson BJ, LaGreca A, Marrero D, Johnson SB, Rubin RR, Cox DJ. Behavioral science in diabetes: contributions and opportunities. Diabetes Care. 1999;22:832-843.

75. Charman D. Burnout and diabetes: reflections from working with educators and patients. J Clin Psychol. 2000;56:607-617.

Suggested Readings and Resources

Anderson B, Funnell M. The Art of Empowerment. Alexandria, Va: American Diabetes Association; 2000.

Anderson B, Rubin RR, eds. Practical Psychology for Diabetes Clinicians: How to Deal With the Key Behavioral Issues Faced by Patients and Health Care Teams. Alexandria, Va: American Diabetes Association; 1996.

Bradley C. Handbook of Psychology and Diabetes. Chur, Switzerland: Harwood Academic Publishers; 1994.

Cox D, Gonder-Frederick L. Major developments in behavioral diabetes research. J Consulting Clin Psychol. 1992;60:628-638.

Feste C. The Physician Within, 2nd ed. Alexandria, Va: American Diabetes Association; 1992.

Guffey L, ed. American Diabetes Association Complete Guide to Diabetes, 2nd ed. Alexandria, Va: American Diabetes Association; 1999.

The Health Literacy Network has information on the internet, which is available at: *http://www.healthliteracy.net*. Accessed April 2001.

Peyrot M, Rubin RR. Living with diabetes: the patient-centered perspective. Diabetes Spectrum. 1994;7:204-205.

Peyrot M, Rubin RR, Psychosocial aspects of diabetes care. In: Leslie D, Robbins D, eds. Diabetes: Clinical Science in Practice. Cambridge: Cambridge University Press; 1995:465-477.

Plotnick L, Henderson R. Clinical Management of the Child and Teenager with Diabetes. Baltimore, Md: Johns Hopkins University Press; 1998.

Learning Assessment: Post-Test Questions

Psychosocial Assessment

1. Which of the following contextual factors need to be assessed to determine a person's ability to effectively manage diabetes:
   A Self-care ease, financial stability, and educator's concerns
   B Cultural influences, socioeconomic factors, and learning barriers
   C Organizational factors, regimen simplicity, and ego strength
   D Learning style, regimen complexity, and cultural biases

2. Based on the Locus-of-Control Theory, ML exhibits a "powerful others" orientation. Which of the following behaviors would be consistent with this orientation?
   A He blames his poor glucose control on his wife's pasta meals
   B He claims he knows more about what's good for his health than the doctors do
   C He states that diabetes runs in the family and that he knows from being with his mother and brother who have diabetes that managing this condition is out of his hands
   D He compares his outcomes with others in the doctor's waiting room

3. Issues of psychosocial adjustment are critical regarding diabetes management because they:
   A Assess emotional well-being and mental illness presentation
   B Point out specific problems posed in self-management skills
   C Are essential to successful efforts in improving self-care
   D Allow the diabetes educator to not teach mentally unstable people

4. A diagnosis of clinical depression is made when:
   A A patient reports feeling depressed
   B A patient exhibits 2 specific symptoms on a consistent basis for at least 4 weeks
   C Laboratory data confirm the diagnosis of depression
   D Patient exhibits 5 or more specific symptoms over a minimum 2-week period

5. In relationship to Health Beliefs, there are 4 perceptions that influence a person's behavior in diabetes self-care. These include:
   A Self-care benefits, social supports, susceptibility, and cost
   B Susceptibility, severity, self-care activity benefits, and cost
   C Severity, self-care cost and limitations, and susceptibility
   D Social supports, severity, susceptibility, and limitations

6. JP is considered to have an internal locus of control. Which of the following responses related to an elevated blood glucose value is more reflective of this type of orientation?
   A "I overate at my last meal without taking an adequate amount of insulin to cover the carbohydrate"
   B "My mother gave me a piece of regular cake with icing and ice cream because it was my sister's birthday"
   C "My primary care practitioner did not raise my insulin dosage so I couldn't take extra; it's not my fault"
   D "I guess that my blood sugar is high because it is winter now; that's the way it's supposed to be"

7 A stated intention to change behavior made by a person who has diabetes is:
   A A poor predictor of behaviors
   B More likely to occur if it involves self-management behaviors
   C More likely to result in positive outcomes if achieved within 6 to 12 weeks
   D More likely to occur if it involves lifestyle changes

Please answer the next 2 questions based upon the following case scenario.

LJ was recently diagnosed with type 2 diabetes mellitus after her ophthalmologist found advanced retinopathy in both her eyes. In addition to her problem with vision, she is grieving the death of her husband of 40 years. Since his death 4 months ago, she has become exceptionally concerned and frustrated dealing with the losses in her life: living alone, being unable to drive at night due to poor vision, generally poor appetite, and having to structure meals around medication and blood testing.

8 At this time, which psychological presentation is LJ most at risk for?
   A Anxiety disorder
   B Eating disorder
   C Depressive disorder
   D Personality disorder

9 Which approach is best for the educator to use with LJ?
   A Uncaring and politically correct
   B Caring and actively listening
   C Distant and matter of fact
   D Structured and firm

10 A diagnosis of clinical anxiety (Generalized Anxiety Disorder) is made when
   A A patient expresses fear of needles and injecting insulin
   B A patient manifests at least 3 of 6 specific symptoms of anxiety and worry for more days than not for at least 6 months
   C A patient manifests symptoms of anxiety following a traumatic experience
   D A patient reacts to most aspects of diabetes-care in a worrisome and self-doubting manner

11 According to Self-Efficacy Theory, a patient's sense of self-efficacy or confidence is important because
   A A doctor might not be available in an emergency
   B Diabetes-care will be less expensive
   C The more confident a patient feels about performing self-care behaviors, the more likely that person is to engage in those behaviors
   D Self-confidence eliminates the need for many coping skills

12 The transtheoretical model of behavior change postulates 5 stages of readiness in implementing new health-enhancing behavior, which are
   A Precontemplation, contemplation, choice, practice, maintenance
   B Precontemplation, contemplation, preparation, action, maintenance
   C Crisis, rumination, choice, action, evaluation
   D Contemplation, problem-solving, decision-making, action, maintenance

13 In the contemplation stage of readiness, the patient is
   A Seriously considering change in the near future
   B Choosing among various behaviors to change
   C Contemplating whether or not to change
   D Considering change in the foreseeable future

14 Which of the following is not a symptom of anorexia or bulimia nervosa?
   A Obesity
   B Exercises excessively to stay fit
   C Omits or reduces insulin doses
   D Misses at least 3 consecutive menstrual cycles

15 Which of the following statements about stress is not true?
   A Stress, acute or chronic, can impair a patient's ability for self-care and diabetes control
   B Complications or the anticipation of complications can cause symptoms of stress
   C A stressor is a symptom of stress
   D Stress is a physical and emotional reaction to a situation that is perceived to be threatening and unmanageable

16 All but one of the following abilities are fundamental self-management skills, which one is not?
   A Solving problems
   B Utilizing family, social, and professional support
   C Coping with an interpersonal conflict
   D Setting and pursuing health-care goals

17 Health literacy is defined as
   A The age at which an individual can read independently
   B The degree to which someone can obtain, process, and understand basic health information and services needed to make appropriate health decisions
   C The absence of a learning disorder or other cognitive impairment
   D The age at which children understand the seriousness of diabetes

18 With regard to family and social support, which of the following statements is not correct?
   A The amount and type of family and social support provided to the patient may powerfully affect the patient's self-care behavior
   B Patients whose support networks are practically or emotionally nonsupportive are often less motivated to take care of their diabetes
   C While parents are the major social influence for diabetes self-care, peers are likely to be the major influence for adolescents with the disease
   D When the patient has high levels of self-esteem and self-efficacy, the absence of a support network is likely to be of little consequence or value

See next page for answer key.

Post-Test Answer Key

Psychosocial Assessment

1. B
2. A
3. C
4. D
5. B
6. A
7. A
8. C
9. B
10. B
11. C
12. B
13. D
14. A
15. C
16. C
17. B
18. D

A Core Curriculum for Diabetes Education
Diabetes Education and Program Management

Behavior Change 3

Richard R. Rubin, PhD, CDE
The Johns Hopkins University School of Medicine
Departments of Medicine and Pediatrics
Baltimore, Maryland

Joseph P. Napora, PhD, LCSW-C
The Johns Hopkins University School of Medicine
The Johns Hopkins Diabetes Center
Baltimore, Maryland

Introduction

1 Self-care behavior is critical for attaining and maintaining physical and emotional health for people who have diabetes. Although technological advances in recent years have offered the promise of tighter glycemic control and improved quality of life, the trade-off of additional self-care demands has been considerable.

2 The key to helping persons with diabetes achieve their desired level of self-care is understanding the psychosocial and behavioral determinants that may influence self-care and a person's capacity and resources for change. These factors are organized into 4 categories: 1) attitudes, beliefs, and intentions; 2) physical and mental health status; 3) skills; and 4) family and community factors. Assessing these factors in individual patients is addressed in detail in Chapter 2, Psychosocial Assessment, in Diabetes Education and Program Management.

3 The effective control of diabetes may depend on the individual's ability to make adjustments with regard to 1 or more of these determinants of self-care. Adjustment to any of these factors usually requires behavior change.

4 Supporting efforts by persons with diabetes to make behavioral changes is important because it may be essential for improving metabolic control, weight, and lipid levels, which, in turn, reduce the risk of long-term complications and resulting costs.

5 In recent years there has been a growing awareness that behavior change and improved glycemic control may also contribute to improved quality of life.

6 The educator's role is to facilitate the motivation and empowerment of individuals for optimum self-care by developing their self-efficacy, promoting their autonomy, and providing them appropriate support.

7 The individual with diabetes and the educator need to work together to develop an individualized education and management plan designed to foster and maintain patterns of self-care and self-management that the individual has chosen to follow.

8 The educator's efforts may be limited by time or economic restrictions, in which case prioritizing treatment and educational objectives would be essential.

9 The individual's ability to maintain behavior change may be influenced by family, environment, culture, and other external factors (see Family and Community Factors, Chapter 2, Psychosocial Assessment, in Diabetes Education and Program Management).

10 The overall objective of this chapter is to provide the diabetes educator with a comprehensive view of the issues and processes of behavior change.
  A At times, some readers may perceive the scope of the material—for example, the case studies—as unrealistic because of time constraints and limited contact with patients. However, with this broad perspective, each educator can select what is most relevant and useful for each patient.

B The ability to prioritize educational and treatment goals is essential, and it is consistent with the principle that a realistic expectation for an individual and educator is some change, not perfection.

Objectives

Upon completion of this chapter, the learner will be able to

1 Explain the role of behavior in diabetes education and management.
2 Identify various perspectives on behavior change.
3 Apply the results of a comprehensive psychosocial assessment to help individuals develop an effective self-care plan, including goal setting, contracting, and skills training.
4 Identify strategies and interventions for facilitating behavioral change consistent with the objective of empowering individuals for maximum self-care.
5 Incorporate strategies in the individual's self-care plan for maintaining change and, thus, preventing relapse.

The Role of Behavior in Diabetes

1 Self-care is a multidimensional construct that requires the individual to adopt and maintain a variety of behaviors in response to numerous influences, including health beliefs, opposing motivations, economic conditions, and life events.

2 Patients may follow some aspects of their regimen, but not others. Levels of self-care vary across areas of the regimen, being highest for medical aspects such as taking medications, and being lowest for lifestyle aspects such as eating choices and exercise.[1]
   A Levels of self-care in different areas of diabetes management are often uncorrelated.[2] Consequently, until recently, it has been difficult to formally establish relationships between specific self-care behaviors and physiologic outcomes.
   B Adherence tends to be lower for regimens that are complex, lifelong, and prophylactic.[3] For example, it can be very difficult for a young person to be motivated to maintain a complex regimen over time when the reward for the effort is as indefinite as reducing the risk of a complication of diabetes that might occur many years in the future.

3 While the relationships of self-care behavior, quality of life, metabolic control, and complications are complex, evidence supporting the existence of relationships among these variables has been increasing in recent years.
   A The results of the Diabetes Control and Complications Trial (DCCT)[4] and the United Kingdom Prospective Diabetes Study (UKPDS)[5] confirm the benefits of intensive treatment, including active self-management for both type 1 and type 2 diabetes.
   B Other research reinforces some of the findings of the DCCT.[6,7] For example, in one study,[8] people who increased the frequency of their self monitoring of blood glucose (SMBG) or exercise lowered their glycosylated hemoglobin levels by an average of 1.3%. Those who improved the frequency of both exercise and SMBG or improved their insulin administration (skipping fewer shots or adjusting doses more often) lowered their glycosylated hemoglobin levels by an average of 2.9%.

4 Burgeoning technology and therapeutic advances affect diabetes self-care behavior.
  A Examples of such advances include SMBG, intensive insulin therapy (ICT) involving multiple daily insulin injections, and insulin pump therapy.
  B The impact of this progress is greatest for patients who take insulin, although the availability of new classes of oral antidiabetes medications may increase the impact of technology on people who do not take insulin.
  C The impact of technology on diabetes education and care is increasing, with developments such as electronic patient records, telemedicine, and the use of computers for assessment and education.
  D These advances are like a two-edged sword: they offer hope for better health, but often involve greater self-care demands.

5 Diabetes self-care requires substantial effort.
  A People who develop diabetes are often asked to make major lifestyle changes:
   - Practice SMBG
   - Follow an often-complex medication regimen
   - Plan and manage nutritional composition and timing of meals
   - Engage in ongoing physical activity
   - Manage hypoglycemia and hyperglycemia and associated mood swings
   - Engage in regular foot care and other preventive health practices
   - Stop smoking
   - Maintain reasonable body weight
   - Manage acute illnesses
  B Research and clinical experience suggest that the behavior change required for maintaining diabetes self-care is difficult for most people.[9-12] The regimen required for managing the disease is formidable and pervasive; it often involves changes in long-established habits or lifestyles that are resistant to modification; and the best effort does not always have the desired outcome.
  C In one study,[13] individuals reported that although most changes were difficult they were not impossible; most of the individuals noted that maintaining change was much harder than making changes initially.

Motivation and Behavior Change

1 Motivation is essential for making the behavior changes that are necessary for living well with diabetes. The demands for change are formidable and relentless, and the individual's need and desire for control of the disease may be the critical factor for success.

2 Two theories of human behavior are useful in motivating diabetes-related self-care behavior: 1) the self-determination theory of human motivation[14] and 2) the transtheoretical model of change.[15]

3 Self-determination theory predicts that when patients with diabetes are given autonomy (a sense of volition and self-initiation) in managing the disease as opposed to being controlled (feeling pressured to behave in an expected manner), they will be more motivated to regulate glucose levels, feel more able to regulate glycemia, and show improvements in their A1C values. These predictions were supported in a study of 128 patients between 18 and 80 years of age.[14]

4 In addition to proposing 5 stages of readiness to change (see Importance of Readiness to Change in Chapter 2, Psychosocial Assessment, in Diabetes Education and Program Management) the transtheoretical model of change identifies 2 intervening variables for change: decisional balance and self-efficacy.[15]

  A *Decisional balance* involves weighing the advantages and disadvantages of a particular action. A patient would be motivated to do blood glucose testing if the results were valued more than the time, discomfort, and inconvenience of the behavior.

  B *Self-efficacy* is the patient's confidence in making and maintaining behavior changes; diabetes-specific self-efficacy pertains to confidence in making and maintaining diabetes-related changes. The more confident the patient feels about doing something, the more likely it will be done.
  - According to the Self-Efficacy Theory,[16] self-efficacy or self-confidence affects self-care behavior.
  - One study[17] suggests that people with diabetes who have a high degree of self-efficacy are more active in the care of their diabetes and have better emotional well-being and glycemic control than people who have a low degree of self-efficacy.

5 In a weight reduction program for women with type 2 diabetes, *motivational interviewing*—defined as a "directive, client-centered counseling style for eliciting behavior change by helping clients explore and resolve ambivalence"[18]—achieved a significant rate of adherence and improved glycemic control.[19]

  A The basic elements of motivational interviewing[20] are consistent with the principles of empowerment theory (see below) and include
  - Elicit, do not impose, a motivation to change.
  - Enable, encourage, and allow the individual to identify and resolve ambivalence.
  - Avoid pressuring the individual to resolve ambivalence.
  - Be aware that readiness to change is not a trait of the individual, that it fluctuates over time.
  - View the relationship with the individual as more of a partnership than as an expert to recipient.

6 A protocol for promoting behavior changes that improve the individual's ability to live with and care for their diabetes has been identified.[21] See Table 3.1.

Perspectives on Behavior Change in Diabetes

1 The compliance perspective[22] is a traditional medical view of the relationship between health professionals and their patients.

  A The compliance perspective assumes that the healthcare professional is responsible for the diagnosis, treatment, and outcome of diabetes care, while the patient is a recipient of this care.

  B The compliance perspective assumes that change occurs as a result of the professional's efforts to get the patient to follow or comply with the prescribed treatment regimen.

Table 3.1. Protocol for Promoting Behavior Change[21]

Consistent with a process of patient-centered decision making, these questions are intended to help patients consider how they can improve their diabetes care. The educator needs to consider the patient's knowledge of diabetes as the protocol is utilized.

1 What part of living with diabetes is most difficult or unsatisfying for you?
2 How does that (the situation described above) make you feel?
3 How would this situation have to change for you to feel better about it?
4 Are you willing to take action to improve the situation for yourself?
5 What are some steps you could take to bring you closer to where you want to be?
6 Is there one thing you will do when you leave here to improve things for yourself?

---

2 Challenging the usefulness of a compliance or adherence approach to behavior change, Glasgow and Anderson[23] noted 2 other perspectives.
   A The first approach is psychologically based and derives from self-determination theory.[14] Principal concepts include autonomy motivation (the psychological process that drives patient behavior change) and autonomy support (actions by healthcare providers that enhance patient autonomy motivation).
   B The second approach[24] comes from a healthcare delivery and medical systems perspective and is based on the concept of "collaborative" or comanagement of chronic illnesses. This model emphasizes collaborative goal-setting and ongoing self-management support as essential to effective disease management.
   C Note that these 2 perspectives are consistent with the principles of the empowerment perspective.

3 The empowerment perspective[22] assumes that most of the responsibility for diabetes care rests with the person who has the disease. Therefore, final decisions regarding diabetes-related behavior are the right and responsibility of the individual.
   A The empowerment perspective holds that the costs and benefits of diabetes care must be seen in the broader personal and social context of a person's life and that persons must be seen as experts in their own lives, while professionals are experts in the clinical aspects of diabetes. Self-care requires an effective coalition that incorporates each party's expertise.
   B The empowerment perspective incorporates the fact that more than 99% of diabetes care is self-care. The vast majority of diabetes care takes place not 2 to 4 times a year in the provider's office, but literally countless times every day in the places where people with diabetes live, work, eat, and play.
   C According to the empowerment perspective, behavior change takes place as healthcare professionals help individuals make informed decisions about self-care. In addition to providing essential knowledge and skills training, efforts to understand the patient's perspective, acknowledge the patient's feelings, and offer relevant information to help the patient make decisions are the cornerstone of the diabetes educator's role in facilitating empowerment.[25]
   D Working with the individual's perspective involves identifying the level of readiness to change and using it as the starting point for further interventions.

E Another foundation of the professional's role is to provide the ongoing support and encouragement that the patient needs to sustain behavior changes that maximize diabetes care and quality of life.[21]

F People with diabetes have always chosen what to do with recommendations they receive from healthcare professionals. Accordingly, the empowerment perspective seeks to clarify the patient's role as an informed, equal, active partner in formulating and maintaining the treatment program. This approach avoids the dilemma in which patients exercise their power to choose by vetoing recommendations made by healthcare providers and educators without effectively using their expertise to develop a more workable plan.

G Not all patients seek to be the primary decision-maker in their care. Professionals must respect different styles. Some people are more comfortable in a less active role, some of the time preferring to follow the recommendations of the providers. Sometimes self-directed care may be achieved in steps.[8] For example, patients who present in very poor control or with limited knowledge may at first prefer a set treatment plan. Once they have experienced self-care, they may choose to take a more active role in self-management.

H Similarly, not all patients are ready to change, and the care provider must respect the level of readiness that exists and work from there (see Importance of Readiness to Change and Assessing Readiness to Change in Chapter 2, Psychosocial Assessment, in Diabetes Education and Program Management).

The Empowerment Approach for Facilitating Behavior Change

1 Facilitating the empowerment of individuals for self-directed behavior change is gaining increased support in diabetes education.[21,26,27] Given the fact that patients make many important and often complex self-care decisions every day, the goal is to enable people to make informed decisions (see Table 3.2).

Table 3.2. Four-Step Patient Empowerment Counseling Model[26]

1 *Help patient identify diabetes-related problems and issues on which they want to work.*
"What problem are you having with diabetes that you want to work on now?"

2 *Help patient identify thoughts and feelings associated with the issue.*
"What are you thinking and feeling when you are struggling with the problem?"

3 *Help patient identify health-related attitudes and beliefs underlying the problem and establish diabetes self-care goals.*
"What deeper attitudes and beliefs lead you to think and feel as you do when you are struggling with the problem?"
"What is your ultimate goal for dealing with the problem?"

4 *Help patient develop and commit to a plan for achieving the goal.*
"What would be the steps, one by one, that would lead to reaching your ultimate goal?"

2 Several key concepts are basic to an empowerment-oriented practice.
  A Emphasizing the whole person.
  - People are more than patients. They are physical, emotional, social, and spiritual beings.
  - The different aspects of a person's life are interrelated and must be taken into account in making diabetes self-care decisions.
  - Practitioners' perspectives tend to be rooted in a clinical context, emphasizing technical considerations, whereas patients' perspectives exist within a life-world context based on practical and experiential considerations.[28]
  - In a qualitative study of women with type 2 diabetes who were judged by diabetes experts as exemplars of self-management, becoming an effective self-manager involved a process from *management-as-rules* to *management-as-work* to *management-as-living*. Patients who achieved the perspective of management-as-living saw taking control of their diabetes as having taken control of their lives and as being guided by something personally meaningful. These exemplars of self-management wanted healthcare providers to serve first as guides and then as safety net when necessary.[29]
  - Recognizing, respecting, and supporting this holistic dynamic helps the educator play a constructive part in the process of change.
  B Acknowledging the patient's role in decision-making.
  - Recognize that it may be impossible to solve problems for the patient or to impose a solution.
  - The effective educator assumes the role of an advisor to the patient on subjects related to the treatment of diabetes. Offering options and supporting the generation of potentially useful approaches to a given problem increase the educator's effectiveness.
  - It is the patient's right and responsibility to make decisions. In one model of diabetes education, the purpose was changed from providing information about why behaviors have to change to providing information that the patient can use to make informed decisions about behavior.[30]
  C Educating for informed choice about treatment options. Three types of education are crucial to empowerment:
  - *Specific self-care skills training.* The first type of education involves providing information about diabetes and its treatment to enable the patient to make wise decisions about diabetes self-care options.[26]
  - *Self-management skills training.* The second type of education involves the ability to coordinate a variety of specific tasks to promote physical well-being and quality of life (eg, coordinating the amount and timing of food, medication, and exercise when attending a party or sick-day management); the ability to effectively utilize family, social, and professional support; and the ability to set and pursue goals. The foundation of self-management skill is the ability to solve problems by coordinating activities and using information and experience to make decisions.
  - *Coping skills training.* The third type of education is designed to facilitate patients' self-awareness and skills for dealing with diabetes-related stressors and the emotional, social, intellectual, and spiritual components of their lives as they relate to the daily decisions patients must make about their diabetes.
  D Taking into account readiness to change.
  - Different approaches to facilitating behavior change are appropriate depending on the patient's stage of readiness to change.[31] The educator should keep in mind

that patients may be at different stages of readiness to change regarding different aspects of self-care and self-management. (See Chapter 2, Psychosocial Assessment, in Diabetes Education and Program Management, for guidelines for assessing readiness to change.)
- For patients in stage 1, the *precontemplation stage* (ie, not planning to change a particular behavior in the foreseeable future), approaches which emphasize providing patients with personalized information and allowing them to express feelings about diabetes may be most effective. For example, the patient may have a negative attitude about diabetes that is associated with a parent or grandparent who had serious complications. Allowing a venting of emotions followed by informing the patient about advances in medical technology and the implications of the DCCT[4] or UKPDS[5] may facilitate a shift to the contemplation stage.
- For patients in stage 2, the *contemplation stage* (ie, seriously thinking about changing behavior in the next 6 months), approaches which encourage patients to develop support networks, provide positive feedback for patients' capacity to make changes, and help patients clarify ambivalent feelings concerning behavior change while emphasizing expected benefits may be most effective.
- For patients in stage 3, the *preparation stage* (ie, intending to change behavior in the next month), approaches that encourage the patient to set specific, achievable goals (eg, walking briskly for at least 15 minutes 3 or more times a week) and that reinforce small changes already made may be most effective.
- For patients in stage 4, the *action stage* (ie, already modifying behavior), approaches that include referral to a diabetes self-management program and providing relevant self-help materials may be most effective.
- In stage 5, the *maintenance stage* (ie, continued in action stage for at least 6 months), approaches that encourage patients to anticipate and plan for potential difficulties (eg, maintaining healthy eating habits while on vacation) and that provide information on community resources such as support groups may be most effective.

E Viewing treatment plans as ongoing experiments.
- Treatment plans need to be refined periodically to reflect changes in a person's life and state of diabetes. It is critically important that both the educator and patient recognize this fact and use it to their advantage.
- The beauty of an experiment is that it produces information, not success or failure. This information is used to refine the treatment plan and produce more information, which is then used to support further refinement, and so on.
- Because this process mirrors life with a chronic disease, it is an excellent model for positive coping with diabetes.

F The educator's focus is to help patients find their optimum way of self-management.

Twelve Specific Steps for Facilitating Patient Empowerment

1 Ask questions.

A The educator can use specific concrete techniques such as asking questions and using other approaches listed in Table 3.3 to facilitate patient empowerment. History-taking questions such as "Have you been having any low blood sugars lately?" or "How often are you checking your blood sugar these days?" are not particularly effective in facilitating empowerment and self-management.

Table 3.3. Twelve Steps for Facilitating Patient Empowerment

1. Ask questions.
2. Start with the patient's agenda.
3. Work with the patient to individualize the treatment plan.
4. Define the problems as specifically as possible.
5. Take a step-by-step approach.
6. Facilitate problem-solving skills.
7. Focus on behaviors, not outcomes.
8. Use contracts.
9. Involve the family and other people who are important to the patient.
10. Maintain contact between visits.
11. Nourish emotional coping skills.
12. Get help from colleagues and refer to specialists as needed.

    B Open-ended questions like "What's the hardest thing for you right now about dealing with your diabetes?" are more likely to generate the kind of information the patient and educator need to develop self-care strategies that will actually work for a given patient.

    C Asking questions can actually save time for healthcare professionals and patients. It is a waste of valuable time when the educator attempts, visit after visit, to offer recommendations without knowing what is actually bothering the patient most. The educator often ends up making suggestions that have little meaning for the patient, so that both the professional and patient become frustrated.

2. Start with the patient's agenda.

    A Educators often feel they know what their patients need to do to improve their health, as well as the order in which these things need to be done.

    B Unfortunately, operating as if patients will follow the agenda an educator sets almost never works. Patients simply veto any suggestions that do not make sense to them.

    C Veto power may not be expressed directly in words. Patients may express this veto power by simply not doing what the educator has recommended.

    D Resistance to treatment suggestions may be expressed directly or indirectly, and the technique of "rolling with resistance" (in which the educator demonstrates listening and empathy while eliciting further reflection on the part of the patient) may be effective in overcoming resistant behavior.[18]
- Example of resistance: "Not testing my blood is not the problem. It is the stress of not having time for everything I need to do."
- Example of rolling with resistance: "So it's hard to find time for a lot of things including testing, and all of these demands are causing you a lot of stress."

    E Starting with the patient's agenda increases the likelihood that patients will reach critical self-care goals. A more positive relationship is established, and patients are likely to become more open when they see that their needs are the educator's primary concern.

3 Individualize the treatment plan.
  A Everyone is different, so there is no single plan that works for every person with diabetes.
  B The key to successful individualization is a fundamental tool: good questions. If the patient's goal is weight loss, for example, the educator might ask how much weight the person wants to lose, what success the patient has had losing weight in the past, what facts of life will facilitate or hinder weight-loss efforts, and what the patient would like the healthcare professional to do when it comes to facilitating the weight-loss process.
  C One model[32] utilizes 3 criteria for matching patients to treatment regimens:
  • Program decisions consistent with the patient's physiological, psychological, and environmental states.
  • Assessing the safety of each intervention in the context of these states.
  • Weighing possible interventions in terms of the success of other patients with similar profiles.

4 Define the problem as specifically as possible.
  A The more specifically the patient and educator define a problem, the more likely they are to solve the problem.
  B Questions, again, are the key to success. For example, if a patient complains about changing eating habits, the educator should help the patient define the problem more specifically. Most patients have specific "sticking points" and are aware of them. In this situation, the sticking point might turn out to be a problem resisting late-night snacks.
  C Two benefits result from identifying specific sticking points.
  • First, both patient and educator can see that the problem they face is more manageable than they originally believed (eg, snacking after dinner is less overwhelming than overall failure to follow an eating plan). Thus, the patient's ability and motivation is greater to make changes.
  • Second, problem-solving for specific problems is usually much easier than problem-solving for general problems.

5 Take a step-by-step approach.
  A Problems that seem insurmountable as a whole can often be solved a step at a time.
  B Most diabetes-related problems are daunting. Educators can help their patients simplify a problem by taking a step-by-step approach. Consider the task of establishing an exercise program. The educator knows that a healthy exercise plan for most people would involve a minimum activity level equivalent to 3 brisk 30-minute walks per week or more frequent activity of shorter duration. Yet many patients who want to start exercising would feel overwhelmed starting at this level.
  C The patient needs to identify a first step in reaching his or her goal, such as initiating an exercise program by walking for 15 minutes twice a week. The role of the educator is to help the patient generate a list of possible strategies, assist in using the list to create a meaningful plan, and provide emotional encouragement and practical support for the patient's efforts to change behavior.
  D This process provides 4 benefits:
  • It establishes a cooperative working relationship between the educator and patient in dealing with a goal the patient has chosen.

- The first step the patient has suggested regarding exercise is a meaningful one. If the strategy is meaningful, the patient is more likely to implement it.
- A patient who succeeds in taking a first step is likely to have the confidence to take a second step and a third.
- If the plan does not work, the educator can ask what the patient learned from the experience.

6 Facilitate problem-solving skills.
  A Living well with diabetes requires a high level of problem-solving skills. Diabetes makes life more complicated, so people with diabetes have more decisions to make and problems to solve on a day-to-day basis than people who do not have diabetes.[33]
  B Patients develop diabetes-related problem-solving skills through trial and error, training, and continuous practice. As one young man said, "I hate having diabetes, but it's forced me to be a really good problem-solver, and I wouldn't give that up for anything in the world."
  C One classic problem-solving model[34] consists of 6 steps:
  - Define the problem.
  - If a family member or other caregiver is involved, verify that everyone agrees with the problem definition.
  - Brainstorm possible solutions.
  - Evaluate suggested solutions.
  - Develop a goal-driven action plan.
  - If not successful, evaluate and refine action plan.

  D Anticipating and preventing common problems is an effective problem-solving strategy.[35]
  E The educator can support the patient's effort to solve a problem by asking what lesson was learned from the experience, whether the effort was successful or not.[35]

7 Focus on behaviors, not outcomes.
  A When an educator helps a patient work on behaviors, desired outcomes are likely to follow.
  B It is easier for patients to achieve their chosen goals, such as improved blood glucose control or reduced weight, when they focus on the behaviors required to reach these goals (eg, attending to nutritional values on commercial food products or starting a walking program).
  C Behavior is something the patient can work on and ultimately control directly, while outcomes such as blood glucose levels are often influenced by factors outside the individual's control.
  D Focusing only on physiologic outcomes can lead to feelings of frustration and even helplessness. Although focusing on behavior is not a panacea, it increases the patient's sense of control.

8 Use contracts.
  A Helping patients formally specify what they will do to reach goals can facilitate self-management.
  B A useful behavioral contract might include the following elements:[36]
  - Goals that are realistic, ambitious, and achievable and that are salient to the patient.

- Goals stated in specific, measurable, behavioral terms.
- Goals represented in terms of successes and not simply the absence of a problem.
- Rewards for achieving the goal. These rewards may be anything the patient chooses, ranging from sleeping through the night (less need to awaken and urinate, improved blood glucose control) to being alive to see a grandchild graduate from high school to feeling good about oneself for improved self-care.
- Plans for dealing with the first sign of slipping, such as to whom the patient will turn to for assistance in achieving a goal. The patient could choose the educator or any other appropriate person for this role.
- Although the educator's objective is to empower the patient for self-reliance and self-care, goal setting is a collaborative effort to the extent the patient needs or prefers assistance.

9 Involve the family and others who are important to the individual.
 A Diabetes is a family disease powerful enough to affect the lives of everyone who loves, lives with, or cares for a person with diabetes.
 B Family members and other important people in the patient's life can significantly affect the way a person with diabetes lives with the disease.
 C Involving the family and significant others may take several forms.
  - Include important family members and significant others in office visits if at all possible, and with the patient's permission. Getting the perspective of family members can be helpful to the patient and the educator.
  - When it is not possible to include family members, ask questions about how the family members are involved in diabetes care. These questions include queries concerning what family members do to facilitate and hinder self-care and what the patient needs from family members and others to make life with diabetes easier (see Chapter 2, Psychosocial Assessment, in Diabetes Education and Program Management).
  - Family and social support have many levels and types, and one model[37] proposes a holistic approach that involves the patient's total life space. This model notes that "support" in the form of advice (however well intentioned and caring) can be problematic when it is perceived as judgmental or blaming.
  - Diabetes support groups allow for exchanges in a setting of common understanding and reduce the risk of inappropriate value judgments that are commonly made about health behaviors. [37]

10 Maintain contact between visits.
 A Research and clinical experience show that even brief, occasional contact with a healthcare professional (between regularly scheduled visits) can powerfully affect people struggling with a chronic disease.
 B Some potentially effective approaches for maintaining patient contact are through phone calls, postcards, newsletters, e-mail messages, and office-based support groups.
 C Maintaining contact helps patients feel cared for, enhances motivation, and provides the educator with an invaluable early-warning system for problems that might otherwise get worse before the patient called about them.

11 Nourish emotional coping skills.
   A One of the things that people with diabetes need most is a strong emotional foundation. Educators need to be prepared to help their patients deal with emotional issues. The assessment of patient coping skills is discussed in Chapter 2, Psychosocial Assessment, in Diabetes Education and Program Management.
   B Books are available to help healthcare professionals,[35] parents,[36] and people with diabetes[12,38-40] cope with the emotional side of diabetes.
   C Persistent emotional distress needs to be assessed to determine if the symptoms meet the criteria of a clinical disorder, such as a Depressive or Anxiety Disorder (see Chapter 6, Psychological Disorders, in Diabetes Education and Program Management).

12 Get help.
   A Educators also need help and support because caring for people with diabetes can be as hard as living with it, though in different ways.
   B Following the empowerment approach will avoid considerable frustration and distress (see Potential Benefits to Educators for Facilitating Patient Empowerment below).
   C Getting help may mean consulting with a colleague to get suggestions for dealing with a difficult issue. Sometimes just talking things out or getting someone else's perspective can help.
   D Getting help may also mean referring a patient for specialized services for which the educator is not trained or does not have the time to provide.

Facilitating Self-Care

1 To control diabetes, patients need a variety of skills. Developing and maintaining healthy patterns of self-care requires 3 basic sets of skills: specific self-care skills, self-management skills, and coping skills. Educational interventions need to facilitate the development of each set of skills (the assessment of these skills is discussed in Chapter 2, Psychosocial Assessment, in Diabetes Education and Program Management).

2 Specific self-care skills training:
   A *Self-care skill* involves the patient's ability to accomplish the specific tasks of metabolic control, including SMBG, insulin administration and dose adjustment, taking medications on time, using a food/meal plan, and managing hypoglycemia and hyperglycemia.
   B *Meta-analyses*, a method of statistically combining the results of many different studies, reveal that active diabetes education that involves demonstration of skills, practice, and direct practical feedback for efforts is the most effective approach for improving self-care skills and metabolic control.[41-43]
   C More didactic approaches are less effective because they tend to increase knowledge without increasing skill or improving glycemia. Skill acquisition requires an emphasis on modeling, practice, and feedback.[18]
   D The key approach for facilitating behavior change is clear: do not talk; teach behavior. Although these findings may seem obvious, their implications for the design of educational interventions are profound and often not adequately taken into account.

E To make the inherently difficult process of behavior change as manageable as possible, educators can help individuals learn to make the best use of their skills and resources, which may mean pursuing incremental change. If the goal is improved glycemic control, some studies show that performing just one new behavior (eg, situational adjustment of insulin) can lead to significantly improved glycosylated hemoglobin levels even in the absence of changes in such basic aspects of lifestyle as food planning and exercise.[44]

3 Self-management skills training:

A With this training the individual learns to continually manage the relationships among food intake, medications, physical and emotional states, activity level, and a variety of life events to achieve and maintain the most desirable metabolic control. The foundation of self-management skill is the ability to solve problems by coordinating activities and using information and experience to make decisions.

B In helping individuals to develop their self-management skills, various psychosocial determinants of self-care behavior should be considered: health beliefs, attitudes, and intentions; self-efficacy; locus of control orientation; cognitive maturity; health status; and various contextual factors (see Chapter 2, Psychosocial Assessment, in Diabetes Education and Program Management).

C Self-management skill also involves the ability to coordinate a variety of specific tasks to promote physical well-being and quality of life (eg, coordinating the amount and timing of food, medication, and exercise when attending a party or managing sick days); the ability to effectively utilize family, social, and professional support; and the ability to set and pursue goals that fit with other life goals.
- Consistent with the empowerment approach to diabetes education, goal setting and goal contracting are included in various educational programs.[36,45-47]
- Elements of effective goal setting and goal contracting include describing goals in specific, concrete, behavioral terms; setting goals that are realistic, achievable, and pertinent to the patient;[36] and utilizing the patient's support network to prevent relapse or goal failure.[45]

D Rigid adherence to a regimen may be less effective than juggling components of treatment in response to daily events and SMBG results.[8,48]

E Given the demands of life with diabetes, the patient's physical and emotional well-being is most enhanced by flexibility and by skill in problem solving.[33]

F To be effective, diabetes education must incorporate interventions to foster the development of these skills. One productive approach involves discussing potential options for handling situations in which the patient finds diabetes to be problematic. The goal of this approach is to develop, practice, and refine strategies for handling these situations in ways that promote physical and emotional well-being.

4 Coping skills training:

A Diabetes coping skills are behaviors that eliminate or modify the stressors common to diabetes (eg, maintaining a rigid regimen of self-care, fear of complications), stressors that may cause emotional distress and attitudinal barriers that block the successful application of new knowledge and self-care behaviors.

B Cognitive behavioral models, including rational emotive therapy and reframing, can be an effective component of active, individualized coping skills training.[11,12,45]

- In this training, patients learn that certain thoughts or attitudes trigger adaptive behavior in difficult situations, while other thoughts and attitudes (usually linked with irrational beliefs or misinformation) trigger maladaptive behavior.
- Patients are then taught how to cope effectively with troublesome diabetes-related situations by restructuring their beliefs, thoughts, and attitudes.
- A case example of the coping skills training process has been described in detail.[45]

C Other coping skills include
- Anticipating a potentially stressful situation and avoiding it or preparing to deal with it constructively (eg, taking a healthy low-fat dish or low-carbohydrate dessert to a dinner party).
- Practicing a relaxation technique (in one study, patients using guided imagery improved their diabetes self-care behavior).[49]
- Making positive lifestyle choices that adhere to the rigors of the diabetes regimen—eating well, exercising regularly, balancing energy expenditures (work) with energy conservation (play) and replenishment (rest).[50]
- Methodically solving problems that inhibit diabetes self-care behavior[51]—studies indicate that training in problem solving improves metabolic control and quality of life.[52,53]
- Mobilizing and utilizing personal and professional support (a study of patients with type 1 diabetes indicated that following a healthy diabetes-care regimen is associated with good family support and rapport with health professionals).[54]
- The burden of self-care can be formidable, and the use of humor can help to lighten the load. However, using humor to deny the seriousness of a situation can be destructive.

D A final component of coping skills training is relapse prevention, which offers protection against the possibility that the inevitable slips in self-care may trigger a full-blown relapse.[55]
- Some specific relapse prevention techniques include contracting to employ both cognitive and behavioral strategies and mobilizing the support of others.[45]
- The Transtheoretical Model suggests several processes for maintaining self-care behavior, including reinforcement management (using both tangible and intangible rewards to encourage the continuation of positive actions) and stimulus control (changing the environment to promote healthy behavior or to avoid undesirable activity).[56]

The Effects of the Organization and Structure of Educational and Treatment Programs

1 The way in which educational and treatment programs are organized or structured can facilitate or hinder the degree to which individuals participate as well as their ability to make changes.

2 Educators can incorporate specific structural issues into the interventions they design.
A Multidisciplinary staff:
- Given the complexity of life with diabetes, patients will generally benefit from educational and treatment interventions that allow them to consult with multidisciplinary staff that includes physicians, nurses, dietitians, mental health specialists, exercise specialists, and pharmacists.

- Because few clinics can support such a staff, a viable alternative is a referral network of experienced specialists in each field. Access to specialists tends to facilitate self-care, so developing an effective and coordinated referral network is helpful to educators and their patients.

B Educators can consider helping patients to prepare before visits with their physicians. Studies[57] show that a brief intervention focused on training patients to be more active and assertive during interviews with a physician leads to improvement in glucose control and quality of life.

C Ongoing professional support:
- Most changes involved in maintaining healthy patterns of self-care require continuing support, yet patients typically go for months without consulting healthcare providers.
- Two options for encouraging more frequent contact (and potentially facilitating behavior change) are on-call availability and follow-up telephone contact.
- Follow-up telephone contact initiated by the patient at set times or as circumstances require or by the educator may also support the patient's self-care efforts.
- These contacts can help patients maintain their motivation to change by addressing specific problems that might lead to relapse and by facilitating a pattern of open communication that makes it easier for the patient to call if problems arise.

D Group support:
- Whenever possible, provide opportunities for group experiences with others who have diabetes. Such opportunities can take the form of group education, formal or informal diabetes support groups, referral to these groups, and other self-improvement activities such as walking groups.
- Groups encourage efforts to improve self-care through mutual sharing and encouragement, modeling, positive reinforcement, and personal goal setting.

E Programs can be augmented with various interactive computer-based resources and automated telephone systems.
- There are many worthwhile, diabetes-oriented programs available on the internet, such as those produced by the American Diabetes Association.
- Hand-held computers for assisting patients in adjusting their insulin, diabetes-relevant video games, and PC-based home learning programs are technologies designed to improve patient's ability to manage diabetes.[58]
- Studies of Automated Telephone Disease Management (ATDM) systems indicate that the technique can increase the effectiveness of diabetes care, including decreasing diabetes crises, decreasing A1C levels, more frequent glucose monitoring, and fewer medication adherence problems.[58,59]

Reevaluating Traditional Teaching Methods to Incorporate the Empowerment Approach

1 Empowering patients requires diabetes educators to evaluate their teaching methods and approaches to patient care.

2 Recognize that patients are in control of their own self-care. This realization often happens indirectly. Every day educators work with patients who refuse to follow the educator's good advice about caring for their diabetes. The first and strongest response to this refusal might be frustration or perhaps disappointment. However, further thought might lead the educator to see that these patients are telling the educator in no uncertain terms that they will decide what they will and will not do.

A Because patients truly have veto power, creating a coalition for care that helps the patient assume an initiating role rather than a defensive one decreases frustration for both patients and educators.

B The role of the educator in such a coalition is not to give advice about the "right" or "best" way to accomplish a particular goal, but rather to help patients explore the range of self-care options available and the consequences of implementing each of these options.

C This type of exploration can be frustrating for the educator when the patient is resistant or in denial. In such a case, educators need to recognize the limits of their ability to effect change.

D The technique of "rolling with resistance" can be effective in overcoming the patient's resistance to change.[18]

3 Many educators have difficulty dealing with the emotional content of patients' problems. This limitation makes it difficult for educators to encourage patients to identify, express, and explore negative emotions that are an inevitable part of living with diabetes. Diabetes educators need to refocus their professional tendency to be problem solvers and support their patients' explorations of emotional issues. Emotions are not problems to be solved; rather, they are feelings to be recognized, identified, expressed, and accepted.

A The educator's role is that of a thoughtful, compassionate, active, well-informed listener.

B Educators are not responsible for fixing their patients' negative emotions. Recognizing this aspect of their role may help educators feel more comfortable in helping their patients recognize and work with uncomfortable feelings.

4 Given the clinical and behavioral aspects of diabetes along with today's healthcare environment, the potential for provider burnout is high. Ten myths have been identified that can contribute to burnout.[60]

A Healthcare providers are responsible for diabetes outcomes.

B Healthcare providers are the experts and know all that is needed to control diabetes.

C Patients should defer to providers, due to providers' superior knowledge and status.

D Diabetes control should be patients' highest priority.

E Patients should do exactly what providers tell them, regardless of cost and effectiveness.

F If patients get enough information, they will take care of their diabetes the way providers recommend.

G Patients who fail to return for care or follow medical advice are noncompliant (ie, lazy, stupid, or self-destructive).

H Patients bring type 2 diabetes on themselves.

I Type 2 diabetes is not serious until the patient requires insulin or has chronic complications, and only patients with serious diabetes require self-monitoring of blood glucose and self-care education.

J Control is lost because patients do not follow directions.

Potential Benefits to Educators for Facilitating Patient Empowerment

1 Accepting that the educator's role is limited to education and counseling can relieve any guilt the educator might feel when patients do not follow healthy, self-care programs. The educator can feel a great relief to be able to say, "I did my job (educating and counseling) as well as I could. My desire was to facilitate meaningful change, but getting the patient to change is not always possible." The educator should keep in mind that being responsible to patients is not being responsible for them.

2 Recognizing that changing an individual's behavior is not part of the job description may help educators feel less frustrated with individuals who choose to manage their diabetes in ways that the educator considers unhealthy.

3 When educators spend less energy trying to change individuals, they relieve themselves of a self-imposed burden and free energy for other, more attainable tasks.

4 Educators will benefit from using the same self-management and coping skills that they offer to their patients.

Key Educational Considerations

1 Supporting patients in their efforts to decide upon, initiate, and maintain healthy patterns of self-care is a critical responsibility of the diabetes educator.

2 The role of the educator is to facilitate change; the role of the patient is to make change. Every encounter with the patient can be directed toward empowerment. The key is to ask questions and offer options rather than to issue directives. However, some individuals require more assistance, and the educator might have to be more directly involved in treatment planning.

3 The patient's personal model of diabetes, including health beliefs, locus-of-control orientation, and diabetes self-efficacy, powerfully influences motivation for change. Both the patient and educator need to learn to identify and understand the effects of these factors and, when necessary, how they can be shifted.

4 The power of thoughts and attitudes can be demonstrated through discussions that reveal how diabetes-related behaviors flow directly from personal beliefs.

5 The support a patient receives from family, friends, coworkers, and medical staff also affects patterns of self-care. The educator can assess and make efforts to influence these factors as well. The educator can assist patients to identify gaps in currently available support and to create plans to fill these gaps.

6 Behavior-based education is far more effective than knowledge-based education in changing patterns of self-care. Therefore, all interventions need to be presented in a practical, experience-based context. Specific self-care and self-management skills (including complex problem-solving ability) can be demonstrated, practiced, observed, and refined in face-to-face interactions.

7 Coping skills training can be an invaluable component of efforts to improve self-care patterns. All too often attitudinal and emotional barriers prevent patients from making needed changes in diabetes-related behavior. Patients can be taught a basic approach for managing the emotional side of living with diabetes that may help them cope more effectively with the many common self-care crises.

8 Autonomy and efficacy are central to a patient's motivation to change diabetes-related behavior.

Learning Assessment: Case Study 1

RT is a 57-year-old man who was diagnosed with type 2 diabetes 3 years ago. At the time of diagnosis RT was hypertensive, overweight, did not exercise regularly, and smoked about 2 packs of cigarettes a day. An oral antidiabetes agent was prescribed by his physician, and RT was given a handout of a calorie-restricted diet, asked to monitor his fasting blood glucose level 3 times a week, offered a smoking cessation program, and advised to begin some form of regular exercise.

Since his diagnosis RT has canceled most of his appointments for medical follow-up of his diabetes, keeping only 4 appointments in 3 years. Last week he called to complain of increased fatigue, blurred vision, and frequent urination. At his appointment today his blood glucose is 220 mg/dL (12.2 mmol/L), his blood pressure is 160/95, his weight is 20 lb (4.5 kg) more than it was on diagnosis, and he acknowledges that he is not monitoring his blood glucose levels nor is he exercising or following the eating plan described in the handout he was given. He is still smoking 2 packs of cigarettes per day.

When questioned about his diabetes-related behavior, RT offers the following explanations: "Other than the little problems I had last week, I feel I'm doing fine. After all, I have the milder type of diabetes." "At my job I'm always on the go. There's no way I could eat the way you say I'm supposed to." "The cigarettes are my way of relaxing, and they haven't killed me yet." "My mother died from diabetes when she was 62 years old. I figure it's fate, and it will get me, too, sooner or later. There's nothing I can do about it." "The exercise, the diet, the blood sugar testing—the whole routine is just more than I can manage. I'm just not a structured sort of person."

"You tell me what to do, like the blood sugar testing, for instance, and I go home thinking I might be able to do it, but when I get home I realize I can't. I can't get the drop on the strip or whatever, so I get frustrated and give up." "Even when I feel like I'm really going to just do it, like start exercising, right away I flop, because it all gets so complicated, with the timing and making sure I don't go low, and all that. It's just too much to think about." "I get so mad. It's just unfair. I ask 'Why me?' When the answer is 'There is no reason', I just say to forget it all. I know that's crazy, but that's just the way my mind works."

Questions for Discussion
1 What factors seem to be creating RT's resistance to self-care?
2 What other factors might you want to assess before beginning to work with RT?
3 What empowerment-based strategies can you use with RT?
4 How would you decide which aspect of self-care to address first?

Discussion

1 RT offers a classic, if all too common, example of resistance to change. His attitudes and his lack of skills interact to create a vicious cycle that leaves him stuck.

2 His motivation to change is limited by the fact that he sees his disease as relatively mild and the consequences of better self-care (coordinating food and work, giving up cigarettes) as too costly. He also believes that diabetes-related health outcomes are controlled by chance or fate, so there is no reason to try to affect these outcomes because 'what will be, will be.'

3 RT is not confident that he can do what is necessary to manage his diabetes, and it is clear that his education to date leaves him without sufficient skill to truly take care of himself. His skills are limited in the realms of specific diabetes self-care skills, self-management skills, problem-solving ability, and coping skills.

4 An effective approach for solving these problems begins by creating a coalition between the diabetes educator and RT. The educator can help RT identify some of his diabetes-related emotions and then acknowledge these feelings (if he is ready to do so). Work may then proceed at both attitudinal and behavioral levels.

5 Using an empowerment approach, the educator can ask RT questions about his fatalistic attitude toward diabetes-related health outcomes and what gets in the way when he tries to care for his diabetes.

6 Asking questions rather than making statements is crucial to this approach.

7 Feelings of inadequacy must be recognized and acknowledged. The practical difficulty of living with diabetes also needs to be acknowledged to keep the issue in perspective and create a therapeutic relationship with RT.

8 To address the behavior directly, the educator might ask RT what aspect of self-care he feels he is handling best right now. This question will usually lead to the acknowledgment that everything is not totally hopeless. It may then be possible for RT to identify sources of strength that facilitate other self-care behavior.

9 RT should be asked if he is ready to identify an issue on which he would like to work. It is important for the choice to be his, and he should be encouraged to be both ambitious and realistic in making his choice and setting his goals. Reaching a goal that is insufficiently ambitious provides little satisfaction, while an overly ambitious goal is generally unsuccessful and discouraging.

10 RT, like so many patients, needs intensive, behavior-based skills training. He could benefit from watching the educator demonstrate important skills, practicing the skills while being observed, using the skills at home, and then demonstrating the skills later to the educator. RT also needs some basic diabetes education including nutritional counseling, so referring him to a diabetes education program may be helpful.

11 RT also needs follow-up. He seems willing to try things, but then seems to run into problems and gives up. An intervention as simple as a follow-up phone call 1 week after a face-to-face meeting might be helpful.

Learning Assessment: Case Study 2

CP has type 1 diabetes. He is in the first year of high school, and things are not going well for him. His attitude about school is very negative, which is reflected in grades that put him at risk of failing the first semester. He says that he hates school and that the kids are stupid and nasty. About diabetes, he says he feels he is a freak and he hates the disease and his life. CP's most recent HbA1c, which covered the first 3 months of high school, was 11.8%.

This dialogue demonstrates the utilization of the empowerment and motivational perspectives in facilitating behavior change.

Diabetes Educator: Entering high school appears to have started a downward spiral for you. Your grades and diabetes control have taken a dive.
CP: Yeah, it's been hard for me . . . a new school system, kids I don't know.
DE: Entering high school can be difficult. What about it has been most difficult for you?
CP: Adjusting to the schedule has been hard. I've had a couple of low blood sugars in school that required the assistance of paramedics. The commotion attracted a lot of attention, and now I feel like everyone is watching me. And the ones not gawking are staying as far away from me as possible.
DE: That has to hurt; anything you want to change?
CP: Yeah, if I could just keep from going low, I think I'd be alright, but my lunch period is much later than it used to be, and 3 days a week I have phys. ed. before I get to eat lunch. I have tried eating more breakfast and I have lowered my insulin, but whatever I do doesn't work all the time.
DE: Is there anything else you could do?
CP: Well, my sister, who is a year ahead of me, says it may be early enough in the semester to get my schedule changed. If my gym class was closer to breakfast or soon after lunch, I think I could avoid having my blood sugar drop too low. I also wonder if I could change my insulin. I have tried reducing the number of units, but I wonder if a different combination of insulins might work for me. Can you help me with that?
DE: Yes, I have some ideas, and we can talk about modifying your regimen. In the meantime, do you intend to talk to your school counselor about changing your schedule?
CP: I have mixed feelings about it. It might work but I'm not keen on bringing more attention to my diabetes.
DE: I can see the conflict for you. Would it help to weigh the pros and cons of changing or not changing your schedule?
CP: Hmm. Certainly, eliminating those reactions would be great. I will talk to my counselor about it.
DE: Good! When do you intend to do it?
CP: Tomorrow.
DE: Anything else you want to work on?
CP: Wish I could make some friends at school.
DE: Is there anyone you've connected with?

CP: There is this one guy in my class who seems to like me. Each time I have hit the skids, he has made the effort to ask me how I am doing and if I'm okay.

DE: Sounds like he could become a good support person for you in school. Any ideas about how you can get a friendship going with the guy?

CP: We have a test coming up next week, and I'm going to ask him if he wants to study for it with me.

DE: Good, when?

CP: I'll do it tomorrow too.

DE: Terrific! You should give yourself a big pat on the back for identifying some possible solutions to a difficult situation and for being willing to try some new behaviors. You have a plan now that is a good start for making school a better, more satisfying place for yourself. Let's meet again in 2 weeks and talk more about what else you can do to get better control of the diabetes and to improve relations with your classmates.

Questions for Discussion

1 Which steps have been taken to facilitate patient empowerment?

2 Which elements of motivational interviewing were employed?

3 Although contracting for behavior change can be very effective, the educator did not initiate the formulation of a contract for CP. What is your reaction to her decision?

4 What might the educator consider in anticipating the next meeting with CP?

Discussion

1 CP is manifesting specific diabetes self-care problems (difficulty accommodating a problematic schedule in order to prevent excessive low blood sugar levels) and emotional distress (anger and dysphoria).

2 The educator addresses the issue of glycemic control first, utilizing several patient empowerment principles including asking questions, starting with CP's agenda, defining problems specifically, taking a step-by-step approach, focusing on behaviors, and nourishing emotional coping skills.

3 Consistent with the empowerment approach, the educator also has employed the techniques of motivational interviewing, including eliciting the motivation to change, helping him to resolve ambivalence, and partnering with CP rather than assuming a dominant, expert role.

4 Contracting for behavioral changes is likely to be useful particularly as the treatment plan develops, but the educator decided to start with a few specific changes with the intention of building on a few successes. In addition, she did not want to overwhelm this young man with too many issues and demands.

5 One of the steps for facilitating patient empowerment is to maintain contact between visits, so the educator will contact CP before the next scheduled meeting.

6 With regard to the next session with CP, the educator intends to offer him coping skills training that includes assistance with assertiveness and esteem building. Also, consideration will be given to informing CP about the insulin pump, which might give him more flexibility in managing his blood glucose levels.

7 Also, the educator will monitor CP's emotional status. If symptoms of depression, anxiety, or anger continue despite the behavior changes, she will screen for the possibility of a clinical disorder such as Dysthymic (Depressive) Disorder or Generalized Anxiety Disorder.

References

1 Kurtz SMS. Adherence to diabetes regimens: empirical status and clinical applications. Diabetes Educ. 1990;16:50-59.

2 Ary DV, Toobert D, Wilson W, Glasgow RE. Patient perspective on factors contributing to nonadherence to diabetes regimen. Diabetes Care. 1986;9:168-172.

3 Ley P. Communicating with Patients. London: Croom Helm; 1988.

4 The Diabetes Control and Complications Trial Research Group. The effect of intensive treatment of diabetes on the development and progression of long-term complications in insulin-dependent diabetes mellitus. N Engl J Med. 1993;329:977-986.

5 UK Prospective Diabetes Study Group. Effect of intensive blood-glucose control with metformin on complications in overweight patients with type 2 diabetes (UKPDS 34). Lancet. 1998; 352:854-865.

6 Lorenz RA, Bubb J, Davis D, et al. Changing behavior: practical lessons from the Diabetes Control and Complications Trial. Diabetes Care. 1996;19:648-652.

7 Clement S. Diabetes self-management education (technical review). Diabetes Care. 1995;18:1204-1214.

8 Peyrot M, Rubin RR. Modeling the effect of diabetes education on glycemic control. Diabetes Educ. 1994;20:143-148.

9 Robiner W, Keel PK. Self-care behaviors and adherence in diabetes mellitus. Semin Clin Neuropsychiatry. 1997;2:40-56.

10 Ruggiero L, Glasgow RE, Dryfoos JM, et al. Diabetes self-management: self-reported recommendations and patterns in a large population. Diabetes Care. 1997;30:568-576.

11 Rubin RR, Walen SR, Ellis A. Living with diabetes. J Rational-Emotive Cognitive/Behavioral Ther. 1990;8:21-39.

12 Rubin RR, Biermann J, Toohey B. Psyching Out Diabetes: A Positive Approach to Your Negative Emotions. 3rd ed. Los Angeles: Lowell House; 1999.

13 Sullivan ED, Joseph DH. Struggling with behavior changes: a special case for clients with diabetes. Diabetes Educ. 1998;24:72-77.

14 Williams GC, Freedman ZR, Deci EL. Supporting autonomy to motivate patients with diabetes for glucose control. Diabetes Care.1998;21:1644-1651.

15 Ruggiero L, Prochaska JO. From research to practice: introduction. Diabetes Spectrum. 1993;6:22-24.

16 Bandura A. Social Foundations of Thought and Action: A Social Cognitive Theory. Englewood Cliffs, NJ: Prentice-Hall; 1986.

17 Rubin RR, Peyrot M. Psychosocial problems and interventions in diabetes: a review of the literature. Diabetes Care. 1992;15:1640-1657.

18 Doherty Y, James P, Roberts S. Stage of change counseling. In: Snoek FJ, Skinner TC, eds. Psychology in Diabetes Care. Chichester, England: John Wiley & Sons, Ltd; 2000:99-139.

19. Smith DE, Heckemeyer CM, Kratt PP, Mason DA. Motivational interviewing to improve adherence to a behavioural weight-control program for older obese women with NIDDM: a pilot study. Diabetes Care. 1997;20:52-54.

20. Rollnick S, Miller WR. What is motivational interviewing? Behav Cogn Psychother. 1995; 325-334.

21. Anderson RM, Funnell MM, Arnold MS. Using the empowerment approach to help patients change behavior. In: Anderson BJ, Rubin RR, eds. Practical Psychology for Diabetes Clinicians. Alexandria, Va: American Diabetes Association; 1996:163-172.

22. Arnold MS, Butler PM, Anderson RM, Funnell MM, Feste C. Guidelines for facilitating a patient empowerment program. Diabetes Educ. 1995;21:308-312.

23. Glasgow RE, Anderson RM. In diabetes care, moving from compliance to adherence is not enough. Diabetes Care. 1999;22:2090-2092.

24. Glasgow RE, Wagner EH, Kaplan RM, Vinicor F, Smith L, Norman J. If diabetes is a public health problem, why not treat it as one? Ann Behav Med. 1999;21:1-13.

25. Hampson SE, Glasgow RE, Foster LE. Personal model of diabetes among older adults: relationship to self-management and other variables. Diabetes Educ. 1995;21:300-307.

26. Anderson RM, Funnell MM, Barr PA, et al. Learning to empower patients: results of professional education program for diabetes educators. Diabetes Care. 1991;14:584-590.

27. Anderson R, Funnell M, Carlson A, Saleh-Statin N, Cradock S, Skinner TC. Facilitating self-care through empowerment. In: Snoek FJ, Skinner TC, eds. Psychology in Diabetes Care. Chichester, England: John Wiley & Sons, Ltd; 2000:69-97.

28. Hunt LM, Arar NH, Larme AC. Contrasting patient and practitioner perspectives in type 2 diabetes management. West J Nurs Res. 1998;20:656-676.

29. Ellison GC, Rayman KM. Exemplars' experience of self-managing type 2 diabetes. Diabetes Educ. 1998;24:325-330.

30. Funnell MM, Anderson RM. Putting humpty dumpty back together again: reintegrating the clinical and behavioral components in diabetes care and education. Diabetes Spectrum. 1999;12:19-23.

31. Curry SJ. Commentary on Prochaska JO, DiClemente CC, Norcross JC. In search of how people change: application to addictive behaviors. Diabetes Spectrum. 1993;6:34-35.

32. Caban A, Johnson P, Marseille D, Wylie-Rosett J. Tailoring a lifestyle change approach and resources to the patient. Diabetes Spectrum. 1999;12:33-38.

33. Toobert DJ, Glasgow RE. Problem-solving and diabetes self-care. J Behav Med. 1991;14:71-86.

34. Wysocki T. The Ten Keys to Helping Your Child Grow Up With Diabetes. Alexandria, Va: American Diabetes Association; 1997.

35. Anderson B, Rubin RR, eds. Practical Psychology for Diabetes Clinicians: How to Deal With the Key Behavioral Issues Faced by Patients and Healthcare Teams. Alexandria, Va: American Diabetes Association; 1996.

36. Davis ED, Vander Meer JM, Yarborough PC, Roth SB. Using solution-focused therapy strategies in empowerment-based education. Diabetes Educator. 1999;25:249-57.

37. Wallhagen MI. Social support in diabetes. Diabetes Spectrum. 1999;12:254-56.

38. Lowe E, Arsham G. Diabetes: A Guide to Living Well. 3rd ed. Minneapolis: Chronimed; 1997.

39. Anderson B, Funnell M. The Art of Empowerment. Alexandria, Va: American Diabetes Association; 2000.

40 Edelman SV. Taking control of your diabetes. Caddo, Okla: Professional Communications; 2000.

41 Padgett D, Mumford E, Hynes M, Carter R. Meta-analysis of the effects of educational and psychosocial interventions on management of diabetes mellitus. J Clin Epidemiol. 1988;41:1007-1030.

42 Brown SA. Effects of educational interventions in diabetes care: a meta-analysis of findings. Nurs Res. 1988;37:223-230.

43 Brown SA. Studies of educational interventions and outcomes in diabetic adults: a meta-analysis revisited. Patient Educ Couns. 1990;16:189-215.

44 Rubin RR, Peyrot M, Saudek CD. Differential effect of diabetes education on self-regulation and lifestyle behaviors. Diabetes Care. 1991;14:335-338.

45 Rubin R. Psychotherapy and counselling in diabetes mellitus. In: Snoek FJ, Skinner TC, eds. Psychology in Diabetes Care. Chichester, England: John Wiley & Sons, Ltd; 2000:235-263.

46 Berkowitz KJ, Anderson LA, Panayioto RM, Ziemer DC, Gallina DL. Mini-residency on diabetes care for healthcare providers: enhanced knowledge and attitudes with unexpected challenges to assessing behavior change. Diabetes Educ. 1998;24:143-150.

47 Glasgow RE, Eakin EG. Medical office-based interventions. In: Snoek FJ, Skinner TC, eds. Psychology in Diabetes Care. Chichester, England: John Wiley & Sons, Ltd; 2000:141-168.

48 Sims D, Sims E. From research to practice: motivation, adherence, and the therapeutic alliance. Diabetes Spectrum. 1989;2:49-51.

49 Wichowski HC, Kubsch SM. Increasing diabetic self-care through guided imagery. Complement Ther Nurs Midwifery. 1999;5:159-163.

50 Pohl SL. Facilitating lifestyle change in people with diabetes mellitus: perspective from a private practice. Diabetes Spectrum. 1999;12:28-33.

51 Grey M. Coping and diabetes. Diabetes Spectrum. 2000;13:167-169.

52 Grey M, Boland EA, Davidson M, Li J, Tamborlane WV. Coping skills training for youth with diabetes mellitus has long-lasting effects on metabolic control and quality of life. J Pediatr. 2000;137:107-113.

53 Grey M, Boland EA, Davidson M, Yu C, Tamborlane WV. Coping skills training for youths with diabetes on intensive therapy. Appl Nurs Res. 1999;12:3-12.

54 Lo R. Correlates of expected success at adherence to health regimen of people with IDDM. J Adv Nurs. 1999;30:418-424.

55 Marlatt GA. Situational determinants of relapse and skill-training interventions. In: Marlatt GA, Gordon JR, eds. Relapse Prevention. New York: Guilford Press; 1985.

56 Ruggiero L. Helping people with diabetes change behavior: from theory to practice. Diabetes Spectrum. 2000;13:125-132.

57 Greenfield S, Kaplan SH, Ware JE Jr, et al. Patients' participation in medical care: effects on blood sugar control and quality of life in diabetes. J Gen Intern Med. 1988;3:448-457.

58 Piette JD. Interactive resources for patient education and support. Diabetes Spectrum. 2000;13:110-112.

59 Meneghini LF, Albisser AM, Goldberg RB, Mintz DH. An electronic case manager for diabetes control. Diabetes Care. 1998;21:591-596.

60 Brackenridge B, Swenson K. Am I toast or is it just hot out here? Lessons from the desert in avoiding diabetes provider burnout. Diabetes Spectrum. 1999;12:23-28.

Suggested Readings

Anderson B, Funnell M. The Art of Empowerment. Alexandria, Va: American Diabetes Association; 2000.

Anderson B, Rubin RR, eds. Practical Psychology for Diabetes Clinicians: How to Deal With the Key Behavioral Issues Faced by Patients and Health Care Teams. Alexandria, Va: American Diabetes Association; 1996.

Bradley C. Handbook of Psychology and Diabetes. Chur, Switzerland: Harwood Academic Publishers; 1994.

Edelman SV. Taking Control of Your Diabetes. Caddo, Okla: Professional Communications; 2000.

Feste C. The Physician Within, 2nd ed. Alexandria, Va: American Diabetes Association; 1992.

Guffey L, ed. American Diabetes Association Complete Guide to Diabetes, 2nd ed. Alexandria, Va: American Diabetes Association; 1999.

Lowe E, Arsham G. Diabetes: A Guide to Living Well. 3rd ed. Minneapolis: Chronimed; 1997.

Peyrot M, Rubin RR. Psychosocial aspects of diabetes care. In: Leslie D, Robbins D, eds. Diabetes: Clinical Science in Practice. Cambridge: Cambridge University Press; 1995:465-477.

Plotnick L, Henderson R. Clinical Management of The Child and Teenager With Diabetes. Baltimore, Md: Johns Hopkins University Press; 1998.

Rollnick S, Mason P, Butler C. Health Behavior Change: A Guide for Practitioners. New York: Churchill Livingstone; 1999.

Rubin RR, Biermann J, Toohey B. Psyching Out Diabetes: A Positive Approach to Your Negative Emotions, 3rd ed. Los Angeles: Lowell House; 1999.

Snoek FJ, Skinner TC, eds. Psychology in Diabetes Care. Chichester, England: John Wiley & Sons, Ltd; 2000.

Learning Assessment: Post-Test Questions

Behavior Change   3

1. How have diabetes self-care behaviors been affected by technological advances?
   A Offers better health but involves greater self-care
   B Has little or no effect on self-care demands
   C Reduces self-care demands on persons with diabetes who are not using insulin
   D Requires less active decision-making skills of patients

2. Which is the most effective way for diabetes educators to facilitate self-management skills?
   A Encourage rigid adherence to a treatment program to maintain better blood glucose control
   B Teach using a didactic approach to enhance patient-knowledge of diabetes-related concepts
   C Work with the patient to set realistic self-care goals
   D Use experiences of other patients to teach coping and self-care skills

3. The main difference between a compliance model and empowerment approach to behavior change is the:
   A Clinical outcomes
   B Financial cost
   C Individual's role in self-management
   D Degree of behavior change

4. A diabetes education program that encourages patients to become active learners focuses on:
   A Skills orientation, practice, and direct feedback
   B Oral instructions supported with written educational materials
   C Checklists, monitoring logs, and self-administered questionnaires
   D Sporadically scheduled practice review sessions and a coping skills assessment

5. The empowerment approach:
   A Focuses exclusively on the strengths of the person with diabetes
   B Offers solutions to problems for the patient to choose
   C Provides education to help patients make informed choices
   D Enables the healthcare team to formulate an intervention plan early in the treatment process and have everyone follow it

6. If a patient makes negative comments about the burden of self-care, admits to feeling overwhelmed, and states he is a failure, the diabetes educator should:
   A Listen and help the individual to focus on specific problem areas
   B Offer solutions
   C Agree with the patient to help him move beyond the negative thoughts
   D Give examples of other patients who have overcome difficulties

7. Which of the following might diabetes educators expect as a result of using the empowerment approach?
   A To experience feelings of guilt when patients do not follow suggestions
   B To accept that patients may choose to ignore their recommendations
   C To hold themselves accountable for patient decisions
   D To expect to invest significant time and energy to motivate patients

8. Which of the following statements is the most accurate?
   A Self-management training is about self-awareness
   B Coping skills training is about providing information and treatment options
   C Empowerment concerns a person's self-management and coping skills and the pace at which they proceed
   D Treatment plans need structure and repetition to be effective

9. The organization and structure of an educational and treatment program can affect a patient's ability to make change. All of the following are components of a program except:
   A Interdisciplinary staff
   B Compliance protocols
   C Group support
   D On-call availability and follow-up contact

10. Taking into account a patient's readiness to change, which of the following is an appropriate action for a diabetes educator?
    A Recommend a support group for patients in the precontemplation stage
    B Encourage patients in the contemplation stage to set specific goals
    C Refer patients in the preparation stage to a self-management program
    D Help patients problem-solve and anticipate difficult situations when they are in the maintenance stage

11. Which of the following actions facilitates patient empowerment?
    A Start with the patient's agenda
    B Focus on outcomes rather than behavior
    C Use a standardized set of questions to elicit information
    D Address general issues with a problem-solving approach

12. The DCCT and the UKPDS:
    A Confirm the benefits of intensive treatment, including active self-management, for type 1 diabetes
    B Confirm the benefits of intensive treatment, including active self-management, for type 2 diabetes
    C Confirm the benefits of intensive treatment, including active self-management, for type 1 and type 2 diabetes
    D Confirm the benefits of intensive treatment were negligible

13. A key element of motivational interviewing is:
    A To establish rewards for compliant behavior
    B To establish penalties for noncompliant behavior
    C To pressure the patient to resolve ambivalencies
    D To elicit, rather than impose, a motivation to change

14. Which of the following statements about the compliance perspective on behavior change in diabetes is not correct?
    A The compliance perspective assumes that the healthcare professional is responsible for the diagnosis, treatment, and outcome of diabetes care
    B It is the only valid perspective for achieving behavior change in patients with diabetes
    C This perspective assumes that compliance with the healthcare professional's prescribed treatment regimen is the key to diabetes control
    D The compliance model is a traditional medical view of the relationship between health professionals and patients

15. Aspects of the empowerment perspective include:
    A Providing skills training, prescribing a treatment regimen, and giving ongoing support and encouragement
    B Providing skills training, giving ongoing support and encouragement, understanding and starting from the patient's perspective
    C Providing skills training, giving ongoing support and encouragement, and increasing frequency of patient visits
    D None of the above

16. A fundamental self-management skill is the patient's ability to:
    A Solve problems by coordinating activities and using information and experience to make appropriate decisions
    B Monitor one's own blood glucose level
    C Cope with diabetes-related emotional distress
    D All of the above

17 Coping skills training is designed to:
  A Educate patients about glycemic control
  B Set and pursue self-care goals
  C Facilitate patients' awareness and skills for dealing with diabetes-related stressors
  D All of the above

18 With regard to the creation of a treatment plan, the empowerment perspective advocates that :
  A There is 1 plan for everyone with diabetes
  B There are 2 standard plans, 1 for patients with type 1 diabetes and another for those with type 2 diabetes
  C Everyone is different, so the treatment plan should be individualized to best suit each patient
  D Everyone is different, but using 1 standard treatment plan is more practical and economical than individualizing a plan for each patient

19 Which of the following actions is not an element of effective goal setting and goal contracting?
  A Describing goals in general and broad terms so they are more achievable
  B Setting goals that are realistic, achievable, and pertinent to the patient
  C Utilizing the patient's support network to prevent relapse or goal failure
  D Describing goals in specific, measurable, behavioral terms

20 Cognitive behavioral models, including rational-emotive therapy and reframing, can be an effective component of:
  A Diabetes-specific self-care skills training
  B Coping skills training
  C Self-management skills training
  D All of the above

21 Which of the following educational program interventions does not facilitate a patient's participation and ability to change?
  A Provide multidisciplinary services
  B Provide on-call availability and follow-up contact with staff
  C Encourage and provide opportunities for group interaction and support
  D Avoid negativity by not addressing the subject of relapse

22 Patients' problems often have emotional content, and educators need to:
  A Take responsibility for fixing their patient's negative emotions
  B Be thoughtful, compassionate, active, well-informed listeners
  C Discourage the exploration of emotional issues
  D Maintain focus on problem-solving

23 One myth that can contribute to provider burnout is:
  A Most of the responsibility for diabetes care rests with the patient
  B Patients must be seen as experts in their own lives
  C If patients get enough information, they will take care of their diabetes the way providers recommend
  D Different aspects of a patient's life are interrelated and must be taken into account in making diabetes self-care decisions

See next page for answer key.

Post-Test Answer Key

Behavior Change

1	A	12	C
2	C	13	D
3	C	14	B
4	A	15	B
5	C	16	A
6	A	17	C
7	B	18	C
8	C	19	A
9	B	20	B
10	D	21	D
11	A	22	B
		23	C

A Core Curriculum for Diabetes Education
Diabetes Education and Program Management

Cultural Competence in Diabetes Education and Care   4

Lynne S. Robins, PhD
University of Washington
Department of Medical Education
Seattle, Washington

Introduction

1 This chapter was originally titled Cultural Appropriateness in Diabetes Education and Care; it has been changed to reflect current usage of definitions and terms, as suggested in a set of National (Health Care) Standards for Culturally and Linguistically Appropriate Services (CLAS).[1]

    A These standards, published by the US Department of Health and Human Services' Office of Minority Health, describe cultural and linguistic competence as "the ability of health care providers and health care organizations to understand and respond effectively to the cultural and linguistic needs brought by patients to the health care encounter."

    B Because the definitions of cultural competence and culturally competent care are congruent with cultural appropriateness and culturally appropriate care, all references to the former set of terms have been replaced by the latter set of terms.

2 Cultural competence is an important consideration in providing diabetes education and care:

    A The incidence of diabetes is increasing disproportionately among various ethnic populations in the United States.

    B The cultural distance between patients and healthcare professionals is increasing as the patient population diversifies.

3 There are benefits to providing culturally competent diabetes education and care:

    A Improved treatment outcomes

    B Increased patient satisfaction

    C Improved communication

    D Increased trust between patients and healthcare professionals

    E Reduced disparities in care related to race/ethnicity

4 The theory behind culturally competent diabetes education and care involves key anthropological concepts:

    A Everyone has a culture of origin and cultures of affiliation.

    B Healthcare professionals are influenced by their own personal cultures and the culture of biomedicine.

    C Cultural competence provides a means of bridging cultural differences.

5 Designing culturally competent diabetes education and care programs requires engaging both the individual and the community.

Objectives

Upon completion of this chapter, the learner will be able to

1 Define culturally competent diabetes education and care.

2 Describe the influence of culture on the beliefs and practices of patients and diabetes educators.

3 Explain strategies for providing culturally competent diabetes education and care.

4 Describe the prevalence of diabetes among people from underserved cultural groups.

5 Explain the principles of providing culturally competent diabetes education and care.

6 Describe specific applications of the principles for providing culturally competent diabetes education and care.

The Importance of Being Culturally Competent

1 The premise of this chapter is that diabetes educators can offer more compassionate and effective care to their patients by becoming culturally competent. Adopting the understandings and conceptual tools of anthropology can foster fuller understanding and appreciation of patients' cultural beliefs, behaviors, and perspectives (worldviews) and their influence on diabetes self-care behaviors.

2 Diabetes educators, more so than many other health professionals, need to understand the cultural contexts in which patients conduct their self-care routines. Daily blood glucose measurement, medical nutrition therapy, use of medications, and physical activity impinge on such culturally defined phenomena as family relationships, food preferences and preparation rituals, and beliefs about health and illness.

3 Helping patients navigate through cultural barriers to self-care requires a recognition of these barriers, an appreciation of their power to impede patients' progress toward health, and an understanding of how these barriers might be negotiated. It is also important to recognize and support strengths that patients derive from their cultural and religious beliefs.

Defining Culturally Competent Health Care

1 *Culturally competent* health care and education acknowledges and strives to accommodate patients' understandings about health and sickness. Questions and concerns, beliefs about death and bereavement, personal hygiene practices, dietary preferences, religious behaviors, modesty norms, family involvement, and language preferences are taken into account in a nonjudgmental fashion.[2]

2 Other terms used to describe this type of care include culturally relevant, culturally sensitive, and culturally appropriate health care.

3 Achieving the cultural competence necessary to provide culturally competent patient education and health care is a developmental learning process that requires time, effort, active awareness, practice, and introspection.

4 The following is a glossary of terms used when referring to culturally competent health care.
   A *Anthropology.* The social scientific discipline that seeks to understand the particulars and universals of human behavior by studying people in their cultural contexts.
   B *Culture.* A set of beliefs and behaviors that are learned and shared by members of a group. Culture serves as a guide for acting and for interpreting experience.
   C *Ethnicity.* A shared cultural identity or cultural heritage that forms a part of the lifestyle and shared sense of identity of the members of a group. Ethnicity is a cultural, not a biological, characteristic and is changeable.

- **D** *Enculturation.* The process of learning or acquiring one's culture of origin.
- **E** *Acculturation.* The process of adapting to a culture other than one's culture of origin or first learned culture.
- **F** *Conventional Medicine.* The officially sanctioned medical system of the United States; also called Western, academic, or scientific medicine, or biomedicine.
- **G** *Worldview.* The metaphorical lens through which human beings view and interpret experience. Worldviews determine the character of what is real or true and how it is reliably to be known.
- **H** *Ethnocentric.* The belief that one's own culture is superior to others. The conscious or unconscious practice of interpreting other cultures or the actions of their members in terms of the values and norms of one's own culture.
- **I** *Ethnographer.* A social science researcher, typically an anthropologist, who collaborates with his/her subjects, respondents, or informants to attempt to understand them and the cultural groups to which they belong by gaining an "insider's" perspective.

Understanding Culturally Competent Health Care

1 Many of the concepts used to describe and provide a theoretical basis for culturally competent diabetes education and care are borrowed from the discipline of anthropology (refer to the glossary in the section above for terms you are not familiar with).

2 Everyone has a culture.
- **A** *Culture* is defined as a set of beliefs and behaviors that are learned and shared by members of a group. Culture shapes the way group members view and experience the world.
- **B** As children, all human beings learn a particular cultural tradition through a process called *enculturation*.
- **C** All people are additionally influenced by the many group cultures to which they belong, in addition to their cultures of origin and rearing.
  - These cultures include religious groups; ethnic, gender, and sexual orientation/identity groups; social classes; and voluntary and professional organizations (eg, American Diabetes Association, American Association of Diabetes Educators).
  - The process of learning, borrowing, and then assimilating values and behaviors from these additional cultural groups into a person's cognitive and behavioral repertoires is called acculturation.
- **D** Providing *culturally competent health care* requires a willingness to listen to patients.
  - Learn from patients about their health beliefs.
  - Incorporate patients' concerns and perspectives into structuring and delivering education and health care.
  - Modify personal thinking and behaviors to facilitate mutual respect and rapport.
  - Develop treatment and prevention plans to meet the patients' needs and goals.
  - Establish a true working partnership with patients.[3]

3 All diabetes education and care is essentially cross-cultural.
- **A** Culture is not a factor of significance only for underserved groups or patients. Cultural differences require at least 2 reference points.[3]

- Anthropologist Robert Hahn[4] observed that patients and professionals may appear to understand one another and communicate effectively because they use a common language and share concepts and behavioral patterns. But he warned that these appearances may be deceptive.
- At least two very different reference points are represented in every professional/patient encounter, and the potential for miscommunication is great unless they are explicitly discussed.

B Diabetes educators can be thought of as a cultural group with a worldview and language that distinguishes them from their patients.

C The intensive training of all healthcare professionals has been likened to the process of acculturation.[5]
- Through the process of education, healthcare professionals acquire a worldview that influences the way they interpret sickness, explain its causes and progression, understand its symptoms, and orchestrate methods of treatment.
- Conventionally trained healthcare professionals, for example, learn a biomedical model of health and illness. In this model, disease is characterized as a biochemical or physiological abnormality. The therapeutic goal of disease treatment is to restore the patient to health by addressing the underlying physiological disorder.[6]
- For example, have you ever described your success with patients by saying: "All my patients have A1C levels in the near-normal range" or "I brought that patient's hemoglobin down into the normal range?"
- A more holistic model of health and illness would also entail an assessment of the patient's experience of his or her illness. This approach entails understanding hidden aspects of illness reality and working to transform that reality.

D Attitudes about how sick people and professionals are expected to interact are also learned in the context of health professional education.
- The traditional medical model of health professional/patient relationships is derived from the acute care model of disease treatment. According to this model, health professionals are characteristically active, in charge of, and responsible for treatment of the patient's illness, while the patient is passive, accepting, compliant, and dependent on the provider's knowledge and good will.[7]
- Perhaps most noticeable is that healthcare professionals acquire a style of speaking that differs in form and content from that of the general public, and a knowledge base and set of skills that are rarely shared by those who have not gone through this acculturation process.

Benefits of Providing Culturally Competent Diabetes Education and Care

1 The practice of culturally competent care has the potential to reduce disparities in care related to culture, race, and ethnicity. One conceptual model suggests that cultural competence can improve communication and increase trust between educators and patients, increase knowledge about differences among racial and ethnic groups in epidemiology, and enhance treatment efficacy and understanding of patients' cultural behaviors and environment.[8]

2 Awareness of one's own professional cultural values and worldview is a prerequisite for becoming culturally competent or able to provide culturally competent health care.[9]

Educators who are aware of the cultural basis of their own biases may be less likely to embrace the ethnocentric belief that there is one right or natural way to view the world or accomplish healthcare goals.

3 Rather than making judgments about the merits of another's worldview, it is more productive to seek common ground through co-learning. In a co-learning framework, patients would be empowered to define and address their healthcare concerns in a spirit of true partnership.[10]

4 Patients are more likely to adopt behaviors that are consistent with their personal and cultural values.

5 Like all individuals, diabetes educators belong to many cultural groups—including the culture of diabetes educators! Organizations like the American Association of Diabetes Educators provide opportunities for socialization and affiliation through which professional values and behaviors specific to diabetes education and treatment are transmitted.
  A The perspective that diabetes is largely self-managed is a predominant cultural belief among diabetes educators, and one that is reinforced through professional meetings, publications, and recommendations.
  B Patients may have a different perspective, as many have been acculturated to the roles and responsibilities associated with the traditional medical model. Some patients expect to turn over their care to their health professionals, preferring to play a more passive role in their treatment. Others may believe it is the responsibility of their spouse, adult children, or other family members. These differences in perspective can lead to problems if not recognized, explored, and addressed.

6 *Cultural relativism* is defined as the attitude that other ways of doing things are different but equally valid and that behavior needs to be understood in its cultural context. Adopting this attitude is a necessary first step toward culturally competent and more effective care and education.

7 Even though culturally different from patients, educators can communicate caring and respect by demonstrating goodwill, professional expertise, and an understanding of the patient's life experiences.[11]

The Prevalence of Diabetes

1 When comparing people with diabetes with people in the US without diabetes, the following tends to be true:
  A People with diabetes are older. In 1989, the median age for the population with diabetes was 63 years as compared with the median age of 40 years for all adults.[12] Diabetes is the ninth leading cause of death for people ages 25 to 44. It rises to the fifth leading cause of death for people 45 to 64 and it is the sixth leading cause for people age 65 and older.
  B A higher proportion of adults with type 2 diabetes are women (58.4%) than men (41.6%). These higher proportions of women are found for non-Hispanic Caucasians, African Americans, and Mexican Americans. The difference is greatest for African Americans with type 2 diabetes.[12]

C People with diabetes are often members of traditionally underserved cultural groups. All of these groups, except natives of Alaska, have a prevalence of type 2 diabetes that is 2 to 6 times greater than that of Caucasian persons. Diabetes-related mortality is higher for non-whites, and both prevalence and mortality rates are rapidly increasing.[13]
- African Americans: In 1998, 2.3 million African Americans were known to have diabetes.[14] On average, African Americans are 1.7 times more likely to have diabetes than Caucasians of similar age. African Americans with diabetes are more likely to develop diabetes complications and experience greater disability from the complications than Caucasian Americans with diabetes. African Americans have a higher incidence of and greater disability from diabetes complications such as kidney failure, visual impairment, and amputations. African Americans are twice as likely to die from diabetes as Caucasian Americans.
- Native Americans: Native Americans comprise more than 500 tribal organizations.[15] High prevalence of diabetes among most Native American tribes has been reported. On average, American Indians and Alaska Natives are 2.8 times as likely to have diagnosed diabetes as non-Hispanic Caucasians of similar age, but this might be an underestimation. For example, data from the Navajo Health and Nutrition survey, published in 1997, showed that 22.9% of Navajo adults age 20 or older had diabetes. The Pima tribe in Arizona has one of the highest rates in the world; 50% of individuals from age 20 to 64 have type 2 diabetes.
- Hispanic Americans: On average, Hispanic/Latino Americans are almost twice as likely to have diabetes as non-Hispanic Caucasians of similar age.[16] In 1998, more than 1 in 10 Hispanic-American adults (1.2 million) have diabetes. About 675,000 Hispanic Americans have diabetes but do not know they have it. Among Hispanic persons living in the US, the prevalence of diabetes is 2 to 3 times greater in Mexican and Puerto Rican Americans adults than in non-Hispanic Caucasians, but lowest in Cubans.
- Asian Americans and Pacific Islander Americans:[17] The Seattle Japanese-American Community Diabetes Study found the prevalence of diabetes to be higher than that reported for the US Caucasian population. Filipinos had the highest prevalence of diabetes among the four largest ethnic Asian groups in Hawaii (Chinese, Filipino, Japanese, and Korean); all groups had higher prevalence than those of Caucasians. Native Hawaiians are twice as likely to have diagnosed diabetes than Caucasian residence of Hawaii.

D People with diabetes are less educated.[18] Even after accounting for age, persons with type 2 diabetes have less education than persons without diabetes.

E People with diabetes are poorer.[11,18,19] According to a Gallup Organization survey, households in the lowest economic group had the highest prevalence of diabetes. At all ages and for both men and women, a greater percentage of persons with type 2 diabetes were at lower income levels than persons without diabetes.

2 The reason these social and cultural characteristics are important is because they are likely to distance patients from the Caucasian, middle-class educators and professionals with whom they often interact unless these professionals make an attempt to bridge the barriers.

Culture and Diabetes Education and Self-Management

1 Understanding patients' cultures is especially relevant for managing a chronic illness such as diabetes because of its lifelong course and influence on culturally embedded behaviors. Diabetes and its self-management affect virtually every aspect of a patient's life, and patients are often asked to substantially reshape the ways in which they live.[20]

2 The cultural distance between professionals and patients becomes an issue when either fails to live up to the expectations of the other. Diabetes educators can acquire the skills in understanding, communicating, and intervening that will help them mediate between the mainly Caucasian, middle-class, healthcare system and the many historically underserved populations with diabetes.[11]

   A Diabetes educators often express frustration when patients fail to live up to their expectations to follow nutritional recommendations.
- A fact often overlooked is that patients may view their educators' expectations about meal planning as unrealistic or culturally insensitive. One assumption that educators often make is that individuals have control over their own food preparation and consumption.

   B Focus group discussions with patients have revealed that this assumption is ethnocentric. In a focus group with Latino patients, Anderson et al[21] learned that for Latino women, barriers to following dietary guidelines included their culturally defined roles as food preparers within the family, and family members' desires to have traditional foods of their culture prepared for them. Latino women explained that their own health was a lower priority than meeting their family's expectations related to food as revealed in the following comments:
- "I cook for my daughter and son and take care of all my grandchildren and cook for them, too. It is too difficult to make time to prepare something different and sometimes I don't have time to eat."
- "What I prepare for my family I also eat because I work a lot and I'm too tired to cook something separate for myself."

The behaviors of the women quoted might have been interpreted as noncompliant or difficult. Viewing these behaviors in a cultural context reveals that they were responding to cultural constraints on their behavior related to food preparation. Asking these women about the meaning of food in their lives would have brought into focus the constraints on their ability to control their meals and may also have reduced frustrations on both sides.

3 Listening to others of all traditions is the hallmark of the anthropological perspective and practice. A central goal is to understand how things look from the other person's point of view. "The best curriculum is one that is based on the patient."[22]

   A Listening serves multiple purposes in the process of education, including establishing rapport with the patient, understanding the patient's condition, recognizing the patient's goals, and assessing effective modes of therapy.[4] Listening enables the diabetes educator to identify "what is close to people's hearts"[23] and the "sparks" and "triggers"[24] that are meaningful to people in terms of their cultural and personal values.

   B Healthcare providers also can strive to understand the context of their patients' healthcare needs and concerns.

4 Avoid making assumptions about patients' beliefs based on ethnic identification.
   A An individual's identification with an ethnic group does not determine his or her beliefs, values, or behavior in line with the norms of that group.
   - Factors that lead to variation among people of the same ethnic group include the length of time they have spent in the US, the age at which they came here, their desire to assimilate, whether they live in ethnic enclaves, whether they are from rural or urban areas, and their level of education.
   - Social and economic class cross-cut ethnic boundaries and may sometimes be more important than ethnic background.[25]
   B It is important to recognize that there is variation within cultural traditions.
   - Knowledge of a pattern of health beliefs common to a given identity-group may provide a useful frame of reference when working with these patients, but it is not predictive.[9]
   - Behaviors, values, or worldviews cannot be categorized by culture. This process fosters the stereotyping and falsely implies that the dominant culture, against which all others are compared, is somehow standard.
   - Avoid making assumptions about patients' behaviors based on cultural background or ethnicity. As examples, not all Hispanic-American patients incorporate ethnic foods and not all Muslim patients with diabetes fast during Ramadan.
   C Rather than make assumptions about cultural beliefs and practices, educators need to take time to ask questions about them.
   D It is important to assess these areas, even when the educator and patient share a cultural or ethnic identity.

5 Asking questions of patients is the best way to find out what is important to them, what explanatory model of diabetes they hold, what goals and expectations they have for treatment, and what personal beliefs and values might affect their responses. It is also critical to elicit information about cultural and religious practices that might affect the patient's diabetes self-management.
   A Most people view health professionals as persons in positions of authority and often as persons with very fixed ideas about what is right or important.[3]
   - Patients become very cautious about revealing anything they feel might jeopardize their access to medical services, having their deeply felt concerns dismissed as trivial, or being made to feel foolish by provoking irritable reactions.
   - Patients manage degrees of disclosure in their encounters according to their own assessments of the situation; they are the ones who make the final decisions about how they will respond to recommendations.
   - As an example, professionals working in African-American communities report that older African Americans may not give their healthcare professionals much information about their diabetes. They believe it is the health professional's job to discern their problems and that it would be insulting to the health professional to offer such information. A diabetes educator who is aware of this belief can ask competent questions to bring this view out into the open.
   - It is important to elicit from patients in a compassionate and nonjudgmental way their important concerns, beliefs, and values that may have implications for their health and health care. Several relevant pieces of information usually can be learned with just a few well-put questions and an accepting manner. This is especially important for brief encounters and when time to spend with a patient is

limited. Findings can be used to jointly develop a treatment plan that will be more likely to succeed.

B Key questions for exploring patients' specific values, beliefs, and practices relevant to health and illness include the following.
- What concerns you most about (caring for) your diabetes?
- What is most difficult for you in (caring for) your diabetes?
- How does your culture affect how you care for your diabetes?
- How do your religious practices and beliefs affect how you care for your diabetes?
- What kinds of home remedies do you use for your diabetes or other health conditions? Are there herbs, medicines, or other treatments you use to care for your diabetes or other health concerns?
- Do you see other health practitioners or healers to help you with your diabetes?
- Tell me a little bit about who you consider family and kin.
- What does your family do to help you take care of your diabetes?
- Who helps you when the going gets tough?
- What is your real passion for living?
- What do you want from your doctor or other providers?
- What can I do to be most helpful to you?

Culturally Competent Diabetes Education Programs

1 To be effective, diabetes education programs must be relevant, acceptable, and understandable to intended learners. There must also be a consonance or agreement of purpose between professional and client for each to take and sustain action.[26] Educational programs that are not meaningful to their intended audiences risk failing to attract, retain, or aid the people for whom they are designed.

2 The notion of cultural relevancy is based on the understanding that cultural subgroups differ from one another on the basis of their worldviews, value systems, behavioral styles, and often languages. Consequently, what may be real and relevant to members of one group may not have the same salience and value in another.[26]
- **A** For example, there is often a strong sense of the present within African-American communities. Orientation toward the future and the necessity of preventive health measures such as annual eye examinations are not consistent with this cultural pattern.[27]
- **B** The problem is compounded by the fact that type 2 diabetes is often a silent disease until complications are quite advanced. Therefore, a program focused solely on blood glucose control to prevent future complications might not be as effective among patients who are focused on the present as a program that also includes immediate benefits.

3 A key to designing culturally competent educational programs is the commitment to doing the work of discovering what learners believe about the world and what they think they need to learn.
- **A** This approach requires educators to enter the community unencumbered by preconceived notions about what communities need or how they need to go about achieving healthcare goals.
- **B** Healthcare professionals may need to put aside the ethnocentric belief that patients should sacrifice now for better health tomorrow. There are cultures in which this

idea does not resonate. For these cultures, it would be more beneficial to highlight the immediate benefits of glucose control (eg, not having to get up at night to use the bathroom) than to focus on future or long-term health benefits.

Culturally Competent Community Outreach

1 "The community engagement process means working with and through constituents to achieve common goals. To ensure that community engagement efforts are culturally and linguistically appropriate, they need to be developed from a knowledge and respect for the targeted community's culture."[28]

2 A set of four tenets has been developed[29] for conducting diabetes community outreach programs specifically designed to address the needs of African Americans.

3 These tenets provide a valuable set of planning principles for designing culturally competent community programs and education for all cultural groups.
  A Involve community members and community leaders. Involve community members in each stage of the planning and implementation of health education and care programs intended to be used by them. Such input will help ensure that diabetes programs will be relevant and credible.
  B Empower people. Empowerment is defined as the process of increasing personal, interpersonal, and political control so that individuals can take action to improve their life situations. Personal empowerment enables individuals in problem situations to use their own skills and abilities to change their own behavior and to influence the behavior of individuals and organizations that affect their quality of life (see Chapter 1, Applied Principles of Teaching and Learning, in Diabetes Education and Program Management, for educational strategies based on an empowerment philosophy). As patients gain a sense of control over their diabetes, they are often better able to become empowered in other aspects of their lives.
  C Respect the cultural diversity of the community. Individuals belonging to the same cultural or ethnic group may be bound together by similar experiences, but they are not monolithic in their attitudes or behaviors.
    • Social and economic class cross-cut ethnic boundaries and may sometimes be more important than ethnic background.
    • Diabetes education programs must seek to optimize the quality of life for cultural group members while respecting their diverse cultural beliefs, traditions, and lifestyles.
  D Provide a service. Research institutions should avoid studying patient populations without providing a competent and adequate service to them. It is unrealistic to expect any group to participate actively in a program whose only goal is to generate new knowledge for the sponsoring institution.

Key Educational Considerations

1 Culture influences the way that people think about and behave in relation to health and illness. Due to cultural differences, professionals and patients may have very different perspectives on how to interpret diabetes, explain its causes and progression, understand its symptoms, and orchestrate methods of treatment.

2 Awareness of one's own professional cultural values and worldview is a prerequisite for becoming culturally competent or able to provide culturally competent diabetes care.

3 Cultural values influence both the choices patients make each day as they care for their diabetes and the ways that diabetes educators interpret and react to their choices. It is helpful to examine how your values influence the decisions you make so that you can better understand your patients' decisions and work with them to achieve their goals.

4 Understanding patients' cultures is especially relevant for a chronic illness such as diabetes because of the lifelong course of the disease and its influence on culturally embedded behaviors.

5 Critical areas to explore as part of the cultural assessment are beliefs about diabetes; role of the patient in self-care; health and healing; values and priorities; communication styles and preferences; and common family, cultural, and religious rituals and practices.

6 While a complete cultural assessment may not be possible in all situations (eg, brief encounter in a busy clinic), treating patients with courtesy, focusing attention on the patient rather than acting in a hurry, sitting at the patient's level, and asking at least one culturally related question (eg, "Do you have any religious, family or cultural practices that influence how you care for your diabetes") conveys concern and sensitivity.

7 Educators can do a great deal to decrease cultural barriers during any encounter by manifesting a caring, concerned, and understanding manner. Respect for patients and their culture can be demonstrated through honoring appointment times, not making assumptions about educational level or profession, asking patients how they would like to be addressed, and being sensitive to historical and current cultural differences.

8 Effective communication is essential for an accurate diagnosis, meaningful discussion of treatment options, and patient education. Determine the patient's primary or preferred language and any secondary languages. Use interpreters as needed and ask patients in what language they would prefer written materials, because some people are better able to read English than the language they typically speak (see Chapter 5, Teaching Persons with Low Literacy Skills, in Diabetes Education and Program Management, for more information).

Learning Assessment: Case Study 1

TM is an Hispanic-American woman with type 2 diabetes. She sees a traditional healer and takes an herbal home remedy to decrease her blood glucose levels. For years she had been seeing her physician about her diabetes, and all that time he had recommended that she begin insulin therapy. TM refused, explaining that she just did not want to go "on the needle." Interpreting her fear as an aversion to the discomfort of insulin shots, her physician never questioned TM further to determine why she would not follow his recommendation. TM is beginning to experience neuropathy and microalbuminuria as a result of her ongoing elevated blood glucose levels.

Questions for Discussion

1 How can the diabetes educator find out what is influencing TM's behavior?
2 What strategies could you use when working with her that demonstrate cultural competence?

Discussion

1 Asking TM directly about her concerns regarding insulin can open the way for discovering why she has been unwilling to begin this therapy. In response to your question, she tells you that her mother and others she has known have died once they started on insulin, so she has decided to use herbs and other alternative medicines instead.

2 TM needs to understand that the insulin taken by injection is very similar to that produced by the body and is therefore safe. It is unlikely, however, that this information will change her deeply held beliefs. Other strategies for helping TM understand the safety of using insulin include the following:
  A Introduce TM to other Hispanic American women who have diabetes and take insulin as well as alternative medicines.
  B Offer referral to a support group.
  C Offer referral to other community health resources.
  D Provide tailored written and video materials that reflect her language, culture, and literacy level.

3 TM may not have spoken with her physician about her insulin concerns for a number of reasons.
  A She holds physicians in general in high esteem.
  B She feels intimidated by him.
  C She distrusts Western medicines.
  D She received advice from her healer telling her not to talk with her physician.
  E She may have difficulty completely expressing herself in English.

4 It would be helpful to find out what is in the herbal medicines that TM is taking to be sure that she is not experiencing any adverse effects.

Learning Assessment: Case Study 2

LC is a 60-year-old European-American man with diagnosed type 2 diabetes who has difficulty using his meal plan. LC is an engineer by profession and is employed in the auto industry. He explains that he knows he needs to limit his food intake but just cannot seem to help himself when he is around food. He says that he knows very little about food and leaves that up to his wife. However, he resents his wife telling him what or how much he should eat and reacts by eating even more. LC has expressed a reticence to begin taking pills for fear that he would feel like he had license to eat everything. Furthermore, he tells you that he has not been testing his blood sugar levels because his diabetes was not that bad.

Questions for Discussion
1 What cultural influences are affecting LC's behavior?
2 What strategies could you use when working with him that demonstrate cultural competence?

Discussion
1 LC's behavior is typical of many European-American men of his generation. Preparing food and caring for the family's health are perceived as a woman's responsibilities; being in charge and in control of situations is viewed as the man's role. One way that this value is expressed is by minimizing the seriousness of illnesses.

2 To address LC's need to be in charge, you might begin each visit by asking about his concerns and asking what he would like to learn about or discuss.
   A Asking LC about his thoughts or concerns about his diabetes will likely be more successful than asking about his feelings.
   B Discuss treatment options, blood glucose monitoring, and use of the results in terms of how they will help him be in control of his diabetes.

3 The process of blood glucose monitoring should be discussed in terms of data collection and conducting experiments with foods to test their effect on blood glucose levels. This approach may appeal to someone with an engineering background and may be more acceptable than trying to teach him about foods and their ingredients. Learning through his own explorations may also help decrease the tensions between he and his wife regarding food issues.

Learning Assessment: Case Study 3
AK is a 53-year-old Asian-American man of Japanese descent who was recently diagnosed with type 2 diabetes. He eats a traditional diet that is high in carbohydrates (eg, rice and starchy vegetables), high in sodium, and low in proteins. AK understood that being on "a diabetic diet" meant eating fewer foods, especially fried foods and desserts. Therefore, he eats 2 large meals that are very high in carbohydrates and low in fat. He was referred to you by his doctor because his glycosylated hemoglobin remains elevated. He comes to you very frustrated because he does not understand why he is always hungry and why his blood glucose levels are high all the time despite the changes he has made.

Questions for Discussion
1 What cultural influences are affecting AK's behavior?
2 What strategies could you use when working with him that demonstrate cultural competence?

Discussion
1 AK's eating pattern is based on traditional Asian foods, and his understanding of his meal plan is based on traditional Western foods.

2 Offer AK nutritional information that is compatible with his preferred food choices.
  A Let him know that he will feel less hungry and be able to lower his blood glucose levels by decreasing the portion sizes of some of the carbohydrate foods he eats and filling in with lean meat or other protein foods.
  B Explain that spreading his food consumption over 3 or more meals per day helps prevent overloading his pancreas and thus promotes more even blood glucose levels throughout the day. He may also notice that he is less hungry and more energetic.

Learning Assessment: Case Study 4

ML is a 58-year-old Navajo woman whose first language is Navajo. She lives with her son, his wife, and their four children on a Navajo reservation. She was diagnosed with type 2 diabetes during a free screening at the mall 1 year ago. She states that the screening people told her that she needed to see her doctor right away because if she did not she might go blind or lose a foot. They also told her that she should go on a diet, exercise, and get some medicine from her doctor. She is in today with symptoms of fatigue, blurred vision, increased thirst, frequent urination, and weight loss. Her HbA1c is 10.8% (normal = 4.0% to 6.0%), cholesterol level is 276 mg/dL, triglyceride level is 240 mg/dL. Current weight is 200 lb (91 kg) and height is 5 ft 4 in tall (160 cm). She states that she did not visit the doctor a year ago as she thought that the diagnosis was wrong because she did not feel sick then.

Questions for Discussion

1 What cultural influences are affecting ML's behavior?
2 Considering ML's culture, how would you explain diabetes to her?
3 What strategies could you use when working with her that demonstrate cultural competence?

Discussion

1 Diabetes, which may be asymptomatic in the early phases, is a condition that can be difficult to explain because in many Native American cultures people do not feel they are ill unless they have visible symptoms or pain.

2 In ML's case, a Navajo interpreter who is knowledgeable about diabetes will be needed for the explanation and visits. The interpreter should be from the same culture as the client (and preferably the same community) since culture and health cannot be separated. The diabetes educator should remain aware of his/her communication style and body language even though an interpreter is being used.

3 ML will need the support and understanding of her family in order to make any needed lifestyle changes to lower her blood glucose levels, so it will help if they participate in the education process. If ML chooses to include a method of healing in addition to Western medicines, the diabetes educator should respect and acknowledge her choice.

4 Along with other aspects of self-care, ML needs to be taught how she can prevent the complications of diabetes, described to her in the third person.

5 In addition the educator can do the following.
  A Explain the importance of regular visits to the clinic even when she feels well.
  B Describe to ML what she can expect during the clinical encounter.
  C Schedule ML for more than 1 appointment per visit, especially if transportation is limited.
  D Offer information to ML and her family about available diabetes resources and sponsored activities such as community diabetes education classes, cooking classes, grocery store tours led by a dietitian, and community-wide walking/fitness programs if they are available.
  E Identify an ongoing source of support and information from a community health worker.

References

1 US Department of Health and Human Services, Office of Minority Health. Assuring cultural competence in health care: Recommendations for National Standards and Outcomes-Focused Research Agenda; 2000 on the Internet. Available at: *www.omhrc.gov/clas*. Accessed February 2001.

2 Barclay J. Shaping the care of the future...meeting the needs of all individuals. Nursing: J Clin Prac Educ Manag. 1991;4(31):20-22.

3 O'Connor BB. Healing Traditions. Alternative Medicine and the Health Professions. Philadelphia: University of Pennsylvania Press; 1995.

4 Hahn R. Sickness and Healing. An Anthropological Perspective. New Haven, Conn: Yale University Press; 1995:265.

5 Pachter LM. Culture and clinical care. Folk illness beliefs and behaviors and their implications for healthcare delivery. JAMA. 1994;271:690-694.

6 Good BJ, Good MJ. The meaning of symptoms: a cultural hermeneutic model for clinical practice. In: Eisenberg L, Kleinman A, eds. The Relevance of Social Science for Medicine. Dordrecht, Holland: D. Reidel Publishing Co. 1992;165-196.

7 Anderson RM, Funnell MM, Arnold MS. Beyond compliance and glucose control: educating for patient empowerment. In: Rifkin H, Colwell JA, Taylor SI, eds. Diabetes. Amsterdam, Netherlands: Elsevier Science Publishers, 1991;1285-1289.

8 Brach C, Fraser I. Can cultural competency reduce racial and ethnic disparities? A review and conceptual model. Medical Care Research and Review. 2000;57:181-217.

9 Galanti GA. Caring for Patients from Different Cultures. Philadelphia: University of Pennsylvania Press, 1991.

10 Minkler M. Using participatory action research to build healthy communities. Public Health Reports. 2000;115:191-197.

11 Murphy FG, Satterfield D, Anderson RM, Lyons AE. Diabetes educators as cultural translators. Diabetes Educ. 1993;19:113-116,118.

12 Centers for Disease Control and Prevention. National Diabetes Fact Sheet. Atlanta: US Department of Health and Human Services, Centers for Disease Control and Prevention, Division of Diabetes Translation; 1998.

13 Carter JS, Pugh JA, Monterrosa A. Non-insulin-dependent diabetes mellitus in minorities in the United States. Ann Intern Med. 1996;125:221-232.

14. National Institutes of Health. Diabetes in African Americans. Bethesda, Md: National Institute of Diabetes, Digestive and Kidney Diseases, 1998; NIH Publication 98-3266.

15. National Institutes of Health. Diabetes in Native Americans. Bethesda, Md: National Institute of Diabetes, Digestive and Kidney Diseases, 2000; NIH Publication 00-4567.

16. National Institutes of Health. Diabetes in Hispanic Americans. Bethesda, Md: National Institute of Diabetes and Digestive and Kidney Diseases, 2001; NIH Publication 01-3265.

17. National Institutes of Health. Diabetes in Asian Americans. Bethesda, Md: National Institute of Diabetes and Digestive and Kidney Diseases, 2000; NIH Publication 00-4667.

18. Cowie CC, Eberhard MS. Sociodemographic characteristics of persons with diabetes. In: National Diabetes Data Group, eds. Diabetes in America. 2nd ed. Bethesda, Md: National Institute of Health, National Institute of Diabetes and Digestive and Kidney Diseases, 1995; NIH Publication 95-1468:85-116.

19. Quenan L, Remington P. Diabetes mortality trends in Wisconsin, 1979-1997: the increasing gap between whites and blacks. Wis Med J 2000;99:44-47.

20. Anderson RM. Patient empowerment and the traditional medical model: a case of irreconcilable differences? Diabetes Care. 1995;18:412-415.

21. Anderson RM, Goddard C, Vasquez F, Garcia R, Guzman R. Using focus groups to identify diabetes care and education issues for Latino people with diabetes. Diabetes. 1998;47(Suppl 1):128.

22. Funnell MM. Lessons learned as a diabetes educator. Diabetes Spectrum, 2000; 13:69-70.

23. Labonte R, Robertson A. Delivering the goods, showing our stuff: the case for a constructivist paradigm for health promotion research and practice. Health Educ Q. 1996;23:431-437.

24. McLean S and Warm Springs Healthy Nations. A communication analysis of community mobilization on the Warm Spring Indian Reservation. J Health Communication. 1997;2:113-125.

25. Harwood A. Ethnicity and Medical Care. Cambridge, Mass: Harvard University Press; 1981.

26. Gilbert MJ. Cultural relevance in the delivery of human services. In: Keefe SE, ed. Negotiating Ethnicity: The Impact of Anthropological Theory and Practice. NAPA Bull. 1989;32:706-716.

27. VanSon AR. Crossing cultural and economic boundaries. In: VanSon AR, ed. Diabetes and Patient Education: A Daily Nursing Challenge. New York: Appleton-Century-Crofts; 1984;160-177.

28. Centers for Disease Control and Prevention (CDC), Public Health Practice Program Office. Principles of Community Engagement: CDC/ASTDR Committee on Community Engagement. Order number 199807722-4178. Atlanta, Ga; 1997.

29. Anderson RM, Herman WH, Davis JM, Freedman RP, Funnell MM, Neighbors HW. Barriers to improving diabetes care for blacks. Diabetes Care. 1991;14:605-609.

Suggested Readings

Anderson LA, Janes GR, Ziemer DC, Phillips LS. Diabetes in urban African Americans. Body image, satisfaction with size, and weight change attempts. Diabetes Educ. 1997;23:301-308.

Anderson RM. Patient empowerment and the traditional medical model. Diabetes Care. 1995;18:412-415.

Bartol GM, Richardson L. Using literature to create cultural competence. Image: J Nurs Scholarship. 1998;30:75-79.

Basso KH. Wisdom Sits in Places: Landscapes and Language Among the Western Apache. Albuquerque, NM: University of New Mexico Press; 1999.

Bradley E. Spiritualcise mind-body exercise program. Diabetes Educ. 1996;22:117-118.

Brach C, Fraser I. Can cultural competency reduce racial and ethnic disparities? A review and conceptual model. Medical Care Research and Review. 2000;57:181-217.

Brown SA, Hanis CL. A community-based, culturally sensitive education and group-support intervention for Mexican Americans with NIDDM: a pilot study of efficacy. Diabetes Educ. 1995;21:203-210.

Burden ML, Burden AC. Management of diabetes mellitus during the holy month of Ramadan. Practical Diabetes Internation. 1998;15(suppl 1):S1-S23.

Carter JS, Gilliland SS, Percy GE, et al. Native American Diabetes Project: Designing culturally relevant education materials. Diabetes Educ. 1997;23:133-139.

Carter JS, Pugh JA, Monterrosa A. Non-insulin-dependent diabetes mellitus in minorities in the United States. Ann Intern Med. 1996;125:221-232.

Corkery E, Palmer C, Foley ME, Schechter CB, Frisher L, Roman SH. Effect of a bicultural community health worker on completion of diabetes education in a Hispanic population. Diabetes Care. 1997;20:254-257.

Duran BM, Curan EF. Assessment, program planning, and evaluation in Indian country: toward a postcolonial practice. In: Huff RM, Kline MV, eds. Promoting Health in Multicultural Populations: A Handbook for Practitioners. Thousand Oaks, Calif: Sage Publications, Inc.; 1999:292-311.

Edwards GJ, Coleman-Burns P. A culturally sensitive approach to patient care. Caring for African American patients. Practical Diabetol. 1996;15(3):4-9.

Fadiman A. The Spirit Catches You and You Fall Down: A Hmong Child, Her American Doctors, and the Collision of Two Cultures. New York: Farrar, Straus, and Giroux; 1997.

Fitzgerald JT, Anderson RM, Funnell MM, et al. Differences in the impact of dietary restrictions on African Americans and Caucasians with NIDDM. Diabetes Educ. 1997;23:41-47.

Gaillard TR, Schuster DP, Bossetti BM, Green PA, Osei K. Do sociodemographics and economic status predict risks for Type II diabetes in African Americans? Diabetes Educ. 1997;23:294-300.

Hahn RA. Anthropology and the enhancement of public health practice. In: Hahn RA, ed. Anthropology in Public Health: Bridging Differences in Culture and Society. New York: Oxford University Press; 1999:3-24.

Hosey GM, Freeman WL, Stracqualursi F, Gohdes D. Designing and evaluating diabetes education material for American Indians. Diabetes Educ. 1990;16:407-414.

Jaber LA, Slaughter RL, Grunberger G. Diabetes and related metabolic risk factors among Arab Americans. Ann Pharmacother. 1995;29:573-577.

Keenan DP. In the face of diversity: modifying nutrition education delivery to meet the needs of an increasingly multicultural consumer base. J Nutr Ed. 1996;28:86-91.

Kretzmann JP, Kretzmann MJL. Building Communities From the Inside Out: A Path Toward Finding and Mobilizing a Community's Assets. Chicago, Ill: ACTA Publications; 1993.

Kulkarni K. Nutrition counseling for Indian and Pakistani patients. Practical Diabetol. 1996;1S(2):19-20.

Labonte R, Feather J, Hills M. A story/dialogue method for health promotion knowledge development and evaluation. Health Educ Res. 1999;14:39-50.

Ledda MA, Walker EA, Basch CE. Development and formative evaluation of a foot self-care program for African Americans with diabetes. Diabetes Educ. 1997;23:48-51.

Magnus MH. What's your IQ on cross-cultural nutrition counseling? Diabetes Educ. 1996;22:57-60, 62.

National Institutes of Health. Diabetes in African Americans. Bethesda, Md: National Institute of Diabetes and Digestive and Kidney Diseases, 1998; NIH Publication 98-3266.

National Institutes of Health. Diabetes in Native Americans. Bethesda, Md: National Institute of Diabetes and Digestive and Kidney Diseases, 2000; NIH Publication 00-4567.

National Institutes of Health. Diabetes in Hispanic Americans. Bethesda, Md: National Institute of Diabetes and Digestive and Kidney Diseases, 2001; NIH Publication 01-3265.

National Institutes of Health. Diabetes in Asian Americans. Bethesda, Md: National Institute of Diabetes and Digestive and Kidney Diseases, 2000; NIH Publication 00-4667.

Oomen JS, Owen LG, Suggs LS. Culture counts: why current treatment models fail Hispanic women with type 2 diabetes. Diabetes Educ. 1999;25:220-225.

Penn NE, Kar S, Kramer J, Skinner J, Zambrana RE. Ethnic minorities, health care systems, and behavior. Health Psychol. 1995;14:641-646.

Pichert JW, Briscoe VJ. A questionnaire for assessing barriers to healthcare utilization, part I. Diabetes Educ. 1997;23:181-191.

Pichert JW, Briscoe VJ. Strategies for overcoming barriers to healthcare utilization, part II. Diabetes Educ. 1997;23:251-256.

Rankin SH, Galbraith ME, Huang P. Quality of life and social environment as reported by Chinese immigrants with non-insulin-dependent diabetes mellitus. Diabetes Educ. 1997;23:171-177.

Resnicow K, Baranowski T, Ahluwalia JS, Braithwaite R. Cultural sensitivity in public health: defined and demystified. Ethnicity and Disease. 1999;9:10-21.

Skelly AH, Marshall JR, Haughey BP, Davis PJ, Dunford RG. Self-efficacy and confidence in outcomes as determinants of self-care practices in inner-city, African-American women with non-insulin-dependent diabetes. Diabetes Educ. 1995;21:38-46.

Smith SE, Willms DG, Johnson NA. Nurtured Knowledge: Learning to Do Participatory Action Research. New York: The Apex Press; 1997.

Stringer ET. Action Research: A Handbook for Practitioners. Thousand Oaks, Calif: Sage Publications, Inc.; 1996.

Tripp-Reimer T, Choi E, Kelley LS, Enslein JC. Cultural barriers to care: inverting the problem. Diabetes Spectrum. 2000;14:13-22.

Wing RR, Anglin K. Effectiveness of a behavioral weight control program for blacks and whites with NIDDM. Diabetes Care. 1996;19:409-412.

Additional information may be obtained from the National Diabetes Education Program, National Institute of Diabetes and Digestive and Kidney Diseases, National Institutes of Health. Telephone: 800-438-5383.

Additional information may be obtained from the National Diabetes Information Clearinghouse, National Institute of Diabetes and Digestive and Kidney Diseases, National Institutes of Health. Telephone: 301-654-3327. Internet: *www.niddk.nih.gov*. Accessed February 2001.

Additional information may be obtained from the Combined Health Information Database (CHID) on the Internet. Available at: *http://chid.nih.gov*. Accessed November 2000.

US Department of Health and Human Services, Office of Minority Health. Assuring cultural competence in health care: Recommendations for National Standards and Outcomes-Focused Research, 2000 on the Internet. Available at: *http://www.omhrc.gov/clas*. Accessed February 2001.

Learning Assessment: Post-Test Questions

Cultural Competence in Diabetes Education and Care   4

1. A goal of cultural competence diabetes care is to:
   A Acknowledge and accommodate the patient's beliefs about health and illness
   B Change the patient's beliefs about health and illness
   C Reinforce the need to abandon "folk remedies" that may be doing harm
   D Help the patient with the acculturation process and self-care management

2. Cultural competence or intercultural sensitivity:
   A Is innate to all human beings
   B Requires active awareness and practice
   C Is not achievable by most people
   D Has a great deal of historic precedent

3. A set of beliefs or behaviors that are learned and shared by members of a group is known as:
   A An ethnicity
   B Cultural relativism
   C A culture
   D A worldview

4. The belief that one's culture is superior to others is known as:
   A Ethnicity
   B Cultural relativism
   C Enculturation
   D Ethnocentrism

5. ZW has recently moved to the US from Thailand. He seeks your advice as he begins to adapt his diet to what is available in his local markets. This process is known as:
   A Enculturation
   B Acculturation
   C Cultural adjustment
   D Ethnocentrism

6. DD is a diabetes educator serving a large multicultural population. She seeks to become more sensitive to the needs of her patients and provide culturally competent care. To do so, she can include all of the following except:
   A Learn about the patient's health beliefs by asking him or her
   B Negotiate mutually acceptable treatment plans
   C Stress the importance of adjusting to new ways of doing things
   D Incorporate patient's concerns and perspectives

7. An example of how DD might demonstrate her understanding and respect for different cultural beliefs and preferences is by:
   A Demonstrating to patients and families how they might adapt their favorite ethnic dishes to the diabetes meal plan
   B Organizing screening programs in high-risk communities
   C Pointing out to patients and families the areas that need improvement in their diet
   D Asking local community agencies to distribute diabetes literature

8. Healthcare professionals in the US who seek to increase their cultural competence recognize that:
   A Barriers such as language and vocabulary can be more easily overcome when English is the common language
   B Their own ethnocentric worldview is based on a biomedical model of health and illness and can be a barrier to improved care
   C Positive patient outcomes are an appropriate indicator that cultural barriers have been addressed
   D The patient's own cultural beliefs are of a less importance than their own

9. African Americans with type 2 diabetes:
   A Have the highest rates of diabetes in the US
   B Have a higher incidence of diabetes and greater disability from complications than Caucasian Americans
   C Are 3 times more likely to have diabetes than Caucasians
   D Are at less risk statistically for the development of complications of diabetes

10. DD has been working with AR, a Hispanic woman with type 2 diabetes, on issues related to her meal plan. In developing a culturally competent intervention, DD would need to consider all of the following factors except:
    A Culturally defined roles within the family
    B Cultural constraints on behaviors related to food preparation
    C Cultural norms of the Caucasian population in the US
    D Cultural differences in the expectations of the patient and healthcare provider

11. DD feels that as a diabetes educator it is her responsibility to learn more about the culture of her patients. One of the most important techniques she can utilize to do this is to:
    A Avoid sensitive areas of religious and political beliefs
    B Ask her patients questions about their specific health beliefs and values
    C Categorize behaviors and beliefs by culture
    D Share with them what she considers to be the main problems with their healthcare practices

12. DD, in her interactions with AR, a Hispanic woman with type 2 diabetes, has encouraged AR to bring in some of her favorite family recipes so that they can review and adapt them to fit her meal plan. This approach is an example of all of the following except:
    A Cultural sensitivity
    B Cultural relativism
    C Patient empowerment
    D Ethnocentrism

13. DD is concerned about AR's use of traditional remedies to help her diabetes. One approach she might use is to:
    A Ask AR to bring in her home remedies and send them to the lab for analysis
    B Ask AR to tell her more about these remedies and how she uses them
    C Explain to AR the potential side effects of many of the natural remedies
    D Impress on AR the importance of adhering to the medical treatment plan

See next page for answer key.

Post-Test Answer Key

Cultural Competence in Diabetes Education and Care   4

1. A
2. B
3. C
4. D
5. B
6. C
7. A
8. B
9. B
10. C
11. B
12. D
13. B

A Core Curriculum for Diabetes Education
Diabetes Education and Program Management

Teaching Persons With Low Literacy Skills   5

James W. Pichert, PhD
Diabetes Research and Training Center
Vanderbilt University School of Medicine
Nashville, Tennessee

James D. Anderst, MD
Medical College of Wisconsin
Milwaukee, Wisconsin

Stephania Miller, PhD
Diabetes Research and Training Center
Vanderbilt University School of Medicine
Nashville, Tennessee

Introduction

1 One reading expert notes that literacy is like money.[1] Persons with little money find it more difficult to meet their basic needs than those with a lot of money. Similarly, persons with limited or no reading ability find it far more challenging to pursue their educational, vocational, and healthcare goals than their literate peers. Even greater challenges confront those whose reading problems are caused or compounded by language barriers, cognitive impairments, or mental handicaps. Fortunately, many low-literate persons succeed despite enormous challenges because they are remarkably resourceful and/or have significant social supports. Unfortunately, low literacy, self-reported poor health, and regimen non-adherence are related.[2,3]

2 Educators help persons with diabetes by understanding the magnitude and health-related implications of the literacy problem, knowing how to assess literacy skills, and teaching in ways that maximize patients' abilities and resources. Doing these things well dramatically affects patients' abilities to achieve their healthcare goals and improve their quality of life.

Objectives

Upon completion of this chapter, the learner will be able to

1 Define functional literacy and health literacy.
2 Explain the magnitude and health-related implications of the literacy problem in the United States.
3 Compare and contrast the strengths and weaknesses of several common strategies for assessing literacy in clinic populations.
4 Examine whether their current teaching strategies meet the needs of persons with low literacy skills.
5 Define criteria for producing patient education materials and evaluating the appropriateness of existing materials for patients with low literacy skills.

Defining Literacy

1 In the National Literacy Act of 1991, *literacy* was defined as "an individual's ability to read, write, and speak in English and compute and solve problems at levels of proficiency necessary to function on the job and in society, to achieve one's goals, and to develop one's knowledge and potential."[1] In simpler terms, *functional literacy* is the ability to use reading, writing, and computational skills at levels adequate to meet the needs of everyday situations. These or similar definitions have been used to guide recent nationwide literacy assessments. The concept of *"health literacy"* refers to an individual's ability to read, write, speak, compute, and solve problems in order to participate in self-care and achieve health goals.

2 Literacy levels extend across a continuum of skills. Individuals exhibit varying degrees of literacy and cannot be strictly classified as literate or illiterate. For example, a patient's literacy skills may be sufficient to function at home or work, but not in healthcare settings or in situations that require self-care and diabetes-related decision making.

3 Grade-level equivalents do not adequately define an individual's level of literacy. Many people read at levels higher or lower than the last grade they completed in school or the level determined by the most common readability formulas. Therefore, functional assessments are more useful than grade equivalents for identifying literacy skills. When their literacy skills permit them to fully function in society, people are said to be functionally competent.

4 Low literacy does not necessarily imply low intelligence or functioning. Large numbers of Americans with low literacy skills hold jobs and live productive lives, demonstrating both intelligence and motivation. Some, it seems, have learned coping systems far more complex than reading itself.

5 Defining literacy levels for persons whose first language is not English poses special challenges. Some will have high literacy levels in all their languages, some will be highly literate in one language but not another, and still others will have low literacy levels in all their languages. Literacy is best assessed not only with respect to a person's ability to understand English-language materials, but also those printed in the native languages(s). Finally, some persons with low literacy simply come from oral cultures where the spoken word is the standard medium of communication and literacy is a non-issue.

Identifying the Magnitude of the Literacy Problem

1 In 1992, the National Adult Literacy Survey,[1] funded by the US Department of Education, assessed the nation's literacy by testing more than 15 000 Americans.[1] Some of the results of this survey are shown in Table 5.1.

2 Based on the 5-point scale used in this literacy survey, just over 20% of study participants (representing approximately 40 million American adults) demonstrated skills at Level 1, the lowest level of proficiency. Another 25% (approximately 50 million adults) performed at Level 2.
  A Persons who perform at Level 1 proficiency can, at best, accomplish routine tasks that involve short, simple documents and texts (eg, locating an expiration date on a drivers license, identifying one piece of information from a brief article, or performing simple addition). Persons at Level 1 usually are not able to comprehend the instructions on a prescription label or written meal plan without assistance.
  B Persons who perform at Level 2 also have important functional literacy limitations, including great difficulty with such diabetes self-care tasks as determining algorithmic insulin adjustments, which require complex mathematical problem solving, and following written sick-day guidelines, which require higher level reading skills.

3 The majority of subjects who performed at Levels 1 and 2 did not perceive themselves as having low literacy skills.
  A Simply asking patients if they can read does not provide an adequate assessment of literacy.
  B When offering low-literacy reading materials to patients, it is important to refrain from describing the materials as simple or "easy to understand." Patients who struggle with so-called "simple" material may feel ashamed of their performance, and this negative feeling can interfere with the patient/educator relationship.[4] Instead,

Table 5.1. Selected Results and Implications from the National Adult Literacy Survey[1]

Literacy Level	Estimated Number of Adult Americans	Probable Diabetes-Related Skills*	Teaching Tips for Diabetes Educators
1	40 million	Capable of calculating total carbohydrates from a meal if number of carbohydrates for each food is provided; some may be able to use a pie graph to determine the percentage of calories that should come from each food group; can identify a sentence in a pamphlet that explains how to test blood glucose, but most likely will not understand the directions; some at Level 1 may not be able to perform any of these skills	Repeated demonstrations and oral instruction may be necessary. Use of audiotapes and videotapes may help those patients who have the necessary playback equipment in their homes. After instructing the patient, ask the patient to repeat or demonstrate what was just taught. Negotiate attainable goals each teaching session and focus on actions and behaviors rather than theories and concepts. Try to identify relatives or friends of the patient who can read and may be able to assist. Be careful not to rush these patients. Be certain fundamental prerequisites have been learned before moving on to more complex concepts.
2	50 million	Capable of underlining the meaning of a term in a diabetes brochure but may not understand the term; some may be able to interpret instructions for a blood glucose meter; may need one-on-one counseling to adequately understand material at elementary school level	Provide Level 2 patients with simple educational material and be prepared to counsel patients on the material. Audiotapes and videotapes may prove useful. These patients have the potential for improving their understanding of educational material if they are taught common diabetes-related terms such as *insulin*, *hypoglycemia*, *glucose*, etc.
3	61 million	Can use glucose log table to determine how carbohydrate intake must be modified; can explain difference between type 1 and type 2 diabetes after reading a brochure; capable of low-level inferences and integration such as understanding the connection between glucose levels, exercise, and insulin; cannot make high-level inferences such as explaining the differences between 2 different regimens for treating diabetes	Provide Level 3 patients with current diabetes material, but be sure they completely understand it. These patients are often high-school graduates or even college educated and are accustomed to understanding written material. If they do not understand something, they may feel particularly reluctant to call it to your attention.
4, 5	40 million	Generally capable of higher level inferences and integration; likely capable of doing some self-education with materials written at a level too complex for the general public	Additional reading and educational materials may be suggested for these patients if they express an interest. Patients at Levels 4 and 5 should be able to progress to independent problem solving with encouragement and support.

*Skills and teaching tips are for illustration only. Assessment results and instructional needs will vary from patient to patient.
Source: Adapted from Kirsch et al.[1]

inform patients that the information contained in the reading material is important and worth taking the time and effort to read and understand.

4 The findings from the 1992 National Adult Literacy Survey[1] are consistent with previous studies and suggest that the literacy problem is not improving.
   A Results from a 1986 study showed that 72 million Americans functioned at marginal or low literacy levels.
   B Results from a 1976 study indicated that 20% of American adults had reading abilities below the 5th grade level and another 30% had only marginally competent reading skills.

5 The literacy proficiencies of young adults assessed in 1992 were, on average, lower than the literacy proficiencies of young adults assessed in 1985.

6 More than one half of all low-literate persons in America are Caucasians. African Americans, Hispanics, Native Americans/Alaskan Natives, and Asian/Pacific Islander adults performed, on average, at lower literacy levels than Caucasian adults.
   A Appearance, race, and speech are poor indicators of literacy.
   B Research[5] shows that some poorly dressed working people tested at far higher reading levels than well-dressed, articulate workers.

Assessing Patients' Functional Literacy

1 The most straightforward way to assess patients' understanding of educational material is to give the patients something to read, then ask them to read and explain the meaning of what they have read.
   A Low-literate patients believe that even though it may cause discomfort, health providers should initiate discussions about literacy, not the patient. Educators must communicate their care for the patient both verbally and nonverbally. Because of the sensitive nature of illiteracy they must also directly assure the patient that their conversations are confidential.[4]
   B Some patients with low literacy do not want their physicians to know about their literacy problems for fear that their doctors will think less of them. The same patients may be willing for other staff to know. Again, patients must be assured that their conversations are confidential.
   C Self-reports of education level often are poor indicators of reading ability.
   D Functional reading abilities of patients in medically related programs generally are four to five grade levels below their reported final education level.[5,6]
   E Many low-literate patients attempt to conceal their lack of skills by making up excuses such as "I forgot (or lost) my glasses." Others may carry magazines or newspapers in hopes of hiding their inability to read.
   F Patients can be asked to independently read a brief text (at home, while waiting in the clinic, or between provider visits) and circle everything in the booklet or brochure that (1) is new to them, (2) is different from what they had previously understood, and (3) raises questions. Following up on this request can provide a lot of information about patients and their literacy skills.

2 Literacy assessment tests may provide a general gauge of a patient's reading level if a reading deficiency is suspected.

    A If a literacy screening test is used, its purpose – to provide appropriate education materials – should be stated up front and the educator should then be ready to provide them.

    B Grade levels, despite their limitations, are a popular unit for characterizing both a patient's literacy level and the difficulty level of reading materials.

    C Once the patient's reading level is approximated, appropriate educational materials may be offered. The patient, however, is the final arbiter of the usability and comprehensibility of the materials.

    D Most general literacy assessment tests are not designed for clinical use and may be too time consuming and complex to administer. Examples of such tests are the SORT-R (Slosson Oral Reading Test), the WRAT-R (Wide Range Achievement Test, Revised), the PIAT-R (Peabody Individual Achievement Test, Revised), and the Cloze procedure.

3 The Test of Functional Health Literacy in Adults (TOFHLA)[6] was specifically developed for use in research studies to assess the health literacy of persons in healthcare settings.

    A The TOFHLA consists of actual materials from hospital settings, such as appointment slips, prescription vials, and informed consent documents.

    B The TOFHLA is administered in 2 parts: reading comprehension and numeracy. Thus, both comprehension and mathematical skills are assessed.

    C A Spanish version of TOFHLA, referred to as TOFHLA-S,[3] has also been developed.

    D The TOFHLA is highly correlated with the WRAT-R and REALM (see below); however, because the TOFHLA can take up to 22 minutes to administer it may be too time consuming for clinical use.

4 Since 1993, 2 other literacy assessment tests[7,8] have been developed for routine clinical use.

    A The Rapid Estimate of Adult Literacy in Medicine (REALM)[7] is a fast, efficient method for evaluating reading ability.

- REALM consists of 66 medically related words that range in difficulty from simple to complex (eg, fat and germs to colitis and impetigo). These words are set in a large print and divided into three columns across the page. The test is administered by asking patients to read the words aloud; scoring is based on their ability to correctly pronounce each word.
- The patient's raw score is then converted to an estimated grade range using a conversion chart. The conversion chart describes types of materials that might be appropriate for patients who read at each grade range.
- REALM can be administered in 2 to 3 minutes; it correlates well with more time-consuming tests such as SORT-R, WRAT-R, and PIAT-R; and it is designed for use in clinical settings.
- REALM has limitations. First, REALM assesses pronunciation rather than comprehension. However, REALM is correlated with the WRAT-R, which, in turn, is correlated with reading comprehension tests such as the Stanford Achievement Test. Therefore, REALM may provide a reasonable gauge of reading comprehension for some patients. The second limitation of REALM is that it does not

assess patients' ability to understand and perform quantitative operations. Finally, since REALM is also obviously a reading test, some patients who want to hide their poor literacy skills may not want to take this or similar tests.[4]

B The Medical Achievement Reading Test (MART)[8] is another rapid test designed for clinical use.
- MART consists of only medically related terms that are set in small print on glossy (light-reflecting) paper, similar to the label on a prescription bottle.
- The format of MART was designed purposefully to provide built-in excuses for not being able to read the words. Patients can avoid admitting that they cannot comprehend the material by blaming the glare from the glossy covering or the small print. Thus, the test is intended to be less threatening.
- MART, like REALM, correlates positively with other tests such as the WRAT-R, which is correlated to standardized reading comprehension tests.
- A limitation of MART, like REALM, is that neither comprehension nor quantitative capabilities are tested directly.

5 Readability formulas have often been used to evaluate the relative difficulty of patient education materials. However, these formulas were originally designed only to rank the difficulty levels of books or booklets that were written for school children taking "reading" classes.[9]

A Formulas that are commonly used to evaluate word and sentence length are the SMOG, Flesch, Fry, and Dale-Chall. The National Cancer Institute (NCI) recommends the SMOG as one tool for assessing readability (the procedure for using the SMOG is available from the NCI – see the Suggested Readings).

B To use readability formulas appropriately, writers and evaluators can follow 3 principles:
- Use readability formulas only in concert with direct testing of materials on target audience members.
- Use formulas only when the intended audience is similar to the group that participated in validating the formula.
- Do not write a text with readability formulas in mind.

C Readability formulas will not help persons who are illiterate; text readability does not matter if the patient cannot read at all.

Teaching Approaches for Persons With Low Literacy Skills

1 Patients with low literacy skills benefit most when educators conscientiously use educational and behavioral strategies that are known to be effective. These strategies help low-literate patients achieve a much-desired sense of involvement in and control over treatment or care decisions.[4]

A Directed questioning and active listening are essential for rapport-building and comprehensive assessment.
- Acknowledge the problem of limited reading skills by saying something like "A lot of our patients have trouble reading prescriptions and education materials. Is that a problem for you?" or "Is there anyone you usually ask to help you read your prescriptions or the booklets and pamphlets we give you?"

- Personalize all messages to patients. Instead of saying "Meal planning is the cornerstone of diabetes management," personalize the message by saying something like "Managing your diabetes begins with keeping track of what you eat."
- Invite and encourage patients to describe their strengths by saying "Ms. Jackson, tell me the ways you prefer to learn, and the strategies you've developed for doing your job/homemaking tasks."
- Assure patients that they are not alone in having reading problems and that they can succeed.

B Tailor objectives for self-management education so that their attainment depends less on reading than on other modes of learning.

C Limit the number of educational objectives and amount of material to be taught in a particular session to what is essential for meeting patients' needs and desires. It is better to set modest goals and teach more if a patient proves able rather than set overly ambitious goals that may result in the patient feeling like a failure.

D Repetition is a key to success. State important points at the beginning of instruction and repeat these points during the instruction process. Patients can then be asked to rehearse the important points at the end of the session. Build on what patients know by tying new information to it.

E Concrete illustrations, demonstrations, and hands-on experiences presented from the patient's point of view are more effective than information-telling. For example, use magazine pictures or food models rather than verbal abstractions like "carbohydrates, proteins, and fats." Emphasize actions and behaviors over theories and concepts.
- Storytelling may help some patients learn because the information is embedded in a memorable structure and may represent a more culturally appropriate way to teach.
- Analogies drawn from a patient's experience may be similarly helpful.

F Be especially sensitive to word usage.
- Most patients can learn any and all diabetes-related terms if, when the terms are introduced, they are repeatedly stated and carefully defined in context, and the patients are shown illustrations of what the words mean and how they look in print. Patients can benefit further by using the terms in return demonstrations.
- Many patients with low-to-moderate literacy skills can improve their functional ability to read patient education publications by several "grade" levels if they are taught the meaning and spelling of the 12 to 20 most common diabetes-related words (eg, diabetes, insulin, blood glucose, hypoglycemia, hyperglycemia, nutrition, hospital).

G Pause frequently to ask patients to repeat what has been said or to perform a return demonstration. Be sure that the prerequisites have been mastered before continuing to teach. Achieving success in one area is better than teaching 5 areas and discovering that the patient is bewildered.

H Being patient is essential; persons with low literacy and other learning problems do especially poorly if they feel they are being rushed.

I Recommend aids to recall, including mnemonic devices such as visualizing, categorizing, and use of associations and acronyms.

J Offer encouragement and specific feedback about patient performance.

K Provide audiotapes or videotapes to reinforce and extend patient learning for those who have the necessary playback equipment at home. Multimedia resources provide patients with the opportunity to learn in a more private, relaxed environment that helps to preserve their dignity. In many cases, homemade videotapes will be better received than professional productions, especially if the people in the video look and sound like the intended viewing audience and model effective diabetes management. If you donate one or more copies of videos to local video rental stores, they will often be happy to lend these videos free of charge.

L Identify family members, friends, or members of community agencies who can read and are willing to help. Such persons are usually the key to achieving diabetes goals when low literacy is accompanied or caused by cognitive dysfunction or mental handicaps.

M Personalize printed materials by placing the patient's name on the cover of each item. Print patient-specific information inside the materials.

N Schedule more frequent, short visits if possible and review what was taught during the previous sessions.

O Simplify patients' regimens; work up to complex goals as patients (and/or caregivers) experience success and become confident.

P Highlight 1 or 2 of the most important take-home messages. Stress their importance and ask patients or family members to repeat them.

Q Insofar as it is possible, provide education materials in both English and the native language for persons whose first language is not English.

R Use small-group methods to encourage storytelling and group brainstorming and problem solving. Persons with low literacy may be more comfortable and successful learning from others' experiences. Groups can offer social support. They may also help their members learn such practical skills as how to talk with their doctors, make appointments, and negotiate insurance/payment issues.

S Help patients anticipate what will happen and what they will experience at subsequent visits. Help them picture what will happen. Doing so will reduce uncertainty and fear, and it will help build some confidence.

2 Both educators and patients with low literacy skills may benefit when the curriculum includes topics not usually taught to literate patients, such as how to access ancillary services. Addressing such topics as a routine part of the content helps those persons with low literacy who feel ashamed of their lack of reading ability. Their shame can be exacerbated by health professionals who become frustrated or angry when a patient cannot find a particular location in the medical center, complete a form, or read even the most straightforward instructions.[10] Community outreach programs that assist with these needs can be very helpful. Good relationships with patients can be solidified by being sensitive to their needs for the following assistance:

A Many patients do not show up or are chronically late for appointments because they need help navigating around the medical building(s) in which they receive their care.
- Familiar words (diabetes rather than endocrinology) should be used on hallway signs.
- Color coding for hospital/clinic floors and parking levels can help identify locations.
- Strategically placed information desks staffed by persons attuned to the needs of low-literate clients should be considered in larger institutions.

B Completing forms and registering for care can be the most difficult and embarrassing tasks for persons with low literacy levels.

- Simplify forms as much as possible.
- Advise clerks, receptionists, social workers, and other staff to be sensitive and alert for someone struggling to a complete a form. Support can be offered by saying something like "Many of our patients have trouble with these forms. Would it help if I read the questions to you?" Some large clinics with significant numbers of low-literate patients employ surrogate readers for this purpose.

C Medication and other self-care errors due to patients' inability to read or understand the instructions are among the most troubling and life-threatening problems for low-literate persons.
- Simplify medication and self-care regimens as much as possible (eg, use combination drugs rather than separate pills, or avoid multi-drug regimens that require patients to take different drugs on different schedules).
- Include family members, friends, or agency workers identified by patients as surrogate readers when providing medication and treatment instructions.
- Ability to follow a meal plan is especially challenging for persons with low literacy. Many such persons benefit from educator-led "field trips" to neighborhood groceries. Those who cannot base food selection on nutrition labeling can, if they wish, be taught to make appropriate choices based on characteristics of food packaging, such as colors and shapes of the items.

D Many patients with low literacy skills say they have little or no difficulty understanding appointment reminders if the card or slip of paper is identified as such. Most will then keep the reminder card and obtain assistance from others if they cannot decipher the date, time, and location messages.

E Many patients with low literacy express an interest in attending adult literacy classes. Be prepared to make referrals to such courses by having and posting a list of telephone numbers of literacy classes available in your area; help patients locate these courses if necessary.

3 Review and prepare educational materials for use with patients.

A The National Cancer Institute's publication *Clear and Simple: Developing Effective Print Materials for Low Literate Readers* provides a description of 5 tests that can be used to create educational materials or evaluate those made by others.[11]
- Define the target audience by identifying the segment of the population to be reached.
- Know the target audience by learning about behaviors that help or hinder prevention or self-care; knowledge and attitudes; utilization of existing services; cultural habits, preferences, and sensitivities related to the message(s) being communicated; and common barriers and motivators.
- Develop a concept for the item by defining behavioral objectives; determining a limited number of points that are key to achieving those objectives; selecting the best presentation methods (eg, audio, audiovisual, print, interactive computer); estimating the functional reading level appropriate for print materials; and organizing topics in the way they will be used by the target audience.
- Develop content and visuals using the guidelines presented in Table 5.2.
- Pretest and revise draft materials with the goal of determining whether representative members of the target audience understand the message before going to the expense of publishing and distributing the materials. Besides comprehension, other factors that can be used to assess educational materials are audience attrac-

tion, acceptance, and personal relevance. The materials should be pilot tested with 25 to 50 persons, although results from testing with smaller groups can still provide valuable information. Be sure that the individuals who are participating in the pretest understand that it is the materials, not them, that are being evaluated.

Table 5.2. Checklist for Evaluating/Developing Patient Education Materials

Content/Style	• The material is interactive and allows for audience involvement. • The material presents "how-to" information. • Peer language is used whenever appropriate to increase personal identification and improve readability. • Words are familiar to the reader. Any new words are defined clearly. • Sentences are simple, specific, direct, and written in the active voice. • Each idea is clear and logically sequenced (according to audience logic). • The number of concepts is limited per piece.
Layout	• The material uses advance organizers or headers. • Headers are simple and close to text. • Layout balances white space with words and illustrations. • Text uses uppercase and lowercase letters. • Underlining or bolding rather than all caps give emphasis. • Type style and size of print are easy to read; type is at least 12 point.
Visuals	• Visuals are relevant to text, meaningful to the audience, and appropriately located. • Illustrations and photographs are simple and free from clutter and distraction. • Visuals use adult rather than childlike images. • Illustrations show familiar images that reflect cultural context. • Visuals have captions. Each visual illustrates and is directly related to one message. • Different styles, such as photographs without background detail, shaded line drawings, or simple line drawings, are pretested with the audience to determine which is understood best. • Cues, such as circles or arrows, point out key information. • Colors used are appealing to the audience (as determined by pretesting).
Readability	• Readability analysis is done to suggest the approximate reading level.

Source: Reprinted with permission from the National Cancer Institute.[11]

B An excellent example of low-literacy diabetes materials that were developed using these principles may be found in the "Diabetes Easy-to-Read Library" on the Internet and available at: *http://www.niddk.nih.gov.* Click on "Diabetes" under the "Health Information" heading to find the "Easy-to-Read Publications."[12]

C If the foregoing steps are used to review and prepare educational materials, the use of readability formulas will be largely unnecessary.

D Direct translations of reading materials from English into other languages are rarely successful. Other-language versions of reading materials should also be developed using the steps suggested above.

Key Educational Considerations

1. Nearly one half of all Americans have poor functional literacy. Understanding common diabetes educational materials and dealing with the healthcare system can be frustrating and challenging both for these people and their health professionals.

2. Literacy assessment tools such as REALM and MART may be useful for identifying and evaluating patients with low literacy skills; however, they are best used to approximate someone's ability to comprehend written materials.

3. Diabetes educators can serve low-literate clients most effectively by using teaching strategies that serve patients' specific needs. These strategies may include limiting or simplifying learning objectives, using audiovisual teaching aids, repeating main points, and assessing patient mastery before moving on to new topics.

4. Important considerations for preparing or evaluating patient education materials are knowing the target audience, having a clear concept of the audience's information needs, choosing content and visuals consistent with audience needs, and pretesting the materials with representatives from the target audience.

5. Low-literate patients may experience shame when confronted with written materials commonly found in healthcare environments (eg, forms, reading materials, and insurance papers) that they are unable to read. They may also experience problems accessing healthcare services because of their reading difficulties. Consider examining the extent to which your institution and practices help or hinder low-literate patients.

Self-Review Questions

1. Define functional literacy. Characterize the distribution of functional literacy skills in the general population of the United States.
2. What are the health-related implications of the literacy problem in the United States?
3. Name 3 tools you might use to assess literacy in the population of patients you serve. What are the strengths and weaknesses of each strategy?
4. Describe at least 6 teaching strategies that may help meet the needs of persons with low literacy skills.
5. Describe 5 criteria for producing patient education materials or evaluating the appropriateness of existing materials for your patients.
6. Compare and contrast the utility of different teaching approaches for helping patients with different levels of functional literacy.

Learning Assessment: Case Study 1

PJ is a 45-year-old male recently diagnosed with type 2 diabetes. He is 5 ft 8 in, weighs 190 lb (86.3 kg), body mass index (BMI) = 29, and has a blood pressure of 135/90. PJ holds a daytime job as a housekeeper at a metropolitan hotel where he has been working since he dropped out of high school after the 10th grade. At night he tends bar at a local pub to help his sister pay for their mother's nursing home bills. His mother was placed in the nursing home about 2 years ago after having a stroke. She is 75 years old and has had uncontrolled diabetes for many years. PJ states that when his sister is not busy with her work as an accountant, the two of them often visit their mother together.

PJ was diagnosed with type 2 diabetes at a workplace screening program. He has no symptoms of diabetes, although he does complain of fatigue that he attributes to his rigorous work schedule. PJ expresses that he would like to make an effort to control his diabetes; he is concerned since his mother's physician told him that her stroke was partly due to her uncontrolled diabetes. PJ takes oral diabetes medications exactly as ordered and feels that the pills should be sufficient treatment for his diabetes. He does not understand the relationship between exercise, food, and diabetes.

While asking PJ about his nutritional habits, you discover that he eats many of his meals at the restaurant in the hotel where he works because he gets a big employee discount. He also tells you that his favorite foods are potato chips and hot dogs, and he would really like to continue eating them on a regular basis. PJ states that he does not like exercise and feels he does not have time to cook healthy foods for himself.

You initially give PJ a diabetes education pamphlet designed for the general population. To determine PJ's understanding of the material, you select one sentence in the pamphlet and ask him what it means. You point to a sentence that says, "Reducing cholesterol and fat in your diet, in combination with a regular exercise program, will help you control your diabetes." You ask PJ to read the sentence and tell you what it means. PJ replies that the sentence tells him he should go on a diet to lose fat and that exercise will help control his diabetes. You realize that PJ did not understand the word cholesterol, and that, in this context, he did not really grasp the meaning of most of the words that he read, so you decide to administer the REALM literacy test. PJ scores in the 4th to 6th grade range on the REALM scoring scale, indicating that he should respond well to direct instructions, but may require some additional counseling to adequately understand material written at an elementary school level.

Questions for Discussion
1. How would you characterize PJ's literacy level?
2. What obstacles would you encounter in teaching PJ?
3. What are some strategies for teaching this patient about diabetes and health management?

Discussion

1 The characteristics displayed by PJ place him at a very low literacy level.

- **A** Although PJ completed the 10th grade before dropping out of school, he is an example of a person who reads at a level lower than the last grade completed.
- **B** PJ reads at the 4th to 6th grade level based on the REALM scoring scale and would likely fall into the Level 1 category of literacy proficiency (Table 2.1).
  - Skills common to this level are identifying a country in a short article, locating an expiration date on a drivers license, or calculating a total for a bank deposit entry.
  - Although the Level 1 tasks seem very simple, about 1 of every 5 Americans (40 million people) perform at Level 1 literacy at best and are able to perform "simple, routine tasks involving uncomplicated texts and documents."

2 Much of the educational material designed for the general public is written at a level too complex for many patients to understand.

- **A** PJ's misinterpretation of the pamphlet serves as an example of how patients with low literacy skills may skip words they do not know and use limited meanings for words they know from other contexts.
- **B** These patients often will not make inferences or interpret words in the context in which they are presented.

3 Many obstacles must be overcome to properly teach PJ about diabetes.

- **A** Because of PJ's poor literacy skills, materials such as educational audiotapes and videotapes may be useful.
- **B** Another possibility is to ask whether PJ's sister might assist him in reading and understanding diabetes education material.
- **C** Consistently repeating important information may be useful in working with PJ because many reading-impaired patients use memorization as a coping strategy.
- **D** Competing priorities in PJ's life must also be addressed. It is important to help PJ find a way to make controlling diabetes an important focus in his life while still allowing him to handle his difficult work schedule, his mother and her condition, and the stresses associated with both.
- **E** Finally, PJ may have difficulty forming new habits (eg, eating properly, exercising regularly) and affording some diabetes treatments if his insurance does not cover these expenses.

4 Strategies for teaching PJ include focusing on specific behaviors he agrees to perform and teaching only 1 or 2 essential objectives during each session.

- **A** After discussion with PJ, the 2 of you may decide that the following are some realistic goals for PJ to try to accomplish before his next appointment.
  - Substitute a low-fat variety of hot dogs for his regular brand.
  - Take his mother for walks in her wheelchair for 20 minutes each time he visits her.
- **B** You may also want to ask PJ to see if there is a worksite wellness program at the hotel where he works. If PJ can successfully accomplish his initial goals, he may want to get involved in the worksite wellness program or, if one is not available, to enroll in a diabetes management class. He is more likely to attend if he receives assistance in working these into his schedule.

Learning Assessment: Case Study 2

LM is a 59-year-old female who lost her job as a light machinery operator at a local paper plant due to company downsizing 3 months ago. Her blood pressure is 160/94, she is 5 ft 3 in, and she weighs 160 lb (72.6 kg), BMI = 28.

LM arrived 45 minutes late for her appointment today, and you notice in her chart that she has a history of missing appointments. She states that her family responsibilities often cause her to be late or miss appointments. At her last visit 5 weeks ago, LM started 2 medications in addition to her oral diabetes medication. The 2 medications were an antihypertensive and a drug that inhibits cholesterol formation so as to prevent atherosclerosis. LM has been instructed to take the antihypertensive 2 times per day, the anticholesterol drug once a day, and the oral diabetes medication 3 times per day. LM reports that she has not been feeling well lately. She complains of headaches, sleeplessness, and frequent urination, although the vaginal itching she complained of at the last appointment has since resolved. You also note that she has not yet been accepted to Medicaid, even though she was given application forms immediately after she lost her job and company insurance.

LM's laboratory test results indicate that her blood glucose is 230 mg/dL (12.78 mmol/L) after a 12-hour fast and her cholesterol level is 160 mg/dL, which is down from 240 mg/dL the last time she visited. When you ask LM if she has been taking her medications, she responds that she has taken them exactly as ordered. LM then takes her bag of medications out of her purse so you can look at the bottles. You notice that she has a bottle of antibiotics with her husband's name on it instead of the blood pressure medication that was prescribed. Sensing that LM may not be able to read prescription labels, you decide to give her the REALM reading test. She refuses, stating that she forgot to bring her glasses today.

Questions for Discussion
1. What are LM's physical problems? Why might she be feeling so poorly?
2. What characteristics of poor literacy is LM displaying?
3. What are some strategies for helping LM?

Discussion
1. LM has apparently confused her medications. She appears to be taking her husband's antibiotics instead of her blood pressure pills. In addition, her high blood glucose and very sharp reduction in blood cholesterol since her last visit suggest that she may have switched the dosing for the diabetes pills with the dosing for the cholesterol pills (ie, LM is taking the diabetes pills once a day and the cholesterol pills 3 times per day).

2. Patients with low literacy skills commonly cope by memorizing information about their medications. When confronted with several different medications with different dose directions, some persons may become confused about what they have memorized and take pills in the wrong doses and/or at the wrong times.

3 Patients with low literacy also commonly forget appointments or arrive late. They must often rely on their memories to recall the correct date and time of appointments. Some patients may even get lost on their way to the appointment because they cannot read the road signs or the signs within the hospital/clinic. One reason LM may not have been accepted to Medicaid is that she did not properly complete the forms (or fill them out at all). Accessing health care, from getting to the clinic to taking medications to filling out forms and becoming properly educated about one's diagnoses, requires a fairly high level of literacy. Living with low literacy skills can make navigating the healthcare system a nightmare for some patients.

4 A very important aspect of LM's coping style is the schemes she has created to attempt to hide her poor literacy skills. Claiming she forgot her glasses and blaming others for her poor or late appointment attendance are simple mechanisms to hide the fact that she cannot read very well.

5 All of these characteristics point to the tremendous amount of shame that many people feel about having poor reading skills. Many illiterate people are able to hold jobs for years and function quite well in society even though they cannot read. It is important to not confuse poor reading and writing skills with lack of intelligence; a high degree of intelligence may be necessary to function in society without being able to read.

6 A variety of strategies can be used to help LM cope with her reading problems.
  A Provide telephone reminders of her appointments to improve her attendance.
  B If she is interested, tell her where to obtain and then demonstrate how to use a pill organizer with different containers for her pills each day (some pharmacies provide these free to customers, but, if not, an egg carton may be used if LM cannot afford a pill organizer).
  C Enlist the help of family members, friends, or social services to assist her with the aspects of her life that require literacy, such as filling out Medicaid forms and properly taking her medications.
  D Simplify LM's medications by requesting that her provider prescribe pills that are different colors or sizes to make them easy to identify and distinguish from one another.
  E Assist her in enrolling in an adult literacy class if she wishes to learn to read and can make the time to attend class.
  F Perhaps most importantly, end each teaching session with LM repeating/demonstrating to you what you have taught her that day.

7 When dealing with functionally illiterate patients, be sensitive to the shame they may feel because they cannot read.
  A When you suspect a patient is illiterate, take steps to reduce their embarrassment. For instance, when giving them a piece of literature to read to see if they understand the meaning, a helpful comment might be "many of our patients cannot understand this pamphlet; tell me if you have trouble with it," or "the glossy covering on this prescription bottle makes it hard to read for some patients; tell me if it bothers you." These statements and others like them provide excuses for the patients. They do not have to admit directly that they cannot read the material, but you can still find out if they are functionally illiterate.

B Reduce potential for shame associated with LM having taken the wrong medications: "When two or more family members take several medicines it's pretty easy to get them mixed up, and it looks like that might have happened in your home. It's good that we caught the mix-up early. This time I want to be sure I've been clear about your medications so you can go home and get the medicine you need and your husband gets what he needs…"

References

1. Kirsch L, Jungeblut A, Jenkins L, Kolstad A. Adult Literacy in America: A First Look at the Results of the National Adult Literacy Survey. Washington DC: National Center for Education Statistics, Department of Education; 1993.

2. Kalichman SC, Ramachandran B, Catz S. Adherence to combination antiretroviral therapies in HIV patients of low health literacy. J Gen Intern Med. 1999;14:267-273.

3. Baker DW, Parker RM, Williams MV, Clark WS, Nurss J. The relationship of patient reading ability to self-reported health and use of health services. Am J of Public Health. 1997;87:1027-1030.

4. Brez S, Taylor M. Assessing literacy for patient teaching: perspectives of adults with low literacy skills. J Adv Nurs. 1997;25: 1040-1047.

5. Doak C, Doak L, Root J. Teaching Patients With Low Literacy Skills. 2nd Edition. Philadelphia: JB Lippincott Co.; 1996.

6. Hanson-Divers EC. Developing a medical achievement reading test to evaluate patient literacy skills: A preliminary study. J Health Care Poor Underserved. 1997;8:56-69.

7. Davis TC, Crouch MA, Long SW, et al. Rapid assessment of literacy levels of adult primary care patients. Fam Med. 1991; 23:433-435.

8. Parikh NS, Parker RM, Nurss JR, Baker DW, Williams MV. Shame and health literacy: the unspoken connection. Patient Education and Counseling. 1996;27:33-39.

9. Pichert JW, Elam P. Readability formulas may mislead you. Patient Education and Counseling. 1985;7:181-191.

10. Baker DW, Parker RM, Williams MV, et al. The health care experience of patients with low literacy. Arch Fam Med. 1996;5:329-334.

11. National Cancer Institute, National Institutes of Health. Clear and Simple: Developing Effective Print Materials for Low Literate Readers. Bethesda, Md: National Institutes of Health, undated. Detailed guidelines for writers who wish to communicate effectively to low-literate audiences are available on the Internet at no charge. Available at: *http://rex.nci.nih.gov/ NCI Pub Interface/Clear and Simple/ HOME.HTM*. Accessed November 2000.

12. "Diabetes Easy-to-Read Library" on the Internet and available at: *http://www.niddk. nih.gov*. Click on "Diabetes" under the "Health Information" heading to find the "Easy-to-Read Publications." A series of low literacy booklets on diabetes-related complications can be found on the Internet. Available at: *http://www.niddk.nih.gov/ health/diabetes/pubs/complications/index. htm*. Accessed November 2000.

Suggested Readings

The National Work Group on Literacy and Health. Communicating with patients who have limited literacy skills: Report of the National Work Group on Literacy and Health. J Fam Pract. 1998;46:168-176. Report includes sources of low-literacy education materials.

Health Literacy, Report of the Council on Scientific Affairs, AMA Position Statement. JAMA. 1999;281:552-557.

An excellent series of free low literacy diabetes materials may be found in the "Diabetes Easy-to-Read Library" on the Internet. Available at: *http://www.niddk.nih.gov*. Look under the "Health Information" heading and click on "Diabetes" to find the "Easy-to-Read Publications." Accessed November 2000.

The Indian Health Service has developed a series of easy-reading diabetes booklets for Native Americans. These and other materials are listed among the "Resources for Diabetes Education Material" on the Internet. Available at: *http://www.ihs.gov/MedicalPrograms/Diabetes/index.asp*. Accessed November 2000.

The National Heart, Lung and Blood Institute (NHLBI) offers a variety of educational tools, many of which are aimed at low literacy persons who need help with nutrition and weight control. Check out the materials on the Internet and available at: *http://www.nhlbi.nih.gov/health*. Accessed November 2000.

Searches for materials may be initiated through the Combined Health Information Database on the Internet and available at: *http://chid.nih.gov*. Accessed November 2000.

Diabetes Educational Materials for People With Limited Reading Skills. Searches-on-File, Topics in Diabetes. Bethesda, Md: National Diabetes Information Clearinghouse; Mar 1997. Contact the NDIC at 1 Information Way, Bethesda, MD 20892-3560. Telephone: 301-654-3327.

The Center for Health Care Strategies offers valuable "Health Literacy Fact Sheets" on the Internet and available at: *http://www.chcs.org*. Go to the "Resources" page and click on "Health Literacy Fact Sheets." Each fact sheets deals with one important aspect of health literacy. The Center for Health Care Strategies prepared these documents in collaboration with the National Academy on an Aging Society. Accessed November 2000.

Mettger W. Communicating Nutrition Information to Low-Literate Individuals: An Assessment of Methods. Bethesda, Md: National Cancer Institute, National Institutes of Health; 1989. To order, contact: Office of Cancer Communications, NCI, Building 31, Room 10A03, 9000 Rockville Pike, Bethesda, MD 20892. Telephone: 1-800-4-CANCER.

National Cancer Institute, National Institutes of Health. Detailed guidelines for writers who wish to communicate effectively with low-literate audiences. "Clear and Simple," "Making Health Communications Work," and "Theory At A Glance" are on the

Internet and available free at: *htttp://www.nci.nih.gov* or by calling 1-800-4-CANCER. If you use the Internet, go to the NCI Web site and search the alternatives under "Information for Patients, Public and the Mass Media" in order to find these program planning publications. Accessed November 2000.

Beyond the Brochure: Alternative Approaches to Effective Health Communications (PDF-821K). Free from the Centers for Disease Control and Prevention. On the Internet and may be downloaded from the "cancer" publications section of the CDC: *www.cdc.gov.* Accessed November 2000.

Resources for teaching may be obtained from the Office of Minority Health Resource Center. Telephone: 1-800-444-6472. Available at: *http://www.omhrc.gov.* Accessed November 2000. OMH lists many Spanish language health materials.

Learning Assessment: Post-Test Questions

Teaching Persons With Low Literacy Skills   5

1. Which instrument can be used by the diabetes educator to assess the health literacy of an adult in less than 5 minutes?
   A The Test of Functional Health Literacy in Adults (TOFHLA)
   B The Rapid Estimate of Adult Literacy in Medicine (REALM)
   C The Medical Achievement Reading Test (MART)
   D Slossen Oral Reading Test (SORT-R)

2. Which literacy assessment test is available in Spanish?
   A The Test of Functional Health Literacy in Adults (TOFHLA)
   B The Rapid Estimate of Adult Literacy in Medicine (REALM)
   C The Medical Achievement Reading Test (MART)
   D Slossen Oral Reading Test (SORT-R)

3. The most effective way to determine the medical literacy level of a person with diabetes who is referred to you for counseling is to:
   A Ask the patient how well he or she reads
   B Obtain information about the patient's background since the reading level will be equivalent to the reported final educational level
   C Gauge the patient's reading level from the newspapers and magazines that he or she likes to read
   D Ask the patient to read an educational pamphlet on diabetes and explain the meaning of what was read

4. Health literacy is the ability to read, understand, and act on healthcare information. Which of the following approaches would be best to use with a patient who has an elementary school functional level?
   A Give repeated demonstrations on the use of a glucose meter
   B Have patient read a simple brochure and follow up with one-on-one counseling to ensure the material is adequately understood
   C Have patient complete a glucose monitoring log
   D Provide written materials explaining the connection between food intake, exercise, and insulin on blood glucose levels

5. REALM and MART are designed to gauge a patient's:
   A Intelligence and learning ability
   B Ability to understand and perform quantitative operations
   C Reading ability and comprehension
   D Ability to comply with written instructions

6. FG, a 50-year-old obese man with type 2 diabetes has low health literacy skills. What is likely to be the most effective way to teach him about weight control in diabetes management?
   A Use videos to explain the effects of overweight and excessive body fat on blood sugar levels
   B Give him written information in which key terms are underlined and explained in simple language
   C Provide a low caloric diet menu sheet and ask him to comply with the suggested food pattern
   D Have him maintain a glucose log and a food diary so you can show how food intake influences blood sugar levels

7 You are working with BT, a 60-year-old patient with newly diagnosed diabetes and low literacy skills. Which strategy would NOT be appropriate in the planning, implementation, and evaluation of instruction?
  A Use only short-term learning objectives and limit the number
  B Use audiovisual teaching aids to cover all major conceptual points
  C Repeat major points during the instruction process
  D Use written tests to evaluate learning

8 Strategies for diabetes education should include all of the following except:
  A Limit the number of learning objectives to what is essential for meeting education goals
  B Limit the amount of material taught in a particular session
  C Emphasize the philosophical rationale and general concepts around which the program is designed
  D Emphasize actions and behaviors over theories and concepts

9 A diabetes educator who assesses functional literacy needs to know that:
  A Grade-level equivalents are the best predictor of a person's level of literacy
  B Literacy skills are closely correlated with intelligence and motivation
  C The patient's ability to function in everyday life affects literacy skills
  D Appearance, race, and speech patterns are often useful indicators of literacy level

10 When developing patient education materials for a low-literacy population, it is important to:
  A Employ a passive writing style and use few definitions
  B Use all capital letters in the layout to emphasize key concepts
  C Incorporate commercially produced audio/visual materials
  D Introduce definitions in one section to establish a working vocabulary

See next page for answer key.

Post-Test Answer Key

Teaching Persons With Low Literacy Skills

1. B
2. A
3. D
4. A
5. C
6. A
7. D
8. C
9. C
10. D

A Core Curriculum for Diabetes Education
Diabetes Education and Program Management

Psychological Disorders 6

Richard R. Rubin, PhD, CDE
The Johns Hopkins University School of Medicine
Departments of Medicine and Pediatrics
Baltimore, Maryland

Joseph P. Napora, PhD, LCSW-C
The Johns Hopkins University School of Medicine
The Johns Hopkins Diabetes Center
Baltimore, Maryland

Introduction

1 The relationship between diabetes and both mental disorders and subclinical psychological syndromes has received growing attention over the past 2 decades.

2 Persons with diabetes may suffer disproportionately from certain psychological disorders, and the course and consequences of some of these disorders may be more severe for persons with diabetes.

3 Each *mental disorder* is defined by a distinct group of signs and symptoms that have been specified in the Diagnostic and Statistical Manual of Mental Disorders, Fourth Edition (DSM-IV).[1] Educators should be familiar with criteria for the disorders that are common to patients with diabetes: depressive disorders, anxiety disorders (including specific phobia), eating disorders, and adjustment disorders.

4 Some patients manifest a *subclinical syndrome*, features of a mental disorder that do not meet the criteria for a mental disorder. The distinction between mental disorders and subclinical syndromes is generally one of duration and severity. Degree of functional impairment is often a key measure of severity. Most people with diabetes experience some symptoms of a mental disorder, at least occasionally. However, patients who suffer from a complex of symptoms for a long enough period of time and with debilitating effects usually warrant the diagnosis of a clinical disorder.

5 A goal of the psychosocial assessment described in Chapter 2, Psychosocial Assessment, in Diabetes Education and Program Management, is to identify patients who suffer from either clinical or subclinical psychological problems, since the presence of either clinical or subclinical problems is likely to affect diabetes self-management, physiologic outcomes, and quality of life.

6 Effective approaches for working with patients who have subclinical problems include education in problem solving, goal setting, behavioral contracting, and coping skills training. These and other techniques are described in Chapter 3, Behavior Change, in Diabetes Education and Program Management. When these approaches are successful, they reduce both the likelihood that subclinical symptoms will impair the individual's capacity for self-care and the risk that the emotional strain will worsen and become a full-blown clinical disorder.

7 Educators need to be acquainted with effective treatments for mental disorders and subclinical psychological problems, including information on the side effects of some psychotropic medications that are commonly used with diabetes patients who manifest psychological symptoms.

8 Since the diagnosis and treatment of most mental disorders is outside of the scope of practice of all but a few educators, it is not their responsibility to diagnose or prescribe treatment for serious psychological disorders.

9 A role of the educator is to screen patients and to refer them to a mental health specialist for formal diagnosis and treatment when symptom criteria indicate the presence of a serious disorder. With the medications and counseling interventions that are available, psychological disorders can be treated successfully with the appropriate referral.

Objectives

Upon completion of this chapter, the learner will be able to

1 Explain the relationship between diabetes and mental disorders common to people with diabetes, including depressive disorders, anxiety disorders (including specific phobia), eating disorders, and adjustment disorders.
2 Distinguish among the various psychological disorders that can affect diabetes management.
3 Identify subclinical syndromes that might impair diabetes self-care.
4 Identify current counseling and psychotherapeutic treatments for the psychological problems that are common among people with diabetes.
5 List current pharmacologic treatments for the psychological problems that are common among people with diabetes.
6 Describe indications for referring a patient to a mental health specialist for consultation or treatment.

Depressive Disorder

1 See Table 6.1 for symptoms of clinical depression. Signs and symptoms of depression are also described in Chapter 2, Psychosocial Assessment, in Diabetes Education and Program Management. DSM-IV[1] provides extensive information about the attributes of depression. Dysthymic disorder, dysthymia, and mood disorder are other terms used for clinical depression.

2 Depression appears to be more common among people with diabetes than in the general population.

Table 6.1. Symptoms of Clinical Depression

1 Depressed mood (feeling sad or empty) most of the day, nearly every day
2 Significant weight loss when not dieting or weight gain (eg, a change of more than 5% of body weight in a month), or a decrease or increase in appetite nearly every day
3 Trouble sleeping or sleeping too much nearly every day
4 Feeling very agitated or physically sluggish nearly every day
5 Fatigue or loss of energy nearly every day
6 Markedly diminished interest or pleasure in all or almost all activities most of day, nearly every day
7 Feeling worthless or excessively or inappropriately guilty nearly every day
8 Diminished ability to think or concentrate, or indecisiveness, nearly every day
9 Recurrent thoughts of death (not just fear of dying), recurrent thoughts of suicide, a suicide attempt or a specific plan to commit suicide

A Although estimates of the prevalence of depression vary, at least 1 of every 5 people with diabetes is likely to be affected by depression.[2] Some studies suggest that as many as 40% of patients with diabetes have significantly elevated levels of depressive symptomatology;[3] not all of these individuals are clinically depressed—ie, not all meet the criteria for the diagnosis of a depressive disorder.

B Some populations of people with diabetes have a consistently high prevalence of depression. For example, in a study of older Mexican Americans with diabetes, 31.1% of the subjects reported high levels of depression.[4] In a study of African Americans with diabetes ranging in age from 35 to 75 years, 30% had a prevalence of depressive symptoms.[5]

C Levels of depression (clinical and subclinical) among people with diabetes are 2 to 3 times the estimated prevalence in the population at large.[6]

3 Depression may be more severe in people with diabetes.

A Depression is a recurring condition for many people who have diabetes. Only about 20% of people with diabetes who recover from an episode of depression remain asymptomatic more than 5 years.[7]

B Individual depressive episodes may be more severe as well as more common among people with diabetes.

C The symptoms of depression and diabetes may exacerbate one another at the neuroendocrine level. For example, hormonal disregulation associated with depression may contribute to glycemic disregulation (and vice versa).[8]

D An aspect of diabetes that appears to increase depressive symptomatology is the extent to which the disease intrudes in life (ie, disrupts valued activities and interests due to constraints imposed by the disease) rather than diabetic complications per se or personal control over health outcomes.[9]

4 Depression has especially adverse effects for people with diabetes.

A Clinical depression can severely hamper the management of diabetes. Feelings of helplessness and hopelessness that often are associated with depression can contribute to a disastrous cycle of poor self-care, worsened glycemia, and deepened depression.[10]

B Clinical depression has been associated with poor glycemic control and an increased risk of microvascular and macrovascular complications in part because of its effect on self-care and other health behaviors.[11]

C Type 1 patients with a lifetime history of major depression showed significantly worse glycemic control than patients with no history of psychiatric illness.[12]

D Even subclinical depression (ie, persistent depressive symptoms that fall short of the criteria for diagnosing clinical depression) appears to be associated with diminished functioning and increased medical morbidity.[13] The correlation has been shown across several populations including Mexican Americans,[4] African Americans,[5] and children.[14]

E The results of one study of people with diabetes showed that depressive affect—and, to a lesser extent, anxiety—was associated with lower, self-reported quality of life, independent of the level of physical illness.[15]

5 Depression remains unrecognized and untreated in a majority of cases despite its specific relevance to diabetes.[6]

A Reasons for underdiagnosis of depression in people with diabetes include the perception that depression in the medically ill is secondary to the medical condition and thus not of independent importance, labeling depressed patients as "noncompliant," and concerns about the accuracy of the diagnosis of depression in this patient population.

B Some of the symptoms of depression such as fatigue or changes in libido, appetite, and weight are also symptoms of hyperglycemia.[11]

C Current diagnostic approaches are relatively sensitive for detecting depression in a person with diabetes. The use of tools described in Chapter 2, Psychosocial Assessment, in Diabetes Education and Program Management, can help the educator screen patients who may be depressed.

D The role of the educator is to refer the patient to a mental health specialist for formal diagnosis and treatment when symptom criteria indicate the presence of depression. With the medications and counseling interventions that are available, depression and other mood disorders can be treated successfully with referral to a qualified provider.

6 Depression in diabetes is responsive to psychotherapy.

  A *Cognitive-behavioral therapy* (CBT)[16] is effective in the treatment of depression in diabetes.[17-19]
  - CBT is based on the observation that depressed people tend to think in negative, stereotypical ways ("Nobody likes me, I'm a failure").
  - CBT involves a structured program of cognitive modification or reframing and behavioral changes (identifying negative, self-defeating thoughts and actions and replacing them with more accurate and constructive thoughts and behaviors).
  - In one study of people with diabetes treated with CBT, the presence of complications and the lack of adequate blood monitoring were significant independent predictors of diminished response to this treatment mode.[19]

  B *Interpersonal therapy* (IPT)[20] is a proven treatment for depression in people who have no other medical conditions; the use of this psychotherapeutic approach for people with diabetes has not been studied extensively.
  - According to the model from which interpersonal therapy is derived, stressful and conflicted relationships cause, maintain, and exacerbate depression. IPT helps patients develop and refine specific skills in communication and social interaction that help to relieve depression.
  - When anxiety coexists with depression, the outcome of IPT for depression may be affected adversely.[21]

  C Both IPT and CBT help patients build skills for coping with stressful life circumstances, which may provide more lasting relief from depression than antidepressant medications. This benefit is significant given the recurrent nature of depression in diabetes and the need for ongoing coping skills.[6]

7 Depression in diabetes is responsive to treatment with antidepressant medication.[22]

  A Lustman and colleagues[23] demonstrated that depression in diabetes could be treated successfully with antidepressant medication.
  - In a placebo-controlled trial with diabetes patients, 60% of those treated for 8 weeks with nortriptyline (a member of the tricyclic class of antidepressants) had a complete remission of their depression, while only 35% of those treated with a placebo were free of depression at the end of the study.

- Another important finding from this study was that a complete remission of depression among study participants was associated with a 0.8% to 1.2% reduction in glycosylated hemoglobin levels over the 8-week study period. Sustained reductions in glycosylated hemoglobin of this magnitude could provide the additional benefit of slowing the progression of microvascular complications such as retinopathy by as much as one third.

B Fluoxetine [Prozac®], a selective serotonin reuptake inhibitor (SSRI), has been shown to effectively reduce the severity of depression in patients with diabetes. In a randomized placebo-controlled double-blind trial,[23] patients, who received a daily dose of fluoxetine over 8 weeks, had a significantly greater reduction in symptoms of depression than those who received the placebo. In addition, treatment with the drug over the 8 weeks produced a trend toward better glycemic control.

C Tricyclic antidepressants (amitriptyline [Elavil®], desipramine [Norpramin®], imipramine [Tofranil®], and nortriptyline [Pamelor®]) have some side effects that are especially problematic for people who have diabetes, including dry mouth, sedation, increased appetite, and weight gain. Although nortriptyline has been effective in reducing depression symptoms, it has had significant adverse effects on glycemic control.[23]

D The SSRIs seem to be less sedating and do not lead to weight gain in most people. In fact, there is some evidence that SSRIs may actually decrease appetite in some people. Drugs in this class include fluoxetine (Prozac®), paroxetine (Paxil™), citalopram (Celexa®), fluvoxamine (Luvox®), and sertraline (Zoloft™). Unfortunately, SSRIs are more likely to cause agitation; sexual problems such as anorgasmia, decreased libido, and delayed ejaculation; and gastrointestinal distress than tricyclic antidepressants.

E In a study of Native Americans, who are at high risk of depression, SSRIs have been shown to have significant advantages with more favorable side effect outcomes for the treatment of depressed diabetic patients.[24]

F Venlafaxine (Effexor®) mirtazapine (Remeron®), bupropion (Wellbutrin®), and nefazodone (Serzone®) are other antidepressants which came out after the SSRIs. The medications may be appropriate for some patients who do not respond to SSRIs or who have difficulty tolerating some side effects of the SSRIs such as agitation.

8 Choosing and using an antidepressant medication requires experience with these medications and close monitoring of the individual patient.

A All the medications described have similar antidepressant effects when used in their therapeutic dosage range.
- Depression is relieved in 50% to 60% of patients who complete 8 to 16 weeks of treatment.
- Another 30% of those who do not respond to the initial medication will improve when they change to a second antidepressant.

B Some improvement in mood is often seen within the first 2 to 3 weeks of treatment. Medication dosage changes should not be made for 4 to 6 weeks because many patients respond to these agents slowly and incrementally.

C Unfortunately, many patients experience the side effects of antidepressant agents before they experience any beneficial effects. Side effects tend to diminish over time.

D Potential drug interactions must also be considered when choosing antidepressant medications.

E The effectiveness of all psychotropic (eg, antidepressant, antianxiety) medications is an individual matter. Different medications, even those closely related chemically, affect individuals differently.

F Selection of an antidepressant agent for a given patient is based on such factors as presenting symptoms, coexisting medical conditions, drug interactions, side effects, and cost. SSRIs are generally much more expensive than tricyclic antidepressants.

G Maintenance treatment with antidepressants, which is an increasingly common practice among psychiatrists caring for the depressed population at large, may also improve the prognosis for patients with diabetes. The only indications for stopping an antidepressant medication within the first 6 months of treatment are the absence of a therapeutic effect or severe side effects.

H To maximize the likelihood of selecting an effective depression treatment for a given patient, the patient's specific problems including initial presentation of symptoms and other medical conditions need to be matched to the known benefits of the treatments under consideration. The potential benefits of effective depression management for people with diabetes are shown in Table 6.2.

9 Many patients report flu-like symptoms including headache and fever when they discontinue treatment with any of the SSRIs or venlafaxine or nefazodone. Tapering medications, especially those with the shortest half-life such as paroxetine and venlafaxine, may help to reduce these symptoms.

Table 6.2. Potential Benefits of Effective Depression Management in diabetes

1 Improved mood
2 Improved diabetes self-care
3 Improved functioning in work, social, and family realms
4 Improved glycemic control
5 Restoration of normal sleep and eating patterns
6 Decreased somatic preoccupation
7 Pain relief and increased pain tolerance
8 Enhanced sexual functioning

Bipolar Disorders

1 This group of clinical mood disorders includes Manic, Hypomanic, Mixed, or Major Depressive Episodes.

A A *Manic Episode* involves a period of abnormally and persistently elevated or irritable mood, lasting at least 1 week (or any duration if hospitalization is necessary). The disturbed mood is accompanied by at least 3 other symptoms including inflated self-esteem, significant decrease in the need to sleep, unusual talkativeness, distractibility, or subjective experience that thoughts are racing. The mood disturbance is sufficiently severe to cause marked impairment in functioning or to necessitate hospitalization.

B A *Hypomanic Episode* is a period of persistently elevated or irritable mood, lasting throughout at least 4 days, that is clearly different from the usual nondepressed mood. This mood is accompanied by at least 3 symptoms from a list that includes inflated self-esteem, significant decrease in the need to sleep, unusual talkativeness, distractibility, or subjective experience that thoughts are racing. Unlike manic behavior, hypomania is not severe enough to cause marked impairment in functioning or to necessitate hospitalization.

C For a *Mixed Episode*, the criteria are met for both a manic episode and for a major depressive episode nearly every day during at least a 1-week period. The mood disturbance is sufficiently severe to cause marked impairment in functioning or to necessitate hospitalization.

D A *Major Depressive Episode* involves a cluster of depressive symptoms lasting at least 2 weeks and representing a change from previous functioning, a change that signifies substantial distress or impairment in social, occupational, or other important areas of functioning.

2 Although bipolar disorders can be very debilitating, they respond well to medication, so patients with these problems should be referred to a psychiatrist.

Anxiety Disorder

1 See Table 6.3 for symptoms of clinical anxiety disorder. Signs and symptoms of anxiety disorder are also described in more detail in Chapter 2, Psychosocial Assessment. DSM-IV[1] provides extensive information about the attributes of anxiety. Because anxiety and stress are often confused with one another, it is important to understand that while the symptoms of both states are similar, the source of anxiety is uncontrollable worry associated with an unidentifiable stimulus that is usually unreal or imagined whereas the source of stress is an identifiable, adverse stimulus.

Table 6.3. Symptoms of Clinical Anxiety Disorder

1 Restlessness or feeling keyed-up or on-edge
2 Being easily fatigued
3 Difficulty concentrating or mind going blank
4 Irritability
5 Muscle tension
6 Sleep disturbance (difficulty falling or staying asleep, or restless, unsatisfying sleep)

2 Anxiety disorder appears to be more prevalent among people with diabetes than in the general population.
  A Little is known about the rate of anxiety disorder among people with diabetes. However, the results from one study[3] suggest that people who have diabetes may suffer from anxiety disorder as frequently as from depression and at much higher rates than people who do not have diabetes.

B Prevalence studies[25,26] using structured diagnostic interviews have reported an increased incidence of anxiety disorder, especially Generalized Anxiety Disorder and Specific Phobia (formerly Simple Phobia), in people with diabetes.

3 Anxiety disorder may be more prevalent among people with diabetes because of worries about hypoglycemia and severe complications common to the disease.
  A *Generalized Anxiety Disorder* is characterized by excessive and uncontrollable anxiety and worry (apprehensive expectation), occurring more days than not for a period of at least 6 months, about a number of events or activities. In addition, the intensity, duration, or frequency of the anxiety and worry is far out of proportion to the actual situation. The worrisome thoughts interfere with attention to tasks at hand and are difficult to stop.[1]
  B People with diabetes often live with sources and levels of fear greater than those most people experience.
  C People with diabetes may experience *Specific Phobia*, a marked and persistent fear that is excessive or unreasonable and that is cued by the presence or anticipation of a specific object or situation, such as the needle used to inject insulin.
  - In a group of insulin-treated patients attending a diabetes clinic, 14% reported that injections had been avoided because of anxiety and 42% reported concern at having to inject more frequently. In this study, high injection anxiety was associated with high levels of general anxiety.[27]
  - In a study of diabetes-induced visual impairment, significantly more blind than sighted subjects manifested clinical levels of anxiety and phobic anxiety.[28]
  - Fear of hypoglycemia, complications, and the effects of diabetes on day-to-day life are some of the more common fears reported by people who have diabetes.[28,29] The extent and intensity of symptoms that result from these fears would determine if the level of disturbance warrants a diagnosis of Anxiety Disorder or Adjustment Disorder or a subclinical syndrome (features of a mental disorder that do not meet the criteria for a clinical diagnosis).
  D Anxiety affects quality of life[15] and may affect metabolic control indirectly by interfering with diabetes self-care.
  E In one study,[3] the only diabetes-related factor found to be associated with increased risk for symptoms of anxiety disorder was the presence of two or more complications. Type of diabetes, duration of diabetes, and glycosylated hemoglobin level were not associated with an increased risk for anxiety symptomatology.
  F Pregnant women with preexisting diabetes were found to manifest more anxiety and hostility in comparison to nondiabetic women; however, no association was found between emotional state and glycemic control.[30]

4 Anxiety disorder, like depression, remains largely undiagnosed and untreated in patients with diabetes.
  A Difficulty in distinguishing symptoms of anxiety or phobia from those of hypoglycemia might delay or prevent the delivery of psychological interventions warranted in the presence of anxiety or phobia.[31]
  B The role of the educator is to refer the patient to a mental health specialist for formal diagnosis and treatment when symptom criteria indicate the presence of an anxiety disorder. With the medications and counseling interventions that are available, an anxiety disorder can be treated successfully with referral to a qualified provider.

5 Anxiety disorder in people with diabetes is probably responsive to treatment with psychopharmacological agents based on studies of people who do not have diabetes. Unfortunately, very little information is available on the use of these drugs in people with diabetes.
   A Lustman[32] reported improved glycemic control in patients treated with alprazolam (Xanax®), a benzodiazepine, regardless of whether they had a formal diagnosis of anxiety disorder.
   B Treatment with fludiazepam (Erispan), a benzodiazepine, resulted in decreased anxiety ratings as well as an increase in high-density lipoproteins in a small group of patients with type 2 diabetes.[33]

6 Commonly prescribed anxiolytics (antianxiety agents) include benzodiazepines such as alprazolam (Xanax®), lorazepam (Ativan®), oxazepam (Serax®), and clorazepate (Tranxene®). Buspirone (BuSpar®), which is not a benzodiazepine, is also sometimes prescribed for the treatment of anxiety. The antidepressants, paroxetine (Paxil™) and sertraline (Zoloft™) are often prescribed for anxiety.

7 There is little research to indicate which anxiolytic agent is best for people with diabetes.
   A The possibility of oversedation, its effects on self-care, and potential for addiction need to be considered when prescribing any benzodiazepine. Buspirone is associated with minimal sedative and cognitive effects. Its potential for addiction is unknown.[34]
   B Medications with short half-lives such as alprazolam and lorazepam may be the best choices for patients who have renal impairment.

8 The potential benefits of effective anxiety management for people with diabetes are similar to the benefits noted for the effective management of depression.

9 *Obsessive-Compulsive Disorder* is an anxiety disorder characterized by obsessions (recurrent and persistent thoughts, impulses, or images that are intrusive and inappropriate) or compulsions (repetitive behaviors or mental acts that the person feels driven to perform in response to an obsession, or according to rules that must be applied rigidly) that are severe enough to be time consuming or cause marked distress or significant impairment.

Stress and Related Disorders

1 Signs and symptoms of stress are described in Chapter 2, Psychosocial Assessment, in Diabetes Education and Program Management. DSM-IV[1] provides comprehensive information about Adjustment Disorders, which are specific diagnoses associated with the experience of debilitating stress.

2 There is considerable overlap among anxiety, adjustment disorders, and their corresponding subclinical syndromes. Generally, *anxiety* is associated with excessive apprehensions and worries about a number of anticipated events or activities (eg, worries about developing complications of diabetes) and *stress* is associated with an identifiable stressor or stressors (eg, the actual onset of symptoms of kidney failure).

3 The reaction to stress can be emotional, physiological, and behavioral and may lead to deterioration of glycemic control and general well-being in at least 2 ways.
   A Stress has a direct effect on the neuroendocrine system.
   - In the fight-or-flight mode, the liver produces glucose that is likely to elevate blood glucose levels.
   - In this mode, elevations of blood pressure and heart rate damage the elasticity of blood vessels.

   B Stress can impair self-care behavior and health.
   - In the fight-or-flight mode, the cortex secretes cortisol, which over time can impair cognitive ability and increase fatigue, anger, and depression.
   - In this mode, immune system functioning is diminished, and repeated suppression may ultimately weaken resistance to infection.

4 There are numerous potential stressors in dealing with diabetes: the vigilance required for self-care, food restrictions, complications, the anticipation of complications, the risk and effects of hypoglycemia, having to take insulin injections, a work situation not compatible with effective self-care, negative attitudes of others, lack of support, and the cost of diabetes care.

5 The effects of stress on glycemia in people with diabetes has been the subject of numerous studies.[35-38]
   A The results of research have been contradictory, with some studies reporting hypoglycemic responses and others reporting hyperglycemic responses to stress.[39]
   B Significant evidence of the influence of stress on metabolic control in patients with type 2 diabetes but not in those with type 1 diabetes was noted by Surwit et al.[39]
   - Alterations in sympathetic nervous system activity unique to type 2 diabetes may explain this difference.
   - One study of patients with type 2 diabetes suggested that failure to adhere to medical regimes was a function of stress (a syndrome of chronic and transient stressors.[38]

   C A study of adults with type 1 diabetes indicated that patients whose control deteriorated over time or who remained in poor glycemic control were significantly more likely to report severe personal stressors in the month before A1C measurement compared with subjects who were in fair control or who had improved control. Examples of severe personal stressors included a life event that posed a marked or moderate threat and interpersonal conflict.[40]

6 One of the *Adjustment Disorders*, a class of mental problems defined in DSM-IV,[1] may be a suitable diagnosis for symptoms of stress.
   A The criteria for the diagnosis of an adjustment disorder are described in Table 6.4.
   B There are various subtypes of Adjustment Disorder, each one characterizing predominant symptoms—eg, Adjustment Disorder With Depressed Mood, With Anxiety, With Mixed Anxiety and Depressed Mood, With Disturbance of Conduct.

7 Adjustment disorder and stress in general in some people with diabetes may be responsive to psychotherapy and related treatments such as relaxation training and stress management.

A Improved glucose tolerance and reduced long-term hyperglycemia were reported in studies of people with type 2 diabetes after biofeedback-assisted relaxation training (BART).[41]

B The effectiveness of BART for those with type 1 diabetes is less clear-cut, although some studies have reported positive findings.[42]
- One study of patients with type 1 diabetes indicated that mood may have a contrary impact on the response to BART. Significant correlations were found between high scores on inventories measuring depression, anxiety, and hassles intensity and higher blood glucose levels and smaller changes in blood glucose as a result of BART treatment.[43]

Table 6.4. Criteria for Adjustment Disorder

1 Development of emotional or behavioral symptoms in response to an identifiable stressor(s) occurring within 3 months of the onset of the stressor(s).

2 Symptoms or behaviors are clinically significant as evidenced by either
- marked distress that is in excess of what would be expected from exposure to the stressor
- significant impairment in social or occupational (academic) functioning.

3 The disturbance does not meet the criteria either for another disorder or bereavement.

4 Once the stressor (or its consequences) has terminated, the symptoms do not persist for more than an additional 6 months.

---

8 Diabetes self-management and coping skills may eliminate a stressor common to diabetes or reduce its impact (see Chapter 3, Behavior Change, in Diabetes Education and Program Management).

A The potential benefits of effective stress management for people with diabetes include improved glycemic control (both directly and indirectly as a result of improved self-care), improved emotional well-being, and improved quality of life.

B Some people with diabetes may need more intensive treatment, such as psychotherapy and related treatments that have been described for anxiety disorders.

Eating Disorders

1 See Table 6.5 for signs of an eating disorder. Signs and symptoms of eating disorders and tools for identifying patients who may be suffering from eating disorders are described in more detail in Chapter 2, Psychosocial Assessment, in Diabetes Education and Program Management. DSM-IV[1] provides extensive information about the attributes of eating disorders.

2 Eating disorders appear to be more common in people who have diabetes than in the general population.

A The problem of eating disorders in people with diabetes has received increased attention in the past decade.

B There are 2 primary types of eating disorders: anorexia nervosa and bulimia nervosa. *Anorexia nervosa* involves a severe, self-imposed restriction of caloric intake often combined with extremely high levels of exercise. *Bulimia nervosa* involves binge eating followed by a purging, usually by means of vomiting or the use of diuretic medications or laxatives.
- In DSM-IV,[1] there is a third clinical diagnosis for disorders of eating that do not meet the criteria for anorexia or bulimia nervosa; it is titled Eating Disorder Not Otherwise Specified. For example, the person has recurrent episodes of binge eating in the absence of the regular use of inappropriate compensatory behaviors characteristic of Bulimia Nervosa. (This condition may be referred to as *binge eating disorder*.)

C It is difficult to estimate the actual prevalence of eating disorders in people with diabetes due to the problem of distinguishing between a normal (and even positive) focus on food and the body, which is necessary for diabetes management, and the abnormal concerns and behavior associated with an eating disorder. Some researchers[44] have suggested viewing this problem as an eating continuum with normal at one end, clinical eating disorders at the other end, and subclinical aspects at points in between.

D Research in the field offers widely varying estimates of the prevalence of eating disorders in people with diabetes. A meta-analysis of existing data suggests a prevalence of eating disorders in those with diabetes of 1 to 1.5 times that found in the general population, given the same gender and similar age and educational level.[45]

E All studies[46] have not indicated that people with diabetes are at higher risk for eating disorders, but some studies[47,48] do suggest that adolescents and young women with diabetes have an increased risk, especially for bulimia nervosa, which is more prevalent than anorexia nervosa.
- Aspects of type 1 diabetes, such as weight gain, dietary restraint and food diligence, may make young women with diabetes susceptible to developing a clinical or subclinical eating disorder,[49] which may explain, at least in part, why prevalence of a clinical or subclinical eating disorder in adolescent females with type 1 diabetes is almost twice the frequency of nondiabetic peers[50] and even higher compared to men with the same diagnosis.[51]

3 There are indications that eating disorders in patients with type 1 diabetes are in some ways similar to and in other ways different from these same disorders in those without diabetes.

A Hillard and Hillard[52] note many similarities in the eating-disordered behaviors and etiology of people with type 1 diabetes and people who do not have diabetes. These similarities include the type and symptoms of their eating disorder, underlying personality structure, family history of an eating disorder, and other psychiatric diseases.

B A unique and particularly troubling feature of eating-disordered behavior common to many young people with diabetes is insulin purging.[52] Recent research[53] suggests that between one third and one half of all young women with type 1 diabetes frequently take less insulin than they need for glycemic control as a means of controlling their weight.[54]

4 Eating disorders have especially devastating consequences for people with diabetes.

- **A** Eating-disordered behavior, including manipulation of insulin dosage to control weight,[55] can severely compromise diabetes self-care, glycemic control,[50] and medical management.
- **B** A relationship has been reported between eating problems (especially bulimia) and poor adherence to the nondiet aspects of the diabetes regimen,[56,57] poor glycemic control,[447,54] and complications.[48,58]
- **C** In a multicenter study, patients with an eating disorder manifested a greater psychopathology than patients without the disorder, but the presence of an eating disorder did not appear to have a specific effect on glycemic control.[59]
- **D** In a study of differences between bulimia nervosa (BN) and binge eating (BE) in females with type 1 diabetes, females with BN showed poorer glycemic control as well as significantly more severe depression, anxiety, a higher rate of co-occurring mental disorders, and poorer psychosocial functioning compared to those with BE.[60]
- **E** Even subclinical eating disorders can interfere with glycemic control.[61]
- **F** Insulin manipulation per se is associated with an increased risk for poor metabolic control[62] and microvascular complications.[53,58,63,64]

5 Eating disorders in people with diabetes are often unrecognized and untreated.
- **A** Differentiating between normal concerns with food and body image and pathological concerns can be difficult in people with diabetes.
- **B** Those suffering from eating disorders are often resistant to acknowledging the problem. Controlling eating feels crucially important for many of these patients. They are terrified at the prospect of giving up this control, which they feel they will be pressured to do if they acknowledge their eating disorder.
- **C** It is important for educators to be alert to signs that a patient may be suffering from an eating disorder (see Table 6.5), especially when the patient is a young woman.

6 Most patients with diabetes do not eat in a manner that maximizes their chances for normoglycemia. It can sometimes be difficult to draw clear lines between normal struggles to establish and maintain patterns of healthy eating, subclinical eating disorders such as binge eating and "food addiction," and clinical eating disorders such as anorexia and bulimia.

Table 6.5. Signs of an Eating Disorder in Patients With Diabetes

1. Frequent diabetic ketoacidosis (DKA)
2. Excessive exercise
3. Use of diet pills or laxatives to control weight
4. Anxiety about or avoidance of being weighed
5. Frequent and severe hypoglycemia
6. Binging with alcohol
7. Severe stress in the family
8. Frequent insulin omission

7 The techniques for facilitating behavior change described in Chapter 3, Behavior Change, in Diabetes Education and Program Management, are appropriate for working with patients who appear to have normal problems controlling their eating. These techniques may also be helpful for some people who have subclinical eating disorders.

8 Diabetes educators need to be familiar with strategies for primary prevention of eating disorders in female patients who have diabetes (see Table 6.6). These strategies may be effective in preventing clinical eating disorders and may also be helpful in identifying patients who require the services of a mental health specialist experienced in treating eating disorders.

Table 6.6. Strategies for Prevention of Eating Disorders in Young Women With Diabetes[44]

1 Addressing the drive for thinness and associated body dissatisfaction
2 De-emphasizing dieting
3 Counseling patients about the need to express negative feelings about diabetes management
4 Helping the patient who is experiencing conflict over normal developmental struggles
5 Addressing metabolic reactivity during adolescence
6 Involving the family

9 Ongoing consultation with a mental health professional familiar with eating disorders may help prevent subclinical eating disorders from becoming full-blown clinical disorders. Such a consultation relationship should be established whenever possible. When the mental health specialist is a part of the diabetes team, patients are more likely to accept referral for treatment of emotional problems before they become more severe.

10 Eating disorders may be responsive to psychotherapy and pharmacotherapy.
  A Recent literature[65] suggests that psychoeducation directed toward specific, culturally based cognitive distortions may be effective for individuals with mild to moderate eating disorders in the early stages.
  - Psychoeducational therapy is a highly structured treatment program in which a therapeutic setting and didactic instruction are used to help patients understand the nature, etiology, and complications of disordered eating behaviors.
  - The purpose of this intervention is to foster attitudinal and behavioral change in the patient.[66]
  B Interpersonal therapy (IPT) has been effective in treating bulimia nervosa when there has been a "goodness of fit" between the issues presented by a patient and the treatment model (ie, when problematic relationships are central to the disorder).[67] A detailed "interpersonal inventory" is developed to identify core interpersonal problems that become the focus of therapy as opposed to focusing on bulimic symptoms.

C Because many patients suffering from eating disorders are also depressed, treatment with any of the antidepressants discussed earlier in this chapter may be considered. Some antidepressants in the SSRI class may positively affect compulsive behavior, including eating-disordered behavior, as well as depression. Fluoxetine (Prozac®) has been used successfully for this purpose; other agents in the same class may provide similar benefits.

Other Mental Disorders

1 There are other disorders that have not been detailed here, including the personality disorders, schizophrenia, and other psychotic disorders. These are serious and complex conditions. Personality disorders often involve significant impairments in cognitive functioning, mood, and impulse control. Psychotic disorders may involve serious impairment: delusions or hallucinations, disorganized speech, and disorganized behavior. These may grossly interfere with the capacity to meet the ordinary demands of life.

2 Educators may not be able to make a differential diagnosis among these mental disorders, but they are likely to recognize the highly disturbed thinking and behavior that is common with these disorders. Patients who appear to suffer from a serious mental disturbance should be referred to an appropriate mental health professional.

Psychopathology That Presents as a Medical Crisis

1 In many cases a medical crisis may be the first sign that a patient is suffering from a psychiatric disorder. Examples of such medical crises are recurrent diabetic ketoacidosis; frequent, severe hypoglycemic and hyperglycemic episodes (sometimes called brittle diabetes); and severe disruption of self-care activities, especially insulin administration.

2 These destructive behaviors frequently coincide with severe psychological disturbance, including individual psychopathology,[68] family dysfunction,[69] or both.[70]

3 These psychological disturbances have been effectively treated by intensive individual therapy[71] and family therapy, often conducted at least partly in residential or inpatient settings.

Psychological Disorders as Sequelae of Long-Term Diabetes Complications

1 Developing any of the chronic complications of diabetes could be considered an emotional crisis. However, there is little research to clarify the degree to which any of these complications contribute to psychological distress.

2 Only 2 diabetes-related complications have been studied in terms of their association with psychological distress: sexual dysfunction and visual impairment.
  A The sexual dysfunction most often associated with diabetes is Male Erectile Disorder.
   • Erectile dysfunction in a man with diabetes is almost invariably the result of psychological and organic factors.[72]

- Sexual dysfunction is generally developed and maintained by a reciprocal process in which organic problems lead to psychological distress and the distress in turn heightens the organic problems.

B The study of sexual problems in women with diabetes is a recent undertaking.
- In one of the few substantial investigations in this area, Schreiner-Engel et al[73] found that women with type 2 diabetes reported significantly more sexual problems and less sexual satisfaction than nondiabetic control subjects. The authors speculate that late-onset diabetes may distort a woman's sexual body image, signalling the end of her sexual attractiveness and intensifying concerns about earlier aging.
- Women with type 1 diabetes in the same study did not differ from controls in terms of sexual problems and satisfaction.

C Only a few reports describe psychological interventions for men with diabetes who have sexual problems, and none have been described for women.

D There is some evidence that psychological distress increases dramatically during the first 2 years after diagnosis with proliferative diabetic retinopathy,[74] regardless of the severity of the visual impairment.
- Bernbaum et al[75] reported that those with fluctuating visual impairment actually reported lower levels of psychological well-being than people with more severe yet stable impairment.
- In another study,[76] visually impaired people with diabetes participated in a 36-session self-care training program conducted over a 12-week period. The program staff included a psychologist, and psychosocial support groups and individual counseling were available to participants. At the end of the program participants were in better glycemic control and less depressed.

3 Many people may suffer psychological distress following the onset of a diabetes-related complication and the cumulative impact of several complications may be especially severe. One study[3] revealed that both depression and anxiety symptomatology were dramatically elevated in those with more than 2 diabetes-related complications.

Key Educational Considerations

1 Understanding the relationship between psychological disorders and diabetes is critical for the diabetes educator because of the profound impact of these disorders on the education and treatment process and on a person's capacity to live well with diabetes.

2 To effectively address psychological disorders, apply the following key considerations:

A People with diabetes may suffer disproportionately from certain psychological disorders, and the course and consequences of these disorders may also be more severe.

B It is important for educators to know the signs and symptoms of depression, anxiety disorders, specific phobia, adjustment disorders, and eating disorders and be able to recognize markers for these disorders in their patients. When a psychological disorder is suspected, the educator can refer to Chapter 2, Psychosocial Assessment, in Diabetes Education and Program Management, for ways to draw a more decisive conclusion. If the educator feels the patient may be suffering from a mental disorder at the clinical level, referral to a mental health specialist for a definitive diagnosis and treatment is appropriate.

C It is also important for educators to recognize subclinical syndromes, including mild symptoms of depression, anxiety, or stress that may manifest in errant behaviors that have adverse effects on self-care, metabolic control, and quality of life for people with diabetes.

D Subclinical syndromes can often be effectively dealt with by educators, using some of the techniques described in Chapter 3, Behavior Change, in Diabetes Education and Program Management.

E Mental health professionals are invaluable resources for consultation concerning patients with subclinical syndromes and for comprehensive assessment and treatment of patients who may be suffering from clinical disorders.

F Effective psychotherapeutic, psychoeducational, and pharmacological approaches have been identified for depression, anxiety disorders, adjustment disorders, and eating disorders. Educators need to be familiar with these approaches and have resources available for the provision of these treatments.

G A medical crisis (eg, ketoacidosis), deviant self-care behavior (eg, avoiding insulin injections), or poor metabolic control (eg, recurrent hypoglycemia) may indicate the presence of a psychological disorder.

H People with diabetes who are enduring serious, long-term complications, such as sexual dysfunction, kidney failure, or visual impairment, may develop a psychological disorder.

Self-Review Questions

1 What is the difference between a clinical disorder and subclinical syndrome?
2 What are some effective approaches for helping people with subclinical psychological disorders?
3 Approximately what percentage of people with diabetes suffer from clinical depression?
4 Why is the course of depression more severe for a person with diabetes?
5 Why are the effects of depression especially devastating for a person with diabetes?
6 What forms of psychotherapy are good choices for treating depression in a person with diabetes?
7 What are some advantages of SSRI antidepressants as compared with tricyclic antidepressants for people with diabetes?
8 What are the differences between an anxiety disorder, a specific phobia, and an adjustment disorder?
9 What distinguishes anxiety from stress?
10 In what ways might anxiety or stress affect diabetes control?
11 What are the benefits of biofeedback-assisted relaxation training?
12 Why are eating disorders in people with diabetes often unrecognized and untreated?
13 What approaches may be effective for primary prevention of eating disorders in a person with diabetes?
14 What medical crises may indicate an underlying psychological disorder?
15 What is the role of the mental health specialist in caring for patients with diabetes?

Learning Assessment: Case Study 1

SF is a 64-year-old man whose type 2 diabetes was diagnosed 12 years ago. He had signs of background retinopathy at that time. SF did well taking oral medication for his diabetes and handling self-care tasks for the first 9 years after diagnosis. His glycemic control during that period was good, and his retinopathy was stable. Three years ago SF's wife died suddenly of a heart attack, and within the last 18 months SF began to experience painful symptoms of neuropathy. In the past year microalbumin has begun to appear in his urine and he has shown signs of proliferative retinopathy. SF's glycemic control has steadily worsened as well, to the point that an appointment was scheduled with him to discuss the possibility of initiating insulin therapy.

During this appointment SF appears very sad and questions directed to him reveal that he has been sleeping poorly and that he feels fatigued "all the time." SF says that he has lost touch with most of his former friends because he "doesn't get the pleasure from their company that he used to," and adds that he "is no fun to be around." When asked specifically about the prospect of taking insulin, SF says that while he hates the idea of shots, he feels he's "getting what he deserves," for failing to effectively control his diabetes. He adds, "I'm not much good to anyone these days, including myself."

Questions for Discussion

1 What psychological disorder is likely affecting SF?
2 Why is it hard to be sure SF is suffering from this disorder?
3 What further information would be helpful in assessing SF's condition?
4 What treatments might be appropriate for SF?
5 What do you think about SF beginning to take insulin at this time?

Discussion

1 SF appears to be depressed. He is sad and complains of sleep disturbance and fatigue. In addition, he says he has lost interest in activities he used to enjoy, and he is feeling worthless and guilty.
   A He seems to meet the diagnostic criteria for clinical depression. He has also experienced the loss of his wife and the onset of several diabetes-related complications.
   B Research shows that developing multiple complications dramatically increases a person's risk for depression.

2 While the diagnosis of depression seems reasonable in this case, SF's chronic hyperglycemia is another possible explanation for some of his symptoms.

3 To clarify what is actually going on, SF can be asked about any changes in appetite, problems in concentration, and thoughts of death or suicide. In addition, a verbal screening can be complemented by using an instrument designed to assess depression (see Chapter 2, Psychosocial Assessment, in Diabetes Education and Program Management).

4 If the diagnosis of depression is not clear-cut, a referral to a mental health professional for a comprehensive assessment and definitive diagnosis is appropriate. Treatment options for depression include interpersonal or cognitive-behavioral psychotherapy and/or pharmacotherapy.

5 Initiating insulin therapy might not be indicated for SF at this time, as major treatment changes are generally not advisable for a depressed patient because such

patients often feel overwhelmed by the prospect of making changes. One exception may be the patient who is suffering from severe hyperglycemia.

Learning Assessment: Case Study 2

LP, a single parent of 3 teenage children, was diagnosed with type 2 diabetes 6 months ago at the age of 46. She had a very emotional reaction to the diagnosis (initially crying uncontrollably and so unnerved that the physician had to summon her son to come and take her home). Her immediate association with having diabetes was growing up in a family in which several members had suffered serious consequences of the disease.

Because her mother had diabetes and LP had actively supported her efforts at diabetes care, LP had adequate knowledge of diabetes-specific self-care skills. However, in the 6 months since the diagnosis, her control has been poor. She has had several frightening incidents of hypoglycemia, one requiring her daughter to summon paramedics. In addition, she has been troubled by palpitations, trembling, muscle tension, and a pervasive sense of uneasiness.

As LP spoke with the diabetes educator, it was apparent to the educator that LP had a morbid outlook on her health and general well-being. She said that her situation was hopeless and that she had no one to turn to for support. In addition, she was distressed about her job. She had prided herself in being efficient and reliable, but her performance had slipped considerably. LP was making a lot of errors, and her supervisor had warned her that it could not continue. With 3 children to support, the possibility of losing her job has been very worrisome. Feeling very nervous about making mistakes, she has been checking her work repeatedly, which has the undesirable effect of reducing her productivity. Asked about the incidents of hypoglycemia, she said that the pressures of work and other responsibilities make it difficult for her to eat appropriately; when she isn't working she tends to sleep too much.

Questions for Discussion
1 What clinical disorder is likely affecting LP?
2 What stressors are impacting on LP?
3 What are the symptoms of stress being manifested?
4 What affective condition is complicating LP's struggle with adapting to diabetes?
5 Why is it hard to be sure LP is suffering from this disorder?
6 What further information would be helpful in assessing LP's condition?
7 What treatment interventions might be appropriate for LP?

Discussion
1 The diagnosis of diabetes has triggered several stressors for LP, and she is experiencing a significant amount of emotional stress and symptoms of depression. In addition to impairing her ability to manage her diabetes, the symptoms are interfering with her performance at work. Her condition is consistent with a diagnosis of Adjustment Disorder With Depressed Mood. If LP was enduring the same symptoms but functioning satisfactorily with regard to work and glycemic control, then her condition would be considered subclinical.

2 The stressors that can be attributed to the diagnosis of an Adjustment Disorder include the diagnosis of a disease that she believes is so sinister, frightening episodes of hypoglycemia, a decline in work performance, and a concomitant threat to job security.

3 LP is experiencing a complex of stress symptoms including palpitations, trembling, muscle tension, and a pervasive sense of uneasiness. Also, her fear is manifesting in compulsive checking of her work.

4 LP is experiencing symptoms of depression as indicated by her morbid outlook for the future, her expression of hopelessness, and her tendency to sleep excessively.

5 While the diagnosis of Adjustment Disorder With Depressed Mood seems reasonable in this case, LP has frequent episodes of low glucose levels, and some of the symptoms noted in 3 above are also common to hypoglycemia.

6 Because it is possible that LP is suffering from a depressive disorder, a more thorough assessment of her level of depression is indicated. Also, it would be useful to more fully understand the extent of her stress. Techniques and instruments for assessing levels of stress and depression can be found in Chapter 2, Psychosocial Assessment.

7 Self-management and coping skills training might be adequate for empowering LP to deal effectively with the stressors and consequent adjustment disorder that are troubling her. With regard to depression, if assessment of her affective state indicates that the problem is situational (ie, a reaction to current circumstances), it may be practical to delay action until the patient has reduced some of the stress, as the depression may remit when she is less stressed and the diabetes is in better control. However, if the depression is endogenous (trait-bound as opposed to state-bound) or if the depression is at a clinical level, do not assume that an improvement in metabolic control will eliminate the depression. In these circumstances, antidepressant medication and/or cognitive-behavioral psychotherapy are indicated.

Learning Assessment: Case Study 3

QT is a young woman, 15 years old. Type 1 diabetes was diagnosed when she was 6. Her family has always been actively involved in her diabetes management, and although QT herself is knowledgeable, she has been open to their assistance. She maintained excellent glycemic control until about a year ago. Since then her glycosylated hemoglobin level has risen dramatically, and she has had to go to the emergency room twice for DKA.

During her last 2 appointments with the diabetes educator, QT has been much less communicative, offering little explanation for her worsened glycemic control and associated medical crises. She says she "doesn't really know what's going on," adding, "I guess it's just harder now for me to do everything right with all my activities and such." When asked specifically about the fact that her weight has decreased by 18 lb (8.2 kg) over the past year, placing her weight at 85% of normal for her height, body frame, and age, QT responds, "Don't tell me I need to gain that weight back! Last year I was too fat to make the cheerleading squad, and now I feel like I have a real chance."

Questions for Discussion
1 What psychological disorder is likely affecting QT?
2 Why is it hard to be sure QT is suffering from this disorder?
3 What further information would be helpful in assessing QT's condition?
4 What treatments might be appropriate for QT?

Discussion
1 QT appears to be suffering from an eating disorder. She is a young woman whose glycemic control has worsened dramatically, leading to episodes of DKA and significant weight loss.
   - A Her weight is now 85% of normal for her height, body frame, and age, and she is adamantly opposed to regaining the weight she has lost.
   - B QT seems to meet some of the criteria for a clinical eating disorder.

2 There are a couple of reasons why it is difficult to be sure whether QT has an eating disorder.
   - A First, she is 15 years old, so the insulin resistance of puberty might account for some of her worsened glycemic control.
   - B Second, she is not forthcoming about her situation, so essential information is not immediately available. Although most young women who have eating disorders actively resist acknowledging their problem, the educator needs to ask QT about her exercise, missed menstrual periods, and eating behavior, especially any episodes of binge eating.

3 QT should be questioned about any occasions when she did not give herself a scheduled insulin injection or reduced the dose of insulin she administered. Keep in mind that even subclinical eating disorders may have devastating consequences.

4 If it is determined that QT has an eating disorder, then an ideal treatment would be participation in a structured program of psychoeducation to resolve behaviors associated with the disorder. Unfortunately, this option is not widely available.
   - A One possible alternative would be education and counseling that incorporates some elements of a structured psychoeducation program.
   - B Another alternative would be pharmacotherapy to assist the patient in overcoming behaviors associated with the disorder, especially if it is associated with underlying depression.

5 It is important to recognize that patients with established eating disorders are not likely to change their disorder behavior on an outpatient basis. They generally require hospitalization in an eating disorders program. However, if dramatic deterioration in glycemic control is identified by the educator before a full-blown eating disorder has developed, outpatient treatment may be effective.

References

1. Diagnostic and Statistical Manual of Mental Disorders, 4th ed. Washington: American Psychiatric Association; 1994.

2. Gavard JA, Lustman PJ, Clouse RE. Prevalence of depression in adults with diabetes: an epidemiological evaluation. Diabetes Care. 1993;16:1167-1178.

3. Peyrot M, Rubin RR. Levels and risks of depression and anxiety symptomatology among diabetic adults. Diabetes Care. 1997;20:585-590.

4. Black SA. Increased health burden associated with comorbid depression in older diabetic Mexican Americans. Diabetes Care. 1999;22:56-64.

5. Gary TL, Crum RM, Cooper-Patrick L, Ford D, Brancati FL. Depressive symptoms and metabolic control in African-Americans with type 2 diabetes. Diabetes Care. 2000;23:23-29.

6. Lustman PJ, Clouse RE, Alrakawi A, et al. Treatment of major depression in adults with diabetes: a primary care perspective. Clinical Diabetes. 1997;15:122-126.

7. Lustman PJ, Griffith LS, Clouse RE. Recognizing and managing depression in patients with diabetes. In: Anderson BJ, Rubin RR, eds. Practical Psychology for Diabetes Clinicians: How to Deal With the Key Behavioral Issues Faced by Patients and Healthcare Teams. Alexandria, Va: American Diabetes Association; 1996:143-154.

8. Lustman PJ, Griffith LS, Clouse RE. Depression in adults with diabetes: results of a 5-year follow-up study. Diabetes Care. 1988;11:605-612.

9. Talbot F, Nouwen A, Gingras J, Belanger A, Audet J. Relations of diabetes intrusiveness and personal control to symptoms of depression among adults with diabetes. Health Psychol. 1999;18:537-542.

10. Rubin RR, Peyrot M. Psychosocial problems in diabetes treatment: impediments to intensive self-care. Practical Diabetol. 1994;13(2):8-10,12-14.

11. Lustman PJ, Griffith LS, Clouse RE. Depression in adults with diabetes. Semin in Clin Neuropsychology. 1997;2:15-23.

12. de Groot M, Jacobson AM, Samson JA, Welch G. Glycemic control and major depression in patients with type 1 and type 2 diabetes mellitus. J Psychosom Res. 1999;46:425-435.

13. Frasure-Smith N, Lesperance F, Talajic M. Depression and 18-month prognosis after myocardial infarction. Circulation. 1995;91:999-1005.

14. Lernmark B, Persson B, Fisher L, Rydelius PA. Symptoms of depression are important to psychological adaptation and metabolic control in children with diabetes mellitus. Diabet Med. 1999;16:14-22.

15. Kohen D, Burgess AP, Catalan J, Lant A. The role of anxiety and depression in quality of life and symptom reporting in people with diabetes mellitus. Qual Life Res. 1998;7:197-204.

16. Rush AJ, Beck AT, Kovacs M, et al. Comparative efficacy of cognitive therapy and pharmacotherapy in the treatment of depressed outpatients. Cogn Ther Res. 1977;1:17-37.

17. Lustman PJ, Griffith LS, Clouse RE, Cryer PE. Efficacy of cognitive therapy for depression in NIDDM: results of a controlled clinical trial. Diabetes. 1997;46(suppl 1):13A.

18. Lustman PJ, Griffith LS, Freedman KE, Kissel SS, Clouse RE. Cognitive behavior therapy for depression in type 2 diabetes mellitus. A randomized controlled trial. Ann Intern Med. 1998;129:613-621.

19. Lustman PJ, Freedman KE, Griffith LS, Clouse RE. Predicting response to cognitive behavior therapy of depression in type 2 diabetes. Gen Hosp Psychiatry. 1998;20:302-306.

20 Frank E, Kupfer DJ, Wagner EF, et al. Efficacy of interpersonal psychotherapy as a maintenance treatment of recurrent depression. Arch Gen Psychiatry. 1991;48:1053-1059.

21 Feske U, Frank E, Kupfer DJ, Shear MK, Weaver E. Anxiety as a predictor of response to interpersonal psychotherapy for recurrent major depression: an exploratory investigation. Depress Anxiety. 1998;8:135-141.

22 Depression Guideline Panel. Depression in Primary Care, Vol 5: Detection, diagnosis and treatment. Rockville, Md: Department of Health and Human Services, 1993;AHCPR, publication 93-0550 edn.

23 Lustman PJ, Freedman KE, Griffith LS, Clouse RE. Fluoxetine for depression in diabetes: a randomized double-blind placebo-controlled trial. Diabetes Care. 2000;23:618-623.

24 Warnock JK, Mutzig EM. Diabetes mellitus and major depression: considerations for treatment of Native Americans. J Okla State Med Assoc. 1998;91:488-493.

25 Lustman PJ, Griffith LS, Clouse RE, Cryer PE. Psychiatric illness in diabetes mellitus: relationship to symptoms and glucose control. J Nerv Ment Dis. 1986;174:736-742.

26 Popkin MK, Callies AL, Lentz RD, et al. Prevalence of major depression, simple phobia, and other psychiatric disorders in patients with long-standing type 1 diabetes mellitus. Arch Gen Psychiatry. 1988;45:64-68.

27 Zambanini A, Newson RB, Maisey M, Feher MD. Injection related anxiety in insulin-treated diabetes. Diabetes Res Pract. 1999;46:239-246.

28 Cox DJ, Kiernan BD, Schroeder DB, Cowley M. Psychosocial sequelae of visual loss in diabetes. Diabetes Educ. 1998; 24:481-484.

29 Green L, Feher M, Catalan J. Fears and phobias with diabetes. Diabetes Metab Res Rev. 2000;16:287-293.

30 Langer N, Langer O. Pre-existing diabetics: relationship between glycemic control and emotional status in pregnancy. J Matern Fetal Med. 1998;7:257-263.

31 Green L, Feher M, Catalan J. Fears and phobias in people with diabetes. Diabetes Metab Res Rev. 2000;16:287-293.

32 Lustman PJ, Griffith LS, Clouse RE, et al. Effects of alprazolam on glucose regulation in diabetes. Results of double-blind, placebo-controlled trial. Diabetes Care. 1995;18:1133-1139.

33 Okada S, Ichiki K, Tanokuchi S, et al. Effects of an anxiolytic on lipid profile in non-insulin-dependent diabetes mellitus. J Int Med Res. 1994;22:338-342.

34 Pecknold JC, Matas M, Howarth BG, et al. Evaluation of buspirone as an anti-anxiety agent: buspirone and diazepam versus placebo. Can J Psychiatry. 1989;34:766-771.

35 Barglow P, Hatcher R, Edidin DV, Sloan-Rossiter D. Stress and metabolic control in diabetes: psychosomatic evidence and evaluation of methods. Psychosom Med. 1984;46:127-144.

36 Lloyd CE, Dyer PH, Lancashire RJ, Harris T, Daniels JE, Barnett AH. Association between stress and glycemic control in adults with type 1 (insulin-dependent) diabetes. Diabetes Care. 1999;22:1278-1283.

37 Peyrot M, McMurry JF, Kruger DF. A biopsychosocial model of glycemic control in diabetes: stress, coping and regimen adherence. J Health Soc Behav. 1999;40:141-158.

38 MacLean D, Lo R. The non-insulin-dependent diabetic: success and failure in compliance. Aust J Adv Nurs. 1998;15:33-42.

39 Surwit RS, Schneider MS, Feinglos MN. Stress and diabetes mellitus. Diabetes Care. 1992;15:1413-1422.

40 Lloyd CE, Dyer PH, Lancashire RJ, Harris T, Daniels JE, Barnett AH. Association between stress and glycemic control in adults with type 1 (insulin dependent) diabetes. Diabetes Care. 1999;22:1278-1283.

41. Surwit RS, Ross SL, McCaskill CC, et al. Does relaxation therapy add to conventional treatment of diabetes mellitus? Diabetes. 1989;38(suppl 1):9A.

42. McGrady A, Bailey BK, Good MP. Controlled study of biofeedback-assisted relaxation in type I diabetes. Diabetes Care. 1991;14:360-365.

43. McGrady A, Horner J. Role of mood in outcome of biofeedback assisted relaxation therapy in insulin dependent diabetes mellitus. Appl Psychophysiol Biofeedback. 1999;24:79-88.

44. Rapaport WS, LaGreca AM, Levine P. Preventing eating disorders in young women with type I diabetes. In: Anderson BJ, Rubin RR, eds. Practical Psychology for Diabetes Clinicians: How to Deal With the Key Behavioral Issues Faced by Patients and Healthcare Teams. Alexandria, Va: American Diabetes Association; 1996:133-142.

45. Hall RCW. Bulimia nervosa and diabetes mellitus. Semin in Clin Neuropsychiatry. 1997;2:24-30.

46. Fairburn CG, Peveler RC, Davies B, et al. Eating disorders in young adults with insulin-dependent diabetes mellitus: a controlled study. Br Med J. 1991;303:17-20.

47. Stancin T, Link DL, Reuter JM. Binge eating and purging in young women with IDDM. Diabetes Care. 1989;12:601-603.

48. Steel JM, Young RJ, Lloyd GG, Macintyre CC. Abnormal eating attitudes in young insulin-dependent diabetics. Br J Psychiatry. 1989;155:515-521.

49. Verrotti A, Catino M, De Luca FA, Morgese G, Chiarelli F. Eating disorders in adolescents with type 1 diabetes mellitus. Acta Diabetol. 1999;36:21-25.

50. Jones JM, Lawson ML, Daneman D, Olmsted MP, Rodin G. Eating disorders in adolescent females with and without type 1 diabetes: cross sectional study. BMJ. 2000;320:1563-1566.

51. Friedman S, Vila G, Timsit J, Boitard C, Mouren-Simeoni MC. Eating disorders and insulin-dependent diabetes mellitus (IDDM): relationships with glycaemic control and somatic complications. Acta Psychiatr Scand. 1998;97:206-212.

52. Hillard JR, Hillard PJ. Bulimia, anorexia, and diabetes: deadly combinations. Psychiat Clin North Am. 1984;7:367-379.

53. Rydall AC, Rodin GM, Olmsted MP, et al. Disordered eating behavior and microvascular complications in young women with insulin-dependent diabetes mellitus. N Engl J Med. 1997;336:1849-1854.

54. Polonsky WH, Anderson BJ, Lohrer PA, Aponte JE, Jacobson AM, Cole CF. Insulin omission in women with IDDM. Diabetes Care. 1994;17:1178-1185.

55. Herpertz S, Wagener R, Albus C, et al. Diabetes mellitus and eating disorders: a multicenter study on the comorbidity of the two diseases. J Psychosom Res. 1998;44:503-515.

56. LaGreca A, Schwartz L, Satin W, et al. Binge eating among women with IDDM: associations with weight dissatisfaction, adherence, and metabolic control. Diabetes. 1990;39(suppl 1):164A.

57. Pollock M, Kovacs M, Charron-Prochownik D. Eating disorders and maladaptive dietary/insulin management among youths with childhood-onset insulin-dependent diabetes mellitus. J Am Acad Child Adolesc Psychiatry 1995;34:291-296.

58. Rodin G, Rydall A, Olmsted M, et al. A four-year follow-up study of eating disorders and medical complications in young women with insulin dependent diabetes mellitus. Psychosomatic Med. 1994;56:179.

59. Herpertz S, Albus C, Lichtblau K, Kohle K, Mann K, Senf W. Relationship of weight and eating disorders in type 2 diabetic patients: a multicenter study. Int J Eat Disord. 2000;28:68-77.

60. Takii M, Komaki G, Uchigata Y, Maeda M, Omori Y, Kubo C. Differences between bulimia nervosa and binge-eating disorder in females with type 1 diabetes: the important role of insulin omission. J Psychosom Res. 1999;47:221-231.

61. Wing RR, Norwalk MP, Marcus MD, et al. Subclinical eating disorders and glycemic control in adolescents with type I diabetes. Diabetes Care. 1986;9:162-167.

62. LaGreca AM, Schwartz LT, Satin W. Eating patterns in young women with IDDM: another look (letter). Diabetes Care. 1987;10:659-660.

63. Biggs MM, Basco MR, Patterson G, Raskin P. Insulin withholding for weight control in women with diabetes. Diabetes Care. 1994;17:1186-1189.

64. Olmsted MP, Davis R, Garner DM, et al. Efficacy of a brief group psychoeducational intervention for bulimia nervosa. Behav Res Ther. 1991;29:71-83.

65. Davis R, Dearing S, Faulkner J, et al. The road to recovery: a manual for participants in the psychoeducation group for bulimia nervosa. In: Harper-Giuffre H, MacKenzie KR, eds. Washington, DC: American Psychiatric Press, 1992:281-341.

66. Gill G, Robinson M, Marrow J. Hypoglycaemic brittle diabetes successfully managed by social worker intervention. Diabetic Med. 1989;6:448-450.

67. Apple RF. Interpersonal therapy for bulimia nervosa. J Clin Psychol. 1999;55:715-725.

68. Boehnert CE, Popkin MK. Psychological issues in treatment of severely noncompliant diabetics. Psychosomatics. 1986;27:11-20.

69. Coyne JC, Anderson BJ. The "psychosomatic family" reconsidered: II. Recalling a defective model and looking ahead. J Marital Fam Ther. 1989;15:139-148.

70. Follansbee DJ, LaGreca AM, Citrin WS. Coping skills training for adolescents with diabetes. Diabetes. 1983;32(suppl 1):37A.

71. Moran G, Fonagy P, Kurtz A, et al. A controlled study of psychoanalytic treatment of brittle diabetes. J Am Acad Child Adolesc Psychiatry. 1991;30:926-935.

72. Schiavi PC, Hogan B. Sexual problems in diabetes mellitus: psychological aspects. Diabetes Care. 1979;2:9-17.

73. Schreiner-Engel P, Schiavi RC, Vietorisz D, et al. The differential impact of diabetes type on female sexuality. J Psychosom Res. 1987;31:23-33.

74. Wulsin LR, Jacobson AM, Rand LI. Psychosocial adjustment to advanced proliferative diabetic retinopathy. Diabetes Care. 1993;16:1061-1066.

75. Bernbaum M, Albert SG, Brusca SR, et al. A model clinical program for patients with diabetes and vision impairment. Diabetes Educ. 1989;15:325-330.

76. Bernbaum M, Albert SG, Duckro PN. Psychosocial profiles in patients with visual impairment due to diabetic retinopathy. Diabetes Care. 1988;11:551-557.

Suggested Readings

Anderson B, Funnell M. The Art of Empowerment. Alexandria, Va: American Diabetes Association; 2000.

Anderson B, Rubin RR, eds. Practical Psychology for Diabetes Clinicians: How to Deal With the Key Behavioral Issues Faced by Patients and Healthcare Teams. Alexandria, Va: American Diabetes Association; 1996.

Brackenridge BP, Rubin RR. Sweet Kids: How to Balance Diabetes Control and Good Nutrition With Family Peace. Alexandria, Va: American Diabetes Association; 1996.

Edelman SV. Taking control of your diabetes. Caddo, Okla: Professional Communications; 2000.

Guffey L, ed. American Diabetes Association Complete Guide to Diabetes, 2nd ed. Alexandria, Va: American Diabetes Association; 1999.

Lowe E, Arsham G. Diabetes: A Guide to Living Well. 3rd ed. Minneapolis, Minn: Chronimed; 1997.

Peyrot M, Rubin RR. Psychosocial aspects of diabetes care. In: Leslie D, Robbins D, eds. Diabetes: Clinical Science in Practice. Cambridge, Mass: Cambridge University Press; 1995:465-477.

Plotnick L, Henderson R. Clinical Management of the Child and Teenager With Diabetes. Baltimore, Md: Johns Hopkins University Press; 1998.

Rubin RR. Psychotherapy in diabetes mellitus. Semin in Clin Neuropsychiatry. 1997;2:72-81.

Rubin RR. Working with diabetic adolescents. In: Anderson BJ, Rubin RR, eds. Practical Psychology of Diabetes Clinicians: How to Deal With the Key Behavioral Issues Faced by Patients and Health Care Teams. Alexandria, Va: American Diabetes Association; 1996:13-22.

Rubin RR, Biermann J, Toohey B. Psyching Out Diabetes: A Positive Approach to Your Negative Emotions, 3rd ed. Los Angeles, Calif: Lowell House; 1999.

Rubin RR, Peyrot M. Emotional responses to diagnosis. In: Anderson BJ, Rubin RR, eds. Practical Psychology for Diabetes Clinicians: How to Deal With the Key Behavioral Issues Faced by Patients and Healthcare Teams. Alexandria, Va: American Diabetes Association; 1996:155-162.

Rubin RR, Peyrot M. Psychosocial problems and interventions in diabetes: a review of the literature. Diabetes Care. 1992;15:1640-1657.

Rubin RR, Peyrot M. Psychosocial problems. In: Levin ME, Pfeifer MA, eds. Diabetes Complications. Alexandria, Va: American Diabetes Association; 1998.

Saudek CD, Rubin RR, Shump C. The Johns Hopkins Guide to Diabetes: For Today and Tomorrow. Baltimore, Md: The Johns Hopkins University Press; 1997.

Learning Assessment: Post-Test Questions

Psychological Disorders 6

1. Research indicates that depression may be more severe in persons with diabetes due to:
   A Higher rates of substance abuse
   B Neuroendocrine effects caused by both diabetes and depression
   C Reluctance to seek mental health services
   D Lack of family support with diabetes care

2. Which of the following contributes to the underdiagnosis of depression in persons with diabetes:
   A The lack of reliable, valid tools for diagnosing depression in diabetes
   B The fact that depression manifests itself differently in persons with diabetes
   C The perception that depression is secondary to the medical condition itself
   D The lack of recognized primary–care based interventions for depression

3. Interpersonal therapy (IPT) seeks to help depressed individuals:
   A Sublimate feelings of anxiety and hostility
   B Cognitively reframe and restructure negative thoughts and actions
   C Avoid stressful and conflicted relationships
   D Improve skills in communication and social interaction

4. Which of the following actions taken by the diabetes educator exemplifies application of Cognitive Behavioral Therapy (CBT)?
   A Work with patients to build skills for more effective coping
   B Refer patients with depressive symptoms for treatment with antidepressants
   C Stress the relationship of glycemic control to moods
   D Educate the patient to the prevalence of depression in persons with diabetes

5. The advantages of the selective serotonin reuptake inhibitors (SSRIs) include:
   A Less gastrointestinal side effects
   B Less sedation
   C Less agitation
   D Less sexual dysfunction

6. One of the major barriers to effective treatment with antidepressants is:
   A The lack of sufficient choices among effective agents
   B Patient reluctance to accept medication therapy
   C The length of time between initiation of treatment and improvement in symptoms
   D The high degree of drug interactions with other medications

7. Anxiety disorders are characterized by:
   A Compulsive, repetitious rituals
   B Auditory hallucinations
   C Disjointed thought patterns
   D Exaggerated emotional responses to normal fears

8. SS, a 44-year-old school teacher with type 2 diabetes, has just started an antianxiety agent for her symptoms. During your assessment, what potential adverse clinical concern would you have related to the medication?
   A Skin rash
   B Oversedation
   C Palpitations, tremors
   D Loss of glycemic control

9. Often individuals with eating disorders are reluctant to acknowledge the problem. It is important for the diabetes educator to recognize that to an individual with an eating disorder:
   A Exerting control over eating is extremely important
   B Control of blood glucose is of crucial importance
   C Weight gain is desirable
   D Purging is a means of self-punishment

10 An early indicator that a person with diabetes may be suffering from a psychological/psychiatric disorder is:
   A Recurrent diabetic ketoacidosis
   B Family report
   C Exhibition of obvious clinical symptomatology
   D Referral by other health professional

11 The incidence of psychological disorders in the population of persons with diabetes:
   A Is likely to be detected earlier because of their more frequent interactions with health professionals
   B Has the same incidence as in the general population
   C Has a higher incidence than in the general population
   D Is well understood and effectively treated by healthcare providers

12 Symptoms of depression and anxiety are dramatically elevated in persons with diabetes who:
   A Have 2 or more diabetes-related complications
   B Have elevated blood glucose levels
   C Have less access to medical care
   D Have had diabetes for longer than 10 years

13 The use of psychopharmacological agents in the treatment of persons with diabetes who experience anxiety:
   A Has limited effectiveness in select patients
   B Is the most promising area of treatment and intervention modalities
   C Is supported by a number of studies in persons with diabetes
   D Has the potential to improve metabolic control

14 The primary difference between a mental disorder and a subclinical syndrome is:
   A The person with a mental disorder manifests psychotic behavior
   B The person with a subclinical syndrome has features of a mental disorder that do not meet the criteria for a mental disorder
   C The duration of mental disorders is longer than for subclinical syndromes
   D Individuals with mental disorders have more symptoms

15 The role of the educator whose patient is manifesting symptoms that suggest a mental disorder is to:
   A Diagnose but not treat the condition
   B Seek supervision from a mental health specialist
   C Refer the patient to a mental health specialist for diagnosis and treatment
   D Maintain more frequent contact with the patient

16 Which of the following is not a symptom of clinical depression:
   A Hypomania
   B Fatigue or loss of energy nearly every day
   C Trouble sleeping or sleeping too much nearly every day
   D Feeling worthless or inappropriately guilty nearly every day

17 The potential benefit(s) of effective management of depression with diabetes is:
   A Improved glycemic control
   B Pain relief and increased pain tolerance
   C Enhanced sexual functioning
   D All of the above

18 A bipolar disorder often involves a manic episode. Which of the following symptoms is not characteristic of manic behavior?
   A Abnormally and persistently elevated, expansive, or irritable mood lasting at least 1 week
   B Abnormally and persistently elevated, expansive, or irritable mood that requires hospitalization in less than a week from the onset of symptoms
   C Depressive symptoms that impair social, occupational, or other important areas of functioning
   D Significant decrease in need to sleep

19 Stress may lead to deterioration of glycemic control and to increased risk of diabetes complications by:
   A Affecting neuroendocrine system functioning
   B Damaging the elasticity of blood vessels
   C Impairing cognitive ability
   D All of the above

20 Which of the following symptoms would rule out a diagnosis of an Adjustment Disorder?
   A Disturbing emotional or behavioral symptoms that were caused by a stressor that had occurred 10 weeks prior to the onset of the symptoms
   B The patient is suffering from bereavement
   C There is significant impairment in social and occupational functioning
   D The level of distress is in excess of what would be expected from exposure to the stressor

21 Which of the following is not a sign of an eating disorder for patients with diabetes?
   A Binging with alcohol
   B Normoglycemia
   C Frequent diabetic ketoacidosis (DKA)
   D Frequent and severe hypoglycemia

22 Obsessive-Compulsive Disorder is characterized by:
   A Obsessive thoughts, impulses, or images that are intrusive and inappropriate
   B Repetitive behaviors or mental acts that the patient feels driven to do
   C Debilitating expenditures of time or marked distress or situation functional impairment
   D All of the above

23 A sound strategy for preventing eating-disordered behavior in a young woman is:
   A De-emphasizing dieting
   B Emphasizing dieting
   C Helping her to be independent of her family
   D None of the above

24 The sexual dysfunction most often associated with diabetes is:
   A Hyperarousal
   B Persistent aversion to sexual activity
   C Male erectile dysfunction
   D Lessening of a woman's orgasmic capacity

See next page for answer key.

Post-Test Answer Key

Psychological Disorders

1	B	13	D
2	C	14	B
3	D	15	C
4	A	16	A
5	B	17	D
6	D	18	C
7	D	19	D
8	B	20	B
9	A	21	B
10	A	22	D
11	C	23	A
12	A	24	C

A Core Curriculum for Diabetes Education

Program Management

A Core Curriculum for Diabetes Education
Diabetes Education and Program Management

Management of Diabetes Education Programs 7

Kathryn Mulcahy, RN, MSN, CDE
Fairfax Hospital INOVA Diabetes Center
Fairfax, Virginia

Introduction

1 Diabetes educators often find themselves faced with the challenge of either starting a diabetes education program or being hired to manage one. For many educators who have varying levels of business competence, this venture is one for which they are ill prepared.

2 Developing business skills has become as important for diabetes educators as developing clinical skills. To achieve programmatic success, managers of diabetes self-management education (DSME) programs require skills in the following areas:
  A Program development and planning
  B Financial management
  C Strategic planning
  D Marketing
  E Human resource management
  F Continuous quality improvement (CQI)
  G Outcomes management

3 Applying quality improvement strategies to program services is a new skill for many educators but a necessary function for diabetes self-management education programs.

4 Using outcomes measurements to evaluate program effectiveness has become the norm for all health delivery systems.

5 Identifying appropriate marketing strategies to promote a program may be a significant factor in its success.

6 In this chapter, scientific and practical information are organized into steps for effective management with a focus on the business side of diabetes education.

Objectives

Upon completion of this chapter, the learner will be able to
1 Describe the steps in establishing a diabetes self-management education (DSME) program.
2 Identify the management skills necessary to effectively operate a successful DSME program.
3 Apply quality improvement strategies to achieve more effective programs.
4 Use outcome measurements to measure program effectiveness.
5 Identify marketing strategies to promote DSME programs.
6 Explain the difference between leadership and management and develop strategies for making a transition.

Starting a Diabetes Self-Management Program

1 There are many reasons why a diabetes education program is started.
  A An employee recognizes the need and convinces the organizational decision-makers to take action.

B The organization recognizes that there is a need for the population they serve.

C A diabetes educator sees a need within the community and courageously starts an independent practice.

2 Whatever the reason, the person who assumes responsibility for actually starting the program is most often a diabetes educator. The person may be an expert educator but have no management experience. Unfortunately, it is rare when the person responsible for starting a diabetes education program has both the clinical understanding and the business skills that are necessary for success. Since the majority of program coordinators are diabetes educators, this chapter focuses on business skills. For those who come to this task already well prepared with previous management experience or academic preparation such as an MBA or similar degree, this chapter can serve as a review.

Market Analysis

1 *Market analysis* consists of several different elements.

A A thorough assessment of the organization's ability to operate a diabetes education program is performed, including an assessment of strengths and weaknesses, both internal and external. A strategy is needed for positioning the DSME program for success, beginning with the development of a marketing plan.
- Developing a strategic plan and marketing plan at the start of a DSME program increases the potential for long-term success. These plans are described in detail later in the chapter.

B The need or market for DSME programs in the geographic area is determined based on the following questions:
- Is there sufficient demand for the DSME program to have a high potential for success?
- Is the DSME program equipped to provide it?
- What are the strengths of the existing or proposed DSME program?
- What are weaknesses that will be barriers to success?
- And most importantly, can the program be positioned for success given all that is currently known?

2 These are important questions for the DSME program and the organization to answer. There is likely to be a market for the program services given the number of people with diabetes in the United States. A major challenge, however, may be finding and identifying strengths and determining the best positioning message. The term *positioning* was coined in the 1970s by 2 advertising executives, Ries and Trout, who defined the term in the following way: "Positioning starts with a product. It is merchandise, a service, a company, an institution, or even a person...But positioning is what you do to the mind of the prospect. That is your position, the product in the mind of the customer."[1]

3 A financial analysis of the proposed service is necessary, along with a thorough market analysis. The results of these analyses are presented to the sponsoring organization or community supporter.

Role of the National Standards for Diabetes Self-Management Education

1 When faced with starting a program, the first place to start is with the revised National Standards for Diabetes Self-Management Education (2000).[2] The *National Standards* define quality diabetes self-management education that can be implemented in diverse settings to improve healthcare outcomes for people with diabetes. There are 10 evidence-based standards that address structure, process, and outcomes.

   A The development of a new program requires a clear picture of what is being created. The first national standard states the DSME entity must have documentation that describes its organizational structure, mission statement, and overall goals. It also states that quality must be an integral component of the program.

   B There is strong scientific evidence in the business and healthcare literature that establishing a commitment to a strong organizational infrastructure that supports all of the above elements results in efficient and effective provision of services.[3-6]

2 After the standards have been reviewed and data have been collected from a community assessment, competitive analysis, and resource identification, a simple business plan is developed. This plan, which does not need to be complex, serves as a guide for the leader and the team and outlines realistic goals that can be articulated to others.

   A A plan is not cast in stone; it can be changed as the organization alters its planning in response to the environment.

   B According to the Joint Commission on Accreditation of Health Care Organizations (JCAHO), this type of documentation is important to both small and large organizations.[7]

   C A template for a simple business plan is shown in Table 7.1.

Table 7.1. Template for a Business Plan

1 Mission
2 Objectives
3 Community needs assessment
4 Market analysis
5 Description of services
6 Marketing plan
7 Operational implementation plan, with timeline
8 Resources
9 Budget (3 year)

Assessment and Analysis of the DSME Population

1 Developing a new DSME program first requires an analysis of the population to be served, including both the obvious customers as well as potential customers of the program's service. This completed analysis describes the market community.

A In a physician practice, the patient base comprises the population to be served; demographic data can be obtained from the patient database.

B In a larger organization such as a hospital, health system, or managed-care organization, a planning department that keeps market demographics can probably provide a general description of the community served by the organization.

C Additional geographic information related to local diabetes statistics can also be gathered from a state Diabetes Control Program or the county statistics database. This information can be found in the county library, at the county Web site, or at the local university.

2 It is important to determine the target audience and the needs of the targeted population. This information increases the likelihood of creating services that support the population needs.

Resource Identification

1 A thorough identification of resources includes space, staff, office equipment, and patient education materials.

  A An essential resource that is often overlooked is classroom space.
  - If the population includes Medicare beneficiaries, the program is required to provide most of the services in a small-group format. This requires space for not just the person with diabetes but also for at least one family member.[8]
  - Depending on the potential number of patients, a room set up in a classroom style that accommodates between 10 and 20 people is usually needed.
  - When possible, the classroom should have storage space for patient education materials and monitoring and insulin teaching supplies.
  - Handwashing facilities are important if invasive monitoring and/or insulin skills are to be taught.
  - Local and federal requirements concerning syringe disposal and appropriate cleaning of areas where blood products are used should be checked (OSHA, Joint Commission on Accreditation of Health Care Organizations).

  B Audiovisual (AV) supplies such as an overhead projector, slide projector, flip charts, white board and markers, and computer or LCD projector need to be considered. The AV supplies that are used depend on the choice of teaching styles and available financial resources.

  C An office area also is needed that allows space for the members of the clinical team to see patients individually as well as handle other work responsibilities.
  - The offices can be shared or there can be individual offices for each team member. The space should provide a comfortable area for patient teaching.
  - Cost of space will be a factor in whether individual offices or shared offices can be provided. Classroom space can also be shared with other departments.

2 If the DSME is part of a large organization, it may be possible to move services to an off-site location where better space is available. The benefits of the space and amenities of off-site locations must be weighed against the costs of rent, phones, copy machines, maintenance contract for office equipment, and other overhead costs. The cost associated with travel time also must be considered if staff continue to have responsibilities at the main office or campus of the organization.

Creating a Diabetes Education Team

1 Once the target population, their needs, and the resources needed have been identified, a diabetes education team can be formed. The organization's decision makers must demonstrate their commitment to a multidisciplinary team, along with the resources and infrastructure that enable the team to function.[9] The diabetes education team is the most important resource of the DSME. A program cannot exist without knowledgeable and competent diabetes educators.

2 Studies on diabetes education and diabetes care have rarely evaluated the characteristics of the persons who actually provide the diabetes education and the outcome measures of provider efficacy.[10]

  A The studies have clearly identified the importance of having a team provide the diabetes care and education. The team must include the patient and health professionals who are collectively qualified to provide all aspects of education and clinical management. The model shown in Figure 7.1 illustrates the concept of the patient at the center of a multidisciplinary team with collaboration among team members.[11] The team may consist of a registered dietitian (RD), registered nurse (RN), pharmacist, physician, behavioral specialist, exercise physiologist, and paraprofessional (community health worker).[12,13]

Figure 7.1. Multidisciplinary Team Approach to Diabetes Education

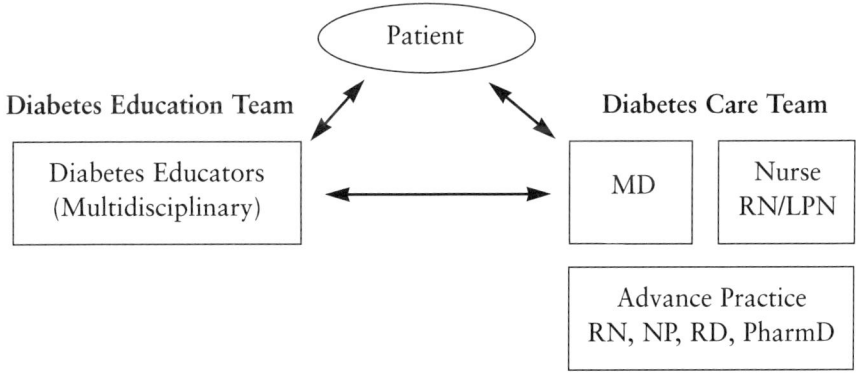

3 The number of staff will depend on the anticipated number of patients and whether the format will include group as well as individual education. The decision about hiring support staff is also based on expected volume as well as available resources. Most programs start first with clinical staff and add support staff as they expand. Financial considerations also are involved in this decision.

4 A desirable ratio of clinical staff to patients has not been well documented, but experience has shown that a good rule of thumb is 5 to 6 (60-minute visits) per day per educator for individual consults and 8 to 10 patients per class for 2 educators.

A Class length is a factor in determining both the number of patients and the capacity per number of staff. For example, 2 full-time educators should be able to handle between 30 and 50 individual patient visits per week depending on the length of the visits and other administrative responsibilities.

B If educators are seeing patients in groups, the capacity significantly increases and the number of patients seen by 2 full-time educators may be as high as 100 or more patients per week, allowing for variation in length of classes and other responsibilities.

5 The National Standards state that DSME must be provided by a multifaceted educational instructional team that may include a behaviorist, exercise physiologist, ophthalmologist, optometrist, pharmacist, physician, podiatrist, registered dietitian, registered nurse, other professional, and paraprofessionals.

A The team must be collectively qualified to teach all content areas and must include at least a registered dietitian and a registered nurse.[14,15] All instructors must be either a certified diabetes educator (CDE) or have recent didactic and experiential preparation in education and diabetes management.[2]

B The research to date has shown that DSME is most effective when delivered by a multidisciplinary team with a comprehensive plan of care.[16-20]

6 If a goal of the program is to earn recognition status in the American Diabetes Association (ADA) Education Recognition Program (ERP), the minimum team as described in the National Standards and adopted by the ADA ERP must be in place.[21]

7 Creating a team includes professional staff as well as support staff and is one of the most critical elements in building a successful diabetes education program.

A The team must understand and be committed to the mission and goals of the program.

B Clear role delineation and professional understanding of the common shared goals among the members must be established.

C Open communication and trust is a high priority for successful teams.

D Mutual respect for each member's professional capabilities must be encouraged.

E People with a "can do" attitude and commitment to excellence are desirable team members.

8 For many educators, coordinating a DSME program is the first time they have been responsible for hiring, evaluating, and supervising staff. The following tips can help the coordinator get started in hiring new staff[22]:

A Prescreening applicants can save time for the coordinator and applicant. Spend 5 minutes on the phone with those candidates who have the most promising resumes.

B Applicants can be asked to describe how they would handle a specific real-life situation. This task can help evaluate their problem-solving skills and provide insight into how they might fit in the DSME team.

C People who have had previous experience as a diabetes educator or who have already acquired CDE status are desirable.

9 As the team is created, it is helpful to have a first draft of job descriptions for the various positions. Reviewing job descriptions can help the candidates understand the job expectations.

   A A new staff can help create or refine the job descriptions after they have developed an understanding of the program mission and goals.

   B Delegating some activities such as writing job descriptions can empower the DSME team and contribute to future cohesiveness.

   C A simple template for a position description is shown in Table 7.2.

   D Other established diabetes education programs can be contacted for information on how they operate. Many are willing to share their job descriptions and other operational and clinical policies with new programs.

Table 7.2. Template for a Position Description

- Department name
- Date
- Approval signature
- Position summary
- Job responsibilities
- Qualifications
- Accountability

10 If it is within the budget, the coordinator may want to consider visiting other established diabetes education programs that are within driving distance. Programs that have been established for several years, have a good reputation in their community, and may have earned the ADA recognition for their education program, can provide useful information.

   A It is also helpful to identify programs that are similar to the planned DSME program in geographic location, population, and organizational structure. Two ways to locate programs in a specific geographic region are through the ADA Web site (*www.diabetes.org*) and by calling the American Association of Diabetes Educators at 1-800-TEAMUP4.

   B In some instances, the DSME team from programs within the same geographic region may view any new programs as potential competition and deny access to their program, or they may not be in a position to share any specific materials due to proprietary rights. Alternatively, programs outside the same market area may be very willing to share information and experience.

Development of Program Services

1 The next step in starting a DSME program is to develop the program services.

   A A common approach to developing program services is to use the National Standards and prepare a curriculum based on Standard 7, which states that programs are required to have a written curriculum with criteria for successful learning outcomes, and that the assessed needs of the individual determine the content areas to be delivered (Table 7.3).[2]

Table 7.3. DSME Education Content Areas

- Describing the diabetes disease process and treatment options
- Incorporating appropriate nutritional management
- Incorporating physical activity into lifestyle
- Using medications (if applicable) for therapeutic effectiveness
- Monitoring blood glucose, monitoring blood or urine ketones (when appropriate), and using results to improve control
- Preventing, detecting, and treating acute complications
- Preventing (through risk-reduction behavior), detecting, and treating chronic complications
- Goal setting to promote health; problem-solving for daily living
- Integrating psychosocial adjustment into daily life
- Promoting preconception care, management during pregnancy, and gestational diabetes management (if applicable)

Source: National Standards for Diabetes Self-Management Education.[2]

B Developing the curriculum should not be a time-consuming activity. A number of curriculums have already been developed that meet the criteria in the National Standards. Determining the target audience and how to deliver the curriculum may require more time and attention.
- The program services must be based on the selected curriculum as well as the needs of the target population.
- Demographics are analyzed for age, type of diabetes, payer mix, and ethnic background; services should be based on this target population.
- The decision about whether to offer classes or individual consults or a combination of both may be influenced by who pays for the services. Medicare and some other insurers mandate the delivery modality, so it is important to understand the payer mix.
- If there is potential for having women with gestational diabetes mellitus (GDM) in the target population, it may be necessary to provide specialized services for these individuals.
- The curriculum may need to account for individuals with type 1 diabetes, unless the numbers are relatively small.

C Clear descriptions of program services are essential for marketing the program. It is best to identify no more than 2 or 3 key services that are likely to be successful. Other services can be added as the need arises and as appropriate resources are developed. The following is an example of a clear description of a program service: Type 2 Diabetes: Getting Started: a small-group program for people with type 2 diabetes who are newly diagnosed or have had no prior diabetes education. A team of certified diabetes educators including a registered nurse and a registered dietitian provides the program. Some of the topic areas include healthy eating, blood glucose monitoring, medications to help you control your diabetes, personal goal setting, how to lower your risk for other health problems, and much more that will help you live a healthy life.

2 Controversy exists over the value of group versus individual education. There is still a widespread belief that one-on-one DSME is the best delivery modality and that group teaching is a compromise made for economic reasons. However, there are data to support the view that group DSME is just as effective as individual education when implemented appropriately.[23] The dilemma is not whether to provide quality DSME programs in a group format, but whether diabetes educators have acquired the skills and strategies to provide effective educational, behavioral, and clinical interventions in a group format.

Budgeting

1 Budgeting is an important aspect of program development and ongoing program management. The elements of creating an initial budget and a 3-year projection are described in this section.

2 Salaries comprise the greatest expense of any program, so the number and composition of staff needed over the first 3 years must be identified.
  A Determine the number of full-time equivalents (FTE) of professional staff and support staff needed. (Example: 1.0 registered nurse (RN), 1.0 registered dietitian (RD), 0.5 secretary for year 1)
  B Project patient volume and program growth over the next 3 years based on a best guess.
  C Determine the average salary for the identified staff and add 25% to 30% for benefits. (Example: RN and RD @ $22/hour ($45 760/year) plus secretary @ $12/hour ($12 480) = total base salary of $104 000 plus 28% benefits ($29 120) = $133 120 annual salary budget for first year)
  D Incorporate an annual cost of living increase for each consecutive year as well as any changes in staff numbers. This amount is probably 2% to 4% annually.

3 The next largest expense is for space if the program will be charged rent. Some programs may be fortunate to have this expense absorbed by their parent organization. However, more organizations are beginning to apply a facilities expense to individual departments.

4 Additional expenses include patient education materials; office supplies such as a minimum of 1 computer, a printer, and a fax machine; AV equipment and supplies such as transparencies or slides; continuing education money for staff; printing; copying; marketing; and phones. Some of these costs may come out of other organizational budgets, but this needs to be verified so the program does not lack some essential resources.

5 If the programs coordinator chooses to purchase an existing diabetes education curriculum or affiliate with an existing educational network, these expenses must be included as well as ongoing costs.

6 If the program has a medical director, appropriate costs must be included in the budget.

7 If the plans include applying for ADA Education Program Recognition sometime during the next 3 years, the application fee must be included in the budget. This information can be obtained from the ADA Web site (*www.diabetes.org*).

8 When all expenses have been considered, income must be projected. This amount is more difficult to quantify because it is based on an educated guess of patient volume and reimbursement. It is best to estimate conservatively for the first several years. The market analysis that has been completed can assist in determining a close estimate of the program's volume. The projections should include who will be underwriting the program until it is self-sustaining.

9 Reimbursement is an ever-changing issue in many healthcare environments. It will depend largely on the percent of Medicare population and whether the parent organization already has some type of contractual arrangement with commercial payers (see Chapter 8, Payment for Diabetes Education, in Diabetes Education and Program Management, for more information on this area of program management).

10 Prepare a spreadsheet with the numbers for all expected expenses and estimated gross revenue and project these numbers over at least 3 years, accounting for cost of living and program growth.

New Program Annual Plan

1 The coordinator and team need to develop an annual or operating plan to serve as a roadmap for the year. It assists in keeping the program directed toward its goals and provides a way to document accomplishments. A template for an annual plan is shown in Figure 7.2.

2 Developing an annual plan is one of the first activities that the team can do together. It helps to bring a unity within the group and is an excellent team-building activity. Everyone begins to feel a sense of ownership in the program and its success. Not only is the team approach important in delivering DSME, it is also important to the success of the program operations. Team members who feel valued and empowered are likely to be more productive.

Figure 7.2. Annual Plan Template

Goal	Fit With Strategic Plan	Activity	Responsible Person or Group	Target Date	Status

Marketing Plan

1 *Marketing* is a social process by which individuals and groups obtain what they need and want through creating and exchanging products and value with others. Many healthcare professionals are uncomfortable with the concept of marketing because they equate it with advertising and may not think it is professional.

2 Marketing is a process of understanding the customers' needs and developing ways of communicating how services can help them meet their needs.

3 A plan needs to be developed to market or promote the DSME services.
  A The customer needs to be identified first, recognizing that different customers have different needs.
  B Regardless of the strategies used to promote the program services, the message has to be matched to the customers and their needs.
  C The following process can be used to develop a marketing plan:
  • Identify customers and their needs
  • Determine appropriate promotional strategies
  • Identify data sources to establish the program's effectiveness
  • Define core messages

4 The program can be promoted to many different customers. It is best to start by defining the top 2 or 3 types of customers and create a marketing plan around them. Examples of some typical customers of a DSME program are shown in Table 7.4.

Table 7.4. Key Customers of a DSME Program

- Physicians (providers)
- Patients
- Insurers
- Community
- Internal organization
- Others

5 When a program is starting, it is important to consider who has the greatest potential to provide the program with business. This is the *primary customer*.

6 Frequently physicians and patients comprise the first target audience. Identify what vehicles already exist that may help get the message to these two potential customer groups.
  A Determine whether there are any physician newsletters or a community newsletter that would publish a notice about the program.
  B Information about the new services can be sent to physicians in a general mailing.
  C Brochures are very helpful because they can be placed in physicians' offices, staff lounges, local grocery stores, and pharmacies, with permission.

D Waiting areas in the hospital and departments are excellent places to display brochures.

E Requesting time on the agenda of physician meetings in local hospitals is another means of alerting physicians to new services. Key physicians can be enlisted as champions of the program; they also may be willing to promote the program at some of the physician meetings.

7 Because time and resources are limited, the target audience must be selected carefully and 1 or 2 strategies must be developed that will get their attention. An example of a simple marketing plan is shown in Figure 7.3.

Figure 7.3. Marketing Plan

Customer	Activity	Responsible Person	Target Date	Status

Managing the Program Effectively

1 Being able to effectively manage the DSME program is just as important as starting the program. The program manager is responsible for assuring high-quality services that are delivered in a cost-effective and efficient manner to the satisfaction of patients, referring providers, staff, and the parent organization.

Organizational Culture

1 The organizational culture is an important aspect of any organization, small or large, and needs to be understood at both the corporate and department levels.

2 A DSME program that is an independent, freestanding program may not have the same complexities as a larger organization but still has a culture that influences every aspect of its functioning.

3 *Culture* implies values, such as aggressiveness or passivity, which set a pattern for an organization's activities, opinions, and actions. This pattern is instilled in the employees by the managers' examples and passed down to succeeding generations of workers. Words alone do not produce culture; rather, it is the actions of the organizational managers.[24]

4 An organization's culture can be its strength when it is consistent with its strategies. The culture can also be a significant barrier to ongoing success when it stands in the way of changes that are necessary in an evolving competitive environment. It can then lead to stagnation and the ultimate demise of a once-successful organization.

5 Because culture is so pervasive, changing it becomes one of the most difficult tasks to undertake. Generally the founder of the diabetes education program contributes greatly to creating the organizational culture whether the program is freestanding or part of a larger organization. The following questions can be used to determine the culture of an organization. The answers are not necessarily right or wrong; they are just the result of the organizational culture.
  A Is there a high level of independence or is it a structured hierarchy?
  B What are the characteristics of the people who have been hired? Are they independent free thinkers, able to change roles easily, or do they look for more specific role definition?
  C Do the employees have a work ethic that conveys a "go-the-extra-mile" attitude, or do they need delineated work hours and days?
  D Were staff hired who had extensive experience in the field or is the program open to hiring novice educators who will develop their competencies as the program develops and likely adopt much of the overall philosophy of management?
  E Are decisions made through a team effort or in a more top-down manner?

6 When the culture of the organization does not fit the work style and personality of an individual, it can cause dissatisfaction on the part of both the employee and the employer. The coordinator influences the culture of the departmental organization and needs to consider carefully the attributes and values that he/she believes will serve to make the program successful.

7 Healthcare providers who deliver care as part of a team and believe that more than one person is needed to provide the clinical interventions necessary for effective diabetes management and diabetes education programs often adopt a more participatory type of organizational structure.

8 An organization that has an operational philosophy that promotes a culture in which individuals and groups at all levels routinely use information in their decision-making is called a *knowledge-based organization*.[25] There are 3 attributes of a knowledge-based organization:
  A A clear sense of direction that brings clarity and supports success
  B Systems, structures, and processes that promote effective and efficient operations
  C Culture and climate based on beliefs, assumptions, and values that encourage behavior that supports the achievement of desired outcomes

Strategic Planning

1 Strategic planning and long-range planning are not the same, although the terms are often mistakenly interchanged. *Long-range planning* refers to the time during which the plan is in place, while *strategic planning* is the approach that is used.[25]
  A Knowledge-based organizations view strategic planning as a process rather than a product. Establishing a clear direction is a fundamental responsibility of the leadership, who must be able to answer the following two questions about the program or organization:
    - Where is this program going?
    - Why is it going there, and what is its purpose and reason for existence?

2 To develop a clear direction, the future must be envisioned and then articulated in an outcomes-focused strategic plan. There are a wide variety of publications about strategic planning as well as strategic-planning experts who can be hired to assist the staff and organization in their planning efforts.

3 Having a clear strategic plan and vision for the future helps create a standard of excellence for everyone to live up to and gives staff the ability to benchmark their own performance. Elements of strategic thinking are
  A Sensitivity to customer views
  B Envisioning the future of program services
  C Developing a capacity for strategic positioning

People Management

1 The first step in people management is hiring the right people.

2 The second step is team building, which is the fuel that runs all successful organizations. Successful teams have pride and sense of accomplishment that comes from striving for and achieving high levels of performance. Employees want to be part of a winning team.[26]
  A Successful teamwork is exciting and offers personal incentives such as status, recognition, and, in some cases, financial rewards.
  B It is not always possible to provide financial compensation for outstanding teamwork. However, people can be given recognition and an opportunity to take on some leadership for different projects.
  C Good teamwork also requires a high level of trust between team members. Examples of some activities that promote teams and also can result in high levels of performance are
    • Regular staff meetings
    • Self-directed work teams
    • Off-site team meetings that bring the team together in a nonwork environment (eg, home, conference center, etc) and are not all work related; these activities help team members develop a better understanding of each other and mutual respect
    • Team-building programs implemented by an external facilitator
    • An opportunity to work with an external facilitator on the Myers-Briggs Type Indicator (MBTI),[27] a self-report personality inventory designed to give people information about their psychological type preference based on 4 dimensions: extraversion or introversion, sensing or intuition, thinking or feeling, and judging or perceiving. The MBTI can be used very effectively for organizational development and team building.
    • Recognition in group meetings and newsletters and through informal acknowledgment

3 *Coaching* is an important responsibility of a leader. It should not be confused with counseling employees who are performing poorly. Coaching is used with staff members who have the potential to be outstanding performers.
  A Coaching is an important skill for leaders to develop to create a climate where personal growth is expected and rewarded.

B To be a good coach, leaders must encourage the staff to explore new options instead of settling for the obvious.

C The best way for a leader to stimulate this type of growth is to ask staff open-ended questions that require thoughtful responses. Samples of such questions are
- What are your recommendations?
- What do you think?
- Can you think of a better way to do this?
- What would you like to accomplish in the next year? (This is a particularly good way to open a performance appraisal.)

D There is considerable payoff in developing leadership skills. In addition to contributing to the success of the program, it also contributes to the growth and development of people, which is often the most satisfying part of a leader's job.[28]

Characteristics of Effective Leadership

1 The nature of leadership depends on the situation, the task to be performed, and the characteristics of the followers.

2 There are differences between management and leadership:
   A Leadership focuses on doing the right things.
   B Management focuses on doing things right.
   C "The leader of the past was a person who knew how to tell. The leader of the future will be a person who knows how to ask."[29]

3 "The first responsibility of a leader is to define reality."[30] There are 6 distinct leadership styles:
   A Coercive
   B Authoritative
   C Affiliative
   D Democratic
   E Pacesetting
   F Coaching

4 Most effective leaders use all styles seamlessly depending on the situation. There is no right or wrong style; rather, the most successful leaders have been found to use a combination of styles.
   A Leadership styles emerge from different components of emotional intelligence. Research has shown that emotional intelligence can be linked to results and it can be learned at any age.
   B *Emotional intelligence* is the ability to manage our relationships and ourselves effectively and consists of 4 capabilities:
   - Self-awareness
   - Self-management
   - Social awareness
   - Social skill

5 Leaders are made, not born. A key to success is becoming as adept at following others as we are at getting others to follow. The following are critical behaviors and skills of effective followers:

A Asking questions instead of giving answers
B Providing opportunities for others to lead
C Doing real work in support of others
D Seeking common understanding instead of consensus

6 The leader of the future will be able to lead and follow, be central and marginal, be hierarchically above and below, be individualistic and a team player, and, above all, be a perpetual learner. Leaders are able to influence the beliefs and behaviors of others to unleash the creative genius of all parts of the organization on a day-to-day basis.

Financial Management

1 The process of budgeting is basically the same for the present and future years. By having a historical perspective on expenses and revenue from previous years, the process does not need to start from scratch. Some helpful tips on the budgeting process are
   A Reviewing the financial activity from the previous year to determine any significant variations from projections
   B Making corrections in the new budget year if there are new trends (either above or below the projection)
   C Determining the impact of new or eliminated services on both expenses and income

2 Financial analysis is just as important as the budgeting process but often is misunderstood or overlooked. The following questions can be used to determine if a financial analysis of existing services has been conducted:
   A Is the cost of a patient visit known?
   B Are all of the components of cost besides staff salary being considered? Examples include administrative overhead; operational overhead such as rent, phones, and office supplies; patient educational materials; AV equipment; nondirect patient time such as documentation and phone time; and employee benefits, which add 25% to 38% to staff salary.
   C If classes are offered, is it known how many attendees are needed to break even?
   D How much of the cost is being reimbursed by insurance?
   E What is the productivity of the staff?
   F What ratio of group to individual education is necessary for the program to operate efficiently and effectively?
   G Has the cost of the patient care processes been analyzed in relation to the overall cost of operating the program?

3 A financial assessment of the program should be undertaken if the answers to any of these questions are unknown. Although the program is not likely to ever be a significant revenue producer for the parent organization, it can provide value in the following ways:
   A Cost avoidance (show how the program affected the self-care behavior of customers, which resulted in decreased hospitalizations, decreased emergency department visits, and decreased hospital length of stay)
   B Improved satisfaction for the patient and provider

4 Understanding the costs of delivering services is the first step in creating a financially viable program.
   A Each service provided needs to be analyzed as to its potential to generate income. This does not mean eliminating services that cannot break even. It does mean that all services should be looked at as a total department and the best mix determined, both to meet the needs of the target audience as well as the economic goals of the organization.
   B Consider this example of an action that resulted from a thorough financial analysis. After a center conducted a financial analysis of their services, they determined that the only way to optimize their services was to increase the number of patients seen at group consults and maintain class sizes of 6 or more participants. This was accomplished by making some adjustments to their current scheduling procedures, developing a staffing template with established educator teams, and developing some alternative group services for patients who had previously been seen only in one-on-one consultations. Their quality monitors showed that patient satisfaction was still high, and clinical and behavioral outcomes were favorable.

5 The program manager must continuously monitor the status of the program's reimbursement and assure that the correct coding is being used to obtain the best reimbursement. Even when coding is correct, there are many roadblocks that can affect the actual dollars reimbursed (see Chapter 8, Payment for Diabetes Education, in Diabetes Education and Program Management, for more information about reimbursement for the delivery of DSME). The following suggestions may help maximize the potential for reimbursement:
   A Become acquainted with the people in the accounts payable department of the parent organization so they can create access to the financial information needed.
   B Request regular financial statements that provide reimbursement data, not just charges. This request may seem simple, but most departmental financial statements provide only gross revenue figures.
   C Be sure that medical record documentation meets Medicare requirements for physician referral and patient eligibility.
   D Confirm that charges are being processed appropriately.
   E Become acquainted with the local Medicare intermediary as well as payer representatives from other key insurers.
   F Contact the case managers from key insurers because they can be a tremendous referral source.
   G Talk with the contracting staff to make sure they are including diabetes education in their negotiations.

Meeting the Standards for Program Recognition

1 Currently the only accrediting body that is approved by the Centers for Medicare and Medicaid Services (CMS), formerly know as the Health Care Financing Administration (HCFA), is the ADA Education Recognition Program. This program is based on the National Standards for Diabetes Self-Management Education.
   A Eligibility requirements for application for ADA Education Program Recognition are
      • Must meet the National Standards for DSME
      • Must be in operation for at least 6 months
      • Data must reflect 6 months of operation

B A DSME program may begin collecting data when the following essential components are in place:
- Established oversight system
- Annual plan
- Coordinator
- Required instructors
- Data tracking system
- Continuous quality improvement (CQI) process
- Curriculum and educational materials

2 A program must have a designated coordinator with academic and/or experiential preparation in program management and the care of persons with chronic disease. The coordinator oversees the planning, implementation, and evaluation of the DSME entity. A written job description that includes these requirements must be developed and available for review.

A A system (committee, governing board, advisory body) must be established that involves professional staff and other stakeholders who participate annually in a planning and review process that includes data analysis and outcomes measurements and addresses community concerns. These criteria are different from the previous standards and ADA Recognition criteria that required predetermined membership and at least 3 meetings per year. The program can determine who is appropriate to carry out the function. It may be an already established collaborative practice committee, a quality team, or the established advisory structure may be kept the same. The frequency of meetings is determined by the program and based on what is needed to carry out the requirements. The advisory group must review the following items annually:
- Operational goal achievement
- Data analysis of operations
- Mission statement
- Organizational structure
- Population served
- Resources
- Outcomes data (behavioral and other)

B The program must have an annual plan that was developed and approved by the advisory body.

C Demographic site information must be documented and tracked on an annual basis. The demographics that are required are
- Total number of participants who received DSME during the data period
- Comprehensive and/or initial (assess, instruct, reassess, measure outcomes pre and post)
- Follow-up (focused teaching or limited consult)
- Average number of hours for comprehensive participants (Example: 100 total patients/640 total hours = 6.4 average hours)
- Average number of hours for follow-up participants (Example: 44 total patients/ 110 total hours = 2.5 average hours)
- Population by age
- Population by types of diabetes
- Population by race/special needs

- Service area, setting/types of educational services
- Number and type of instructors
- Instructor experience, academic preparation, credentials, current time spent delivering DSME, continuing education (CE) credits, and CDE status. CE requirements vary depending on CDE status and number of hours the educator is currently practicing

D It is also important for the group to be actively involved in the program's continuous quality improvement efforts. The program must use a continuous quality improvement process to evaluate the effectiveness of the education experience provided and determine opportunities for improvement.

E Refer to the ADA Web site (*www.diabetes.org*) under Education Program Recognition for more details on the criteria and application process.

Quality as a Management Philosophy

1 *Quality* is a management philosophy that supports a continuous striving for service excellence and an unrelenting commitment to customer satisfaction. It is reflected in the following two questions:

A Are customers (patient, physician, managed care organization, parent organization, etc) receiving what they want?

B Are services provided well (efficiently and effectively)?

2 The quality movement began in Japan in the 1950s when Japanese products were regarded as cheap and of poor quality. Within 30 years, Japanese products had a worldwide reputation for quality while the reputation of American products was slipping in comparison. In the 1980s American companies joined the quality movement, which was led by Deming[31] and Juran,[32,33] the best-known leaders and teachers in the quality movement in the US today.

3 Some examples of the quality philosophy are presented in Table 7.5, contrasting the old ways of doing business with the quality way.

4 As individuals and organizations in healthcare attempted to define quality, hundreds of definitions have come into existence. The definitions include terms such as quality assurance, quality assessment, total quality management, and continuous quality improvement.

5 The two models of quality activities most frequently cited have been the traditional structure, process, and outcome model of quality assurance as described by Donebedian[34] and the industrial model of quality as described by Deming[31] and Juran.[32,33]

6 Quality management focuses on the customer and the goal that customers will become loyal, long-term users of the program products and services. There is a significant focus on the processes that go into the overall delivery of service, or in the case of diabetes education, the delivery of DSME and care and the support processes that go into the entire healthcare delivery model.

Table 7.5. Philosophies of Quality Management

Issue	Old Way	Quality Way
Quality	Quality is fine	Must continuously improve quality
Problems	Employees	Processes/systems
Employees	Motivate employees	• Remove obstacles • Define customer requirements
Processes	Fix problem	Use data/information
Customers	Problems waiting to happen	Partners
Costs	Quality costs more	• Quality costs less • Do it right the first time • Long-term investment
Management	Crisis management	Preventive management

7 Because quality is fundamentally a philosophy, there is no one prescription for application. The concepts need to be applied to the goal of striving for service excellence.

8 There are a number of quality methodologies, with continuous quality improvement (CQI) being one of the most used. Two other frequently used methodologies are quality planning and quality measurement.

Understanding Continuous Quality Improvement (CQI)

1 *Continuous quality improvement* (CQI) is a daily operational philosophy and represents two incremental improvement approaches, quality improvement and process management.
  A *Quality improvement* (QI) is the achievement of higher levels of performance through the application of data analysis and procedure improvement on a continuous, incremental basis.
  B *Process management* is the application of appropriate quality tools to business processes to optimize process performance and increase value to customers.
  C The steps in the CQI process are
   • Identify problem/opportunity
   • Collect data
   • Analyze data
   • Identify alternative solutions
   • Generate recommendations
   • Implement recommendations
   • Evaluate actions
   • Improvement

2 The decision to apply CQI to daily operations is an important organizational decision that needs to be owned by all staff, not just the manager.

3 Implementing a CQI program for DSME has now become one of the national standards for DSME and has been adopted by the ADA Education Recognition Program.

4 Data collection can be an arduous task. Following certain principles can assure that meaningful data are collected. Two questions can guide data collection: What kind of data does the program want to collect and how will the data be obtained?

5 Data can be categorized into one of 3 levels of measurement.

A *Variable data*, also called intervals data, are quantified numeric data stated in standard units of measure (eg, how many, how much, how far, number of minutes waiting, ounces of fluid consumed). Variable data offer the greatest range of possibilities for analysis.

B *Ordinal data* have been quantified using non-numeric standards such as in Likert scales (5 = very satisfied, 4 = somewhat satisfied, 3 = satisfied, etc).

C *Attribute data*, also called nominal data, are categorical data such as sex, race, religion, admitted/not admitted, etc.

6 There are many types of data collection tools. See Table 7.6 for information on data collection tools.

Operational Definitions

1 Since data collection can involve many people, it is important for all measurements to be operationally defined. An operational definition is stated in quantifiable terms that are clear and specify exactly what is to be measured. See Table 7.7 for data collection examples.

Outcomes Measurement

1 *Outcome measures* have been defined as data that describe a patient's health status. Patient health outcomes have been measured for years and their use has been increasing as researchers are beginning to see these outcomes as the best way to improve the performance of providing health care.[35]

2 Outcomes measurement has become somewhat of a buzzword in health care, yet there is significant misunderstanding about what outcomes really are. According to Donebedian, an *outcome* is "a measurable product and is the changed state or condition of an individual as a consequence of health care over time."[34]

3 An outcome is a change that occurs as a result of some intervention; it is not a single point in time. This means that data that are collected without a baseline of comparison or without any other intervention between measures are not really outcomes but rather a single data point.

4 The need to examine outcomes in health care and diabetes care has been reinforced by mandates from the Centers for Medicare and Medicaid Services (CMS), Agency for Health Care Policy and Research (AHCPR), and accrediting bodies such as the Joint Commission on Accreditation of Health Care Organizations (JCAHO), National

Council on Quality Assurance (NCQA), and the ADA Education and Provider Recognition Programs.

5 When determining what outcomes to capture, it is important to recognize that there are different types of outcomes that cross the healthcare continuum. Data are commonly collected on the following outcomes:
   A *Clinical outcomes:* changes in A1C, lipids, blood pressure, and body mass index over time
   B *Health status outcomes* or *education outcomes*: changes in knowledge, attitudes, barriers, and skills over time
   C *Quality-of-life (QOL) outcomes:* patient behavior, functional status, and quality of life assessed through outcomes measurement instruments such as QOL,[36] SF-36,[37] PAID,[38] and Diabetes-Self-Management Assessment Report Tool (D-SMART).[39]
   D *Behavioral outcomes:* physical activity, food/meal planning, medication administration, physical activity, self-monitoring of blood glucose (SMBG), problem-solving (glucose highs and lows), risk-reduction activities (eg, quitting smoking), and coping with diabetes
   E *Patient-centered outcomes:* changes in patient satisfaction and well-being over time
   F *Cost outcomes:* costs of services provided
   G *Cost effectiveness:* ratio of costs of a program or process compared with effects (eg, it costs $1597 per patient to lower the HbA1c by 1.7%)
   H *Cost benefit:* costs and benefits as measured in dollars
   I *Program outcomes:* patient volumes, descriptive characteristics of the patient population, patient-to-staff ratios, program completion rate, and referral patterns over time
   J *Process measures:* identifying processes to improve and facilitate patient care and evaluating change over time

6 Evaluation is critical to the future of DSME programs. The effectiveness of interventions must be documented in order to have a better understanding of which interventions are the most appropriate given a specific population.

7 Diabetes education has long been viewed as the cornerstone of effective diabetes care. Yet, in 1997 when diabetes educators were asked by HCFA to provide specific evidence of the attributes of effective education, diabetes educators had little specific information to offer.

8 At the 1999 AADE Research Summit, a question was posed: "Is diabetes education effective and what methods are the best?"[40] The answer given was "It depends" based on determining what treatment, for what population, delivered by whom, under what set of conditions, for what outcome, and how did it come about.

9 Outcomes measures associated with diabetes education programs include clinical (medical), educational (learning and behavioral), and psychosocial (QOL, coping, efficacy, etc).[41]

10 Pooling outcomes data from many individuals, which is called *aggregate outcomes data*, is useful in determining the performance of a particular program.

Table 7.6. Data Collection Tools

Method	Type of Data Yielded	Easy to Use?	Yields Reliable Data?	High Response Rate?
Survey (method used to question individuals in writing, face-to-face, by phone, or by mail)	Ordinal, variables, attribute	Yes; can be designed to be simple and easy to use	Yes; although respondents' interpretation of survey questions can vary	Depends; telephone or face-to-face surveys can have a high response rate
Chart/file audit (review of closed, open, or computerized medical records to retrieve information)	Variables, attribute	Depends; paper chart review can be labor-intensive and time-intensive	Depends on skill of individuals doing the review	Yes
Checklist (data collection sheet for gathering concurrent information during a study)	Variables, attribute	Yes; can be designed to be simple and easy to use	Depends; all people who will be completing the checklist during the data collection must be trained on how to use the data collection instrument	Depends on the cooperation and availability of the personnel completing the forms
Time study (concurrent information about time to complete a process such as turnaround time)	Variables, attribute	Usually very time-intensive and labor-intensive	Depends; all people who will be completing the time study during the data collection must be trained on how to use the instrument	Depends on the cooperation and availability of the personnel completing the study

Table 7.7 Data Collection Examples

Measurement	Operational Definition
Cycle time to schedule a patient for a visit	Amount of time it takes to schedule a patient appointment; request is measured from the date/time the request is logged as received to the date/time that the appointment occurs
Lab data: A1C, lipids	Validated data from physician or lab; no self-reported data
Patient satisfaction with DSME management	Postintervention patient satisfaction with DSME measured by asking patients to rate their satisfaction on a scale of 1 to 5 (1 = poor to 5 = excellent) immediately and 2 weeks after intervention

11 Measuring outcomes provides the following advantages:
  A Informs the practice about the effectiveness of a program
  B Informs patients about their health status
  C Identifies processes or practice guidelines to improve patient care
  D Provides economic information for the health system
  E Identifies high-risk patients
  F Informs the payer of the effectiveness of a program

12 There are numerous challenges of measuring the outcomes of diabetes education.
  A Appropriate outcomes need to be defined for DSME.
  B Consensus is required on a core set of performance measures for diabetes education.
  C The population needs to be defined and measured independently of other populations.
  D Data need to be captured and reviewed without placing an unmanageable burden on program staff.
  E Data need to be aggregated and analyzed for review to be useful for program management.
  F Outcomes should be reported back to the healthcare provider, patient, and payer so they can also benefit from the knowledge of what interventions have been effective at both the individual and program levels.
  G Educators need to consider the key question: What outcomes do I measure?

13 It has been suggested that education programs should be held accountable for clinical indicators, such as glycemic control, which is the gold standard for effective clinical management. This is an important measure for educators to track. However, educators also need to consider whether it is the only measure and whether they should be held responsible for patients not achieving good glycemic control when this clinical indicator is influenced to a great extent by treatment that may not be within their control.

14 Through an extensive review of the literature and a process of expert consensus, the AADE Outcomes Task Force determined that health-related behaviors are the unique and measurable outcomes of effective diabetes education.[42-45]

15 The paradigm for diabetes education is shifting from a content-driven practice to an outcomes-driven practice. As the profession of diabetes education has evolved, the focus has shifted from delivering the right content to achieving the desirable patient outcomes.

16 Although research in diabetes education has increased and provided valuable evidence to support the value of diabetes education, much more research is still needed.
  A We need to know what specific characteristics comprise best practice in diabetes education.
  B More detail is required about what steps in the process of diabetes education are important, including variables such as characteristics about the providers, population, delivery methodologies, and healthcare environment.
  C While randomized controlled trials (RCT) are the gold standard in study designs, an alternative approach is needed to complement the ongoing research and provide

the ability to better understand the components of what makes DSME effective in real practice settings.

D The process of assessing patient characteristics and determining what interventions are associated with the best outcomes is called *clinical practice improvement* (CPI).[46] CPI in many ways is complementary to the CQI process as well as RCT because it creates a permanent feedback loop aimed at all clinicians involved in the process of care delivery.

- CPI provides clinicians with data about their daily practice and the information necessary to understand and modify their interventions.
- The CPI framework is the basis for the AADE National Diabetes Education Outcomes System (NDEOS), (which is summarized in Figure 7.4) resulted from the work of the AADE Outcomes Task Force.

Figure 7.4. The National Diabetes Education Outcomes System

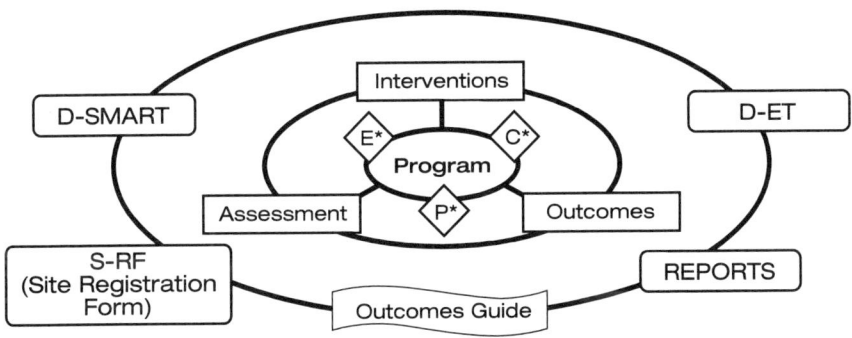

*E = Educator, C = Clinician, P = Person with Diabetes

Source: Reprinted with permission from Mulcahy et al.[39]

Strategies for Capturing Outcomes Data and Reporting Program Outcomes

1 There is increasing demand for diabetes educators to capture outcomes data and report outcomes measures that show evidence of the effectiveness of the DSME they provide. The first step in responding to this demand is to clearly define what outcomes measure the effectiveness of diabetes education, and then develop a system that allows educators to capture outcomes data and report those outcomes.

2 Several major diabetes databases have been developed that capture the data needed to provide outcomes reports for use by diabetes educators.

A Determining which outcomes measurement system is best in a particular situation depends on the specific needs of the program.

B The outcomes measurement system should be selected based on a review of its reporting capability, data fields, data input methodology, cost, expandability, and customer support.

C The diabetes educator needs to determine the specific program requirements before looking at the variety of options in measurement systems.

3 A survey of diabetes educators indicated that they want to have the ability to capture outcomes data and report the effectiveness of the interventions. They also indicated that their greatest barriers to outcomes measurement are time and resources.[47]

4 Since 1997 the AADE Outcomes Task Force has been developing the National Diabetes Education Outcomes System (NDEOS). The NDEOS (summarized in Figure 7.4) is a system that gathers, tracks, and aggregates outcomes measures unique to diabetes education and supports the integration of education into diabetes care.[39] It is intended to complement, not replace, existing automated data systems and, most importantly, to support the diabetes educator in practice.

A Based on expert consensus, a comprehensive review of the literature, and a customer analysis of the AADE membership, the Outcomes Task Force determined that health-related behavior changes are the unique and measurable outcomes of diabetes education.[40,47] These behavior changes can be categorized in the following outcomes areas:
- Physical activity (exercise)
- Food choices (eating)
- Medication administration
- Monitoring of blood glucose
- Problem-solving for blood glucose highs, lows, and sick days
- Risk-reduction activities
- Psychosocial adaptation

B In most circumstances, these outcomes areas can be assessed through self-reported information obtained from individuals with diabetes. However, a variety of clinical and program outcomes measures must also be collected to demonstrate the value of diabetes education in the total system of diabetes care.

C In addition to behavioral outcomes, immediate outcomes of knowledge and skill acquisition need to be assessed as well as long-term outcomes of improved clinical indicators and health status.

D The NDEOS has evolved based on the supposition that improved clinical outcomes are incrementally modified by enhancing patient knowledge and skills and making and sustaining appropriate behavior changes.[48]

E The framework for the NDEOS is assessment, intervention, and outcomes evaluation, which support the National Standards for Diabetes Self-Management Education (2000).[2]
- The system is focused on outcomes rather than content completion and tracks patient and program outcomes longitudinally.
- Additional guiding principles for the NDEOS are to benefit the individual educator and to develop, maintain, and update measurement tools that have validity across multiple practice settings, disciplines, and patient populations.
- By capturing educational (learning), behavioral, and clinical outcomes using valid, reliable, and evidence-based tools, the NDEOS strives to substantially increase the effectiveness and recognition of diabetes educators.[49] This effort supports the mission of AADE, which is to "advance the role of the diabetes educator, and improve the quality of diabetes education and care."[50]

- The NDEOS will enable diabetes educators to identify the specific characteristics of best practice, aid in quality improvement activities, and support AADE's efforts to have a uniform data set from all programs that can be used to influence policy and support reimbursement at both the local and national levels.

F The NDEOS is composed of the 3 unique tools: the Diabetes Self-Management Assessment Report Tool (D-SMART), the Diabetes Educator Tool (D-ET, formerly known as the Diabetes Outcomes Intervention Tool or DO-IT), and the Site Registration Form (SRF).

- The *D-SMART* is the cornerstone of the NDEOS. This self-report instrument captures data on current behavior, priorities for behavior change, and barriers to making appropriate behavior changes. The patients' self-reported responses guide educational interventions by focusing on what patients feel and state are most important to them. By administering the D-SMART prior to and after an educational intervention, changes in behaviors can be measured.

- The *D-ET* serves as the educator's documentation system or data input form and is designed to integrate the educational process with behavioral interventions and clinical management. The D-ET is closely related to the D-SMART in that the different educational domains of knowledge, skills, goals, and barriers are embedded on the form and are meant to help guide educational, behavioral, and clinical interventions. By evaluating the D-SMART, educators can identify deficits in knowledge, skills, goals, and barriers, as well as current behaviors for all 7 behavior areas. This information can be used to prioritize subsequent intervention(s) with the patient.

- The *SRF* is used to assess site characteristics including target populations, educator profiles, program intervention methodologies, and program design. Information from the SRF will enable the AADE to build a better understanding of the settings in which diabetes self-management education is delivered, the populations involved, the methods of delivery, and who provides the education. The SRF will also enable the AADE to identify and establish sets of similar practice settings that can be used for benchmarking.

G A comprehensive analysis of the D-SMART revealed high test-retest reliability. Test-retest reliability was measured by evaluating intraclass correlations and differences in response percentages between the first and second administrations of the D-SMART (patients completed the tool twice within a 2-week period prior to an intervention).

- Chronbach's alpha scores demonstrated high inter-item consistency, with questions related to certain domains (eg, coping with diabetes, barriers to change, and knowledge) being highly correlated (> 0.7).

- Responsiveness of the D-SMART was measured by evaluating both intraclass correlations and response percentages on the second administration (prior to intervention) and the third administration (at least 2 weeks after the intervention). These data were analyzed in the aggregate population and in subpopulations desiring a specific change. The results indicated that the questions and response categories in the D-SMART were sensitive enough to quantify behavior changes for each of the outcome areas.

Benchmarking for Best Practice

1. External organizations can offer models or best practices to which we can aspire or even hope to exceed. This process of comparing current programs against best practices is called *benchmarking*. Benchmarking can begin at any point that has been defined as the best, and the outcomes can be above or below. The following benefits are gained through benchmarking:
   - **A** Breaking paradigms about how a process is functioning
   - **B** Improving understanding of competition
   - **C** Encouraging a search for improvement, practice breakthroughs, and achievement of superior performance
   - **D** Revealing a more accurate picture of customer requirements by comparing similar populations
   - **E** Providing credibility for opportunities for change
   - **F** Helping to provide a view that extends beyond the immediate boundaries

2. By systematically capturing a uniform data set of outcomes measures that are impacted by DSME, we can better understand what makes diabetes education effective. Educators can learn about specific interventions that result in improved outcomes for their patients.

Marketing a DSME Program

1. Choose a customer focus.
   - **A** Look at the payer mix and referral sources.
   - **B** Determine who can provide the most business in the least amount of time.
   - **C** Focus on growth opportunities.
   - **D** Give presentations wherever you are invited.

2. Learn how to influence the decision makers.
   - **A** Learn more about their needs and establish an ongoing relationship.
   - **B** Determine who makes the decisions.
   - **C** Target the message to what customers need.
   - **D** Tell customers how DSME programs can help them meet their needs.

3. Learn how to articulate the role, value, and outcomes (results) of your DSME program.

4. Be prepared to answer the following questions about diabetes education:
   - **A** What is diabetes education?
   - **B** What do diabetes educators do?
   - **C** What is the value and impact of diabetes education on patient outcomes?

5. Find a definition of DSME that conveys your desired message clearly. A commonly used definition is "Diabetes self-management education (including medical nutrition therapy) is an interactive, collaborative, ongoing process involving the person with diabetes and the educator."[51] It is a 4-step process that requires the following:
   - **A** Assessing the individual's education needs
   - **B** Identifying the individual's specific diabetes self-management goals

    C Educating the individual to achieve identified self-management goals
    D Evaluating the attainment of goals

6. Build good customer relations with key customers. Become a reliable source of information so they see diabetes educators as friends and partners in care.
    A Communicate regularly.
    B Keep physicians informed about their individual patients.
    C Report program outcomes to key payers and providers on an annual basis.
    D Advocate for physicians with patients.
    E Advocate for patients with physicians.
    F Offer diabetes updates for referring physicians' staff.
    G Maintain a good relationship with referral staff.

7. Share successful outcomes.
    A Use real success stories when creating marketing materials. The public needs to know that your service is the best they can find in the market area.
    B Use outcomes data and patient stories about how they benefited from DSME services.
    C Prepare messages that are targeted for specific audiences.
    D Use Diabetes Advisory Committee reports to provide helpful information about your services.

8. To emphasize that you have a quality program, tell customers about any awards your program has received, either internally or externally. If you have received ADA Education Program Recognition Status, use that as a way to promote the quality of your program. Share the successes of your staff, who are your greatest assets, because their professional accomplishments are a reflection of the overall quality of the program.

9. When developing a proposal for contracting with a payer or provider, include the following key elements:
    A Cover letter
    B Description of the current situation and challenges of diabetes care
    C Value of DSME
    D National Standards for DSME
    E Studies (2 or 3) on the effectiveness of DSME
    F Specific information about your program
    G ADA Recognition Certificate if you have received it
    H Clinical outcomes data from your program
    I Strong closing statement about the overall benefits of using your services
    J An explanation of what the customer gets out of your program

10. Additional promotional strategies that can be used are
    A Give professional presentations
    B Offer an Open House at the education center
    C Make services portable
    D Attend social functions where customers are
    E Invite customers to lunch
    F Participate in Doctor's Day at your local hospital by planning a special event

G Take snacks to the physicians' lounge at the hospital
H Invite physicians, payers, or their staff to observe a class
I Present your program at nurse practitioner meetings
J Have business cards and brochures available in the emergency department
K Have face-to-face appointments with customers
L Develop a targeted proposal for customers that addresses their needs
M Build an alliance with pharmaceutical representatives

Key Educational Considerations

1 Successful diabetes education programs require the leadership of individuals who have both the clinical knowledge about diabetes care as well the business skills of program management.

2 Applying a systematic approach to starting a diabetes education program is likely to result in desired programmatic and patient outcomes.

3 Using a continuous quality improvement (CQI) process can result in more effective DSME programs.

Self-Review Questions

1 Explain 3 reasons why diabetes self-management programs are started.
2 What is the first step in starting a program?
3 Identify the components of a business plan for a new diabetes education program.
4 What are resources that can be used to conduct a community assessment?
5 How do you identify the resources you will need to start a new diabetes education program?
6 How do you identify the type and number of staff needed to create a diabetes education team?
7 Describe the eligibility criteria for applying to the ADA Education Recognition Program.
8 Explain how to develop a budget for starting a diabetes education program, provide a rationale for the administration, and describe the components that need to be included in developing the budget.
9 Who should be invited to be part of the advisory group?
10 Describe how to conduct a cost analysis of program services.
11 You are planning to apply for ADA ERP status and need to initiate a CQI effort. How would you identify the problem/opportunity for CQI?
12 How do you decide what outcomes data to capture to prove the program's effectiveness?
13 Aside from internal CQI and data review, what are other ways to determine program effectiveness?
14 Describe the difference between a leader and a manager.

Learning Assessment: Case Study 1

MK is an RN in a primary care group practice with a large diabetes patient population. MK has gradually begun providing diabetes education to many of the patients. Over the last 3 years MK has attended several continuing education programs on diabetes and has begun to develop a plan for teaching, as well as acquire many free educational resources. Although MK's knowledge and experience have increased significantly, MK realized that the patients needed more education about the nutritional management of their diabetes than she was able to give them. So MK convinced the physicians to contract with a local registered dietitian, BT, to join her 2 days a week for ongoing patient education. In the last 4 months since BT joined the practice they are seeing more patients. The patients and MK's physician employers are expressing satisfaction with the increasing quality of the service, but they are concerned that patients need to wait as long as 3 weeks to see MK and up to 6 weeks to see BT. Both MK and BT would like to expand the program and add more RD hours, but they realize that they need to show that they can get reimbursed for the service before they can convince the practice to hire a dietitian on a full-time basis. With the support of the physicians, they decide to work toward getting ADA Education Recognition for their diabetes education program, which they need to be eligible to bill Medicare as well as some other commercial payers.

Questions for Discussion

1 How should MK begin the process of getting their program recognized by the American Diabetes Association?
2 What are some key operational steps that MK needs to coordinate to successfully achieve ADA Education Recognition?

Discussion

1 MK begins by downloading the criteria for the application for ADA Recognition from the ADA Web site (*www.diabetes.org*). She also carefully reviews the National Standards for Diabetes Self-Management Education. Realizing there is a considerable amount of work to do, MK begins by creating a checklist of actions that need to occur for their program to meet the requirements. After assessing the existing program, MK determines that they already have many of the components necessary for ADA Recognition. MK knows that they have organizational support and that there clearly is a demand for their services, but they have not really analyzed their population and its needs nor have they evaluated the effectiveness of their services. They have the required minimum team with an RN and an RD. Since neither of them has yet gotten their CDE, they make plans to attend several continuing education programs on diabetes that will give them their required hours.

2 Some of the key activities included on MK's checklist are
   A Analysis of target population. It was difficult to determine an accurate number of patients with diabetes in the practice. However, through querying the database for ICD-9 codes 250.0 to 250.9 for diabetes, MK was able to determine that there were at least 800 active patients in their practice with diabetes. Determining the type of diabetes was more difficult, but because the average age of these patients was 53 MK surmised from personal experience that most of these patients had type 2 diabetes. Many of these individuals work, and MK realized that time away from work could be a potential barrier for people's ability to attend multiple educational sessions.
   B MK asked BT to research how to develop a curriculum as well as review predeveloped curriculums. They found that there were several commercially marketed

programs that met the National Standards and seemed easy to customize to their population. MK decided to recommend using a predeveloped curriculum rather than spend the time developing one.

C As MK and BT began working on the plan for the curriculum, MK began to identify the membership for an advisory group. It was important for the group to be composed of individuals who could fulfill the responsibilities and functions defined in both the National Standards and the ADA Recognition application. The advisory group needed to represent program staff as well as key stakeholders for the program service. After discussing the matter with the physicians and BT, it was decided that the group would consist of MK as program coordinator, one of the physicians from the practice, a patient MK had previously taught, a local endocrinologist, a podiatrist, and a pharmacist from one of the local retail pharmacies.

D At their first meeting, MK presented a draft program plan that included a mission, objectives, and goals for the first year. MK also presented for their review and approval the commercially prepared curriculum that they had customized to their population. The curriculum had included some template chart forms such as an assessment and patient education checklist that they customized for their required documentation.

E At the second meeting of the advisory group, the final touches on the program were reviewed and approved. They were going to offer a series of 4 weekly 2-hour group education programs targeted at persons with type 2 diabetes and based on their new curriculum. Because most of their population worked, they would offer both daytime and evening classes in alternating months. All attendees would receive a 1-hour individual assessment by the dietitian prior to starting class. They would continue to see patients for individual teaching on specific topics such as insulin starts and pattern management based on patient needs and medical necessity.

F The most challenging activity was establishing a data collection process so they could review their services and identify opportunities for improvement. Because their numbers were relatively small, they chose to collect the data manually at first, keeping a record of required elements for each patient. MK developed a tracking form and both she and BT would share responsibility for keeping it current. Their plan was to make it a part of the work process to complete this data-gathering tool at the end of each class or individual visit.

G Through discussion at the third advisory group meeting, MK and the group identified 2 areas that they would monitor as a CQI effort: HbA1c and participants' changes in physical activity behavior. The physicians in their practice were consistent about getting HbA1c measurements on their patients at least every 6 months, so these data would be abstracted from the medical records. They decided to use the D-SMART self-report instrument to capture data on patient behavior. They would have patients complete this form before beginning their education and then again at their 6-month and 12-month office visits. This approach would allow them to capture and report data on behavior change as well as assess patients' needs for additional education on an ongoing basis.

H MK and her team members completed everything on her original action plan in 6 months. As they began their first class under the new structure, MK and BT were already making plans to sit for the CDE exam during the next year since they would both have their required 1000 hours by then. Although there was still much to do before sending in the ADA Education Recognition Program application, they were well on the way to making this happen.

Learning Assessment: Case Study 2
ST is the program coordinator of an ADA recognized education program and has identified the need to implement a formal CQI effort for their program services. Although a variety of data have been collected over the years, they have not really used the data in a coordinated quality improvement initiative. ST has read several articles on CQI and reviewed the JCAHO materials on choosing and evaluating performance measures. After gathering information on the process and some QI tools that would be useful, ST prepares to initiate the CQI. ST has scheduled an end-of-the-year advisory board meeting and prepares to make this effort a major focus of the agenda.

Questions for Discussion
1 What are the essential steps in the CQI process that ST will need to coordinate to address the effectiveness of their services based on one behavioral outcome of participants?
2 Describe the documentation ST may to develop, maintain, and use for analysis and how she would present this plan to the advisory board.

Discussion
1 ST knows that the important first step in the CQI process is to identify the problem or the opportunity (step 1). She begins to collect some data about the program services that will provide a baseline analysis of the program's current status. Fortunately, she had already begun collecting some data and routinely entering the data into the department database. She created a summary report from the data and presented it to the Diabetes Advisory Committee for their review. This allowed the advisory committee to analyze the data and identify 1 or 2 areas of their program that could benefit from some improvement (step 2 in the CQI process).

2 The summary report included the following information:
   A Number of patients and visits by specific service, type of diabetes, and total
   B Financial summary specified by service and total
   C Outcomes
     • Educational: knowledge
     • Behavioral: physical activity, nutrition, medication-taking, monitoring, problem-solving, risk-reduction behavior, and psychosocial adaptation behaviors
     • Clinical: HbA1c, blood pressure, infant birth weights for women with GDM
   D Data on patient satisfaction, hospitalizations, emergency department visits, and days missed from work or school related to diabetes

3 The summary of data revealed that 95% of participants in the program service were satisfied, had experienced significant learning, were making modest but successful changes in behavior, and had an average 1.2% decrease in HbA1c, as well as impressive lack of hospitalizations, emergency department visits, or missed work or school days. Overall, the advisory committee was very pleased with the effectiveness of the services. They noted that the number of people who were performing foot self-exams at 6 months after service was only 23% and that blood pressure was not being

rechecked consistently on patients who had baseline hypertension (step 3). The advisory committee recommended focusing the CQI effort on the group program for type 2 diabetes, the foot care aspect of the program, and the section on risk reduction concerning hypertension. They also asked ST to determine why staff were not rechecking blood pressure and to identify a process change that would improve this situation.

4 ST reviewed the findings and the advisory board's analysis with her staff, and they considered several options for improvement in these 2 areas (step 4).

A The recommended program changes were to begin incorporating the use of monofilaments in teaching foot self-exams and to perform foot exams as part of the session on foot care. The reports from these exams would be shared with both the patient and the patient's physician.

B The second recommendation was to include a more comprehensive educational session on risk-reduction behaviors, such as controlling blood pressure, medication adherence, food choices, participating in weight-management programs, and appropriate physical activity. The staff determined that blood pressure was not being rechecked consistently because of time constraints and the fact that not all of the multidisciplinary staff were confident in their skills in this area. They agreed to consistently recheck blood pressure on all participants who had baseline hypertension, controlled or not (step 5). ST provided competency training in measuring blood pressure for those staff who expressed a lack of confidence and also purchased a blood pressure machine to assist staff in being able to routinely and efficiently perform this procedure. These recommendations were approved by the advisory committee and implemented (step 6).

5 ST and staff started to implement the program changes that had been outlined and captured the data on an ongoing basis so they could evaluate the effect of these changes. At 6 months postimplementation, the staff and the advisory committee reviewed the data again and the program changes were evaluated for their degree of success (step 7). The evaluation showed that 62% of participants now reported they were performing foot self-exams and were using the monofilaments that had been provided by the diabetes center staff. Participants who reported or were assessed to have hypertension at baseline were now being rechecked at follow-up visits 91% of the time, although there had been no appreciable change in their blood pressure readings from baseline. Patients' behavior related to hypertension indicated that 82% returned to their doctor for reevaluation of their blood pressure every 3 months, medication adherence was reported at 89%, and participation in weight-management programs was 53% for appropriate participants.

6 ST, the advisory committee, and the entire staff determined that the program changes had resulted in an overall improvement (step 8) and that they would continue to reevaluate and monitor the effectiveness of their interventions.

References

1. Reis A, Trout L. Positioning: The Battle for Your Mind. 3rd ed. New York: McGraw-Hill; 2000.

2. Mensing C, Boucher J, Cypress M, et al. National standards for diabetes self-management education. Diabetes Care. 2000;23:682-689.

3. Fox CH, Mahoney MC. Improving diabetes preventive care in a family practice residency program: a case study in continuous quality improvement. Fam Med. 1998;30:441-445.

4. Gilroth BE. Management of patient education in US hospitals: evolution of a concept. Patient Educ Couns. 1990;15:101-111.

5. Heins TM, Nord WR, Cameron M. Establishing and sustaining state-of-the-art diabetes education programs: research and recommendations. Diabetes Educ. 1992;18:501-508.

6. Mangan M. Diabetes self-management education programs in the Veterans Health Administration. Diabetes Educ. 1997;23:687-695.

7. Joint Commission on Accreditation of Health Care Organizations. Framework for Improving Performance. Oakbrook Terrace, Ill: Joint Commission on Accreditation of Health Care Organizations; 1994.

8. Health Care Financing Administration. Medicare program: expanded coverage for outpatient diabetes self-management training and diabetes measurements. Federal Register. December 29, 2000.

9. Centers for Disease Control and Prevention. Team Care: Comprehensive Lifetime Management for Diabetes. Atlanta, Ga: US Department of Health and Human Services, Public Health Service, Centers for Disease Control and Prevention, National Center for Chronic Disease Prevention and Health Promotion; 2001.

10. Young-Hyman D. Provider impact in diabetes education: what we know, what we would like to know, paradigms for asking. Diabetes Educ. 1999;25:6(suppl):34-42.

11. Mulcahy K. Architects of the diabetes team. Diabetes Educ. 1999;25:161-162.

12. Humphry J, Jameson LM, Beckman S. Overcoming social and cultural barriers to care for patients with diabetes. West J Med. 1997;167:138-144.

13. Corkery E, Palmer C, Foley ME, Schechter CB, Frisher L, Roman SH. Effect of a bicultural community health worker on completion of diabetes education in a Hispanic population. Diabetes Care. 1997;20:254-257.

14. Aubert RE, Herman WH, Waters J, et al. Nurse case management to improve glycemic control in diabetic patients in a health maintenance organization. Ann Intern Med. 1998;129:605-612.

15. Franz MJ, Monk A, Barry B, et al. Effectiveness of medical nutrition therapy provided by dietitians in the management of non-insulin-dependent diabetes mellitus: a randomized, controlled trial. J Am Diet Assoc. 1995;95:1009-1017.

16. Abourizk NM, O'Conner PJ, Crabtree BF, Schnatz JD. An outpatient model of integrated diabetes treatment and education: functional, metabolic, and knowledge outcomes. Diabetes Educ. 1994;20:416-421.

17. Etzweiler D. Chronic care: a need in search of a system. Diabetes Educ. 1997;23:569-573.

18. Shamoon H, Vaccaro-Olko MI. Diabetes Education Teams. Professional Education in Diabetes: Proceedings of the DRTC Conference. Bethesda, Md: National Diabetes Information Clearinghouse and National Institute of Diabetes and Digestive and Kidney Disorders, National Institute of Health, December 1980.

19. Koproski I, Pretto Z, Poretsky L. Effects of an intervention by a diabetes team in hospitalized patients with diabetes. Diabetes Care. 1997;20:1553-1555.

20. Levetan CS, Salas JR, Wilets IF. Impact of endocrine and diabetes team consultation on hospital length of stay for patients with diabetes. Am J Med. 1995;99:22-28.

21. American Diabetes Association. ADA Education Recognition Program. Available on the internet at: *www.diabetes.org*. Accessed June 2000.

22. Mornell P, Dunnick R. 45 Effective Ways for Hiring Smart! How to Predict Winners and Losers in the Incredibly People-Reading Game. New York: Ten Speed Press; 1998.

23. Rickheim PL, Weaver TW, Flader J. Group versus individual education: A randomized study. Submitted for publication.

24. Ritchie JB. Thompson, P. Organization and People. St. Paul, Minn: West Publishing Company; 1984.

25. Tecker G, Kermit E, Frankel I. Building a Knowledge-Based Culture. Washington, DC: American Society of Association Executives; 1997.

26. Manske FA. Secrets of Effective Leadership: A Practical Guide to Success. Columbia, Tenn: Leadership Education and Development Inc; 1999.

27. Myers B. Introduction to Type. 6th ed. Palo Alto, Calif: Consulting Psychologists Press; 1998.

28. McGinnis AL. Bringing Out the Best in People. Minneapolis, Minn: Augsburg Publishing House; 1985.

29. Drucker P. The Leader of the Future. San Francisco: Jossey-Bass; 1996.

30. DePree M. Leadership is an Art. New York: Dell Publishing; 1989.

31. Deming WE. Out of Crisis. Cambridge, Mass: MIT-CAES; 1986.

32. Juran JM. Juran's Quality Control Handbook. 4th ed. New York: McGraw-Hill; 1988.

33. Juran TM. Reengineering Processes for Competitive Advantage: Business Process Quality Management. Wilton, Conn: Juran Institute; 1994.

34. Donabedian A. The Definition of Quality: A Conceptual Exploration. Ann Arbor, Mich: Health Administration Press; 1980.

35. US Department of Health and Human Services, Agency for Health Care Policy and Research. Washington, DC: US Department of Health and Human Services, 1995; DHHS Publication 95-0045.

36. Anderson RM, Fitzgerald IT, Wisdom K, Davis WK, Hiss RU. A comparison of global versus disease-specific quality of life measures in patients with diabetes. Diabetes Care. 1997;20:299-305.

37. Ware JEJ, Sherbourne CD. The MOS 36-item short-form health survey (SF-36): conceptual framework and item changes. Med Care. 1992;30:473-483.

38. Polonsky WH, Welch GM. Listeing to our patient's concerns: understanding and addressing diabetes-specific emotional distress. Diabetes Spectrum. 1999;9:8-11.

39. Mulcahy KA, Peeples M, Tomky D, Weaver T, Upham P. National Diabetes Education Outcomes System: application to practice. Diabetes Educ. 2000;26:957-964.

40. American Association of Diabetes Educators. Diabetes educational and behavioral research summit. Diabetes Educ. 1999;25(suppl):2-88.

41. Peyrot M. Evaluation of patient education programs: how to do it and how to use it. Diabetes Spectrum. 1996;9:86-93.

42. Brown SA. Predicting metabolic control in diabetes: a pilot study using meta-analysis to estimate a linear model. Nurs Res. 1994;43:362-368.

43. Glasgow R. Evaluating diabetes education. Diabetes Care. 1992;15:1423-1432.

44. McGlynn E. Choosing and evaluating clinical performance measures. Joint Commission. 1998;24:470-479.

45. Peyrot M, Rubin R. Modeling the effect of diabetes education on glycemic control. Diabetes Educ. 1994;20:143-148.

46. Horn SD, Hopkins DSP. Clinical Practice Improvement: A New Technology for Developing Cost-Effective Quality Care. New York: Faulkner & Gray; 1994.

47 Tomky D, Weaver T, Mulcahy K, Peeples M. Diabetes education outcomes: what educators are doing. Diabetes Educ. 2000;26:951-954.

48 Weaver T. Measuring outcomes: what, when, why, and how. On the Cutting Edge [Diabetes Care and Education Practice Group, The American Dietetic Association]. 2000;21(4):6-8.

49 Peeples M, Mulcahy K, Tomky D, Weaver T. National Diabetes Education Outcomes System: a conceptual framework. Diabetes Educ. 2001;27:547-562.

50 American Association of Diabetes Educators. AADE 2000 Member Resource Guide. Chicago, Ill: American Association of Diabetes Educators; 2000.

51 American Diabetes Association Task Force. Report of the Task Force on the Delivery of Diabetes Self-Management Education and Medical Nutrition Therapy. Diabetes Spectrum. 1999;12:44-47.

Suggested Readings

American Association of Diabetes Educators. Diabetes educational and behavioral research summit. Diabetes Educ. 1999;25(suppl):2-88.

American Diabetes Association. ADA Education Recognition Program. Available on the Internet at: *www.diabetes.org*. Accessed June 2001.

Abourizk NN, O'Conner PJ, Crabtree BF, Schnatz JD. An outpatient model of integrated diabetes treatment and education: functional, metabolic, and knowledge outcomes. Diabetes Educ. 1994;20:416-421.

American Diabetes Association Task Force. Report of the Task Force on the Delivery and Diabetes Self-Management and Medical Nutrition Therapy. Diabetes Spectrum. 1999;12:44-47.

Blanchard K. The Heart of a Leader. Tulsa, Okla: Honor Books; 1999.

DePree M. Leadership is an Art. New York: Dell Publishing; 1989.

Drucker P. The Leader of the Future. San Francisco: Jossey-Bass; 1996.

Maxwell JC. The 21 Indispensable Qualities of a Leader. Nashville, Tenn: Thomas Nelson Publisher; 1999.

McGlynn E. Choosing and evaluating clinical performance measures. Joint Commission. 1998;24:470-479.

Mensing C, Boucher J, Cypress M, et al. National standards for diabetes self-management education. Diabetes Care. 2000;23:682-689.

Peyrot M. Evaluation of patient education programs: how to do it and how to use it. Diabetes Spectrum. 1996;9:86-93.

Tecker G, Kermit E, Frankel J. Building a Knowledge-Based Culture. Washington, DC: American Society of Association Executives; 1997.

US Department of Health and Human Services, Agency for Health Care Policy and Research. Washington DC: US Department of Health and Human Services, 1995; DHHS Publication 95-0045.

Learning Assessment: Post-Test Questions

Management of Diabetes Education Programs   7

1. A market analysis for starting a diabetes self-management education program must include which of the following components?
   A Assessment of organization's strengths/weaknesses
   B Marketing plan
   C Competitive analysis
   D All of the above

2. The National Standards for Diabetes Self-Management Education are designed for:
   A Physician office practice settings
   B Hospital-based education programs
   C Home care education programs
   D All of the above

3. A useful resource for determining the target population is:
   A *The Diabetes Educator* journal
   B The county statistics database
   C The ADA Web site
   D All of the above

4. Based on the National Standards for Diabetes Self-Management Education, the team should consist of which of the following healthcare professionals?
   A Physician, registered nurse, and registered dietitian
   B Pharmacist, registered dietitian, and registered nurse
   C Registered nurse, registered dietitian, and community health worker
   D All of the above

5. You have a full-time RD and RN to provide diabetes education for your patient population. The RN has some committee responsibilities that take about 2 hours per week, and she is also responsible for overseeing the QI program, which takes about 4 hours per week. The RD also serves on some required committees that require 1 to 2 hours per week, and she coordinates the department standards, which takes her 2 hours per week. In addition, both educators need approximately 5 hours per week to return patient and physician phone calls and another 5 hours for documentation. Allowing for lunch or dinner breaks, the maximum number of patients that could be seen at this center are:
   A 40 individual 1-hour patient visits per week
   B 100 patients seen in ten 2-hour group sessions, plus 20 individual 1-hour patient visits per week
   C 50 patients seen in five 2-hour sessions, 30 patients seen in three 3-hour sessions, and 21 individual 1-hour patient visits per week
   D All of the above

6. When developing a budget for your program, you should include all of the following except:
   A Staff salaries
   B Continuing education expense
   C Benefits
   D Position descriptions

7. An annual plan should include:
   A Program objectives
   B Action plan
   C Target dates
   D All of the above

8 The culture of an organization has which of the following characteristics?
   A Words rather than the behavior of the CEO produce the organizational culture
   B The culture of an organization is permanent and never changes
   C Changing the organizational culture is one of the most difficult challenges for leaders
   D All of the above

9 Strategic planning provides the following:
   A Clear direction for the organization
   B Purpose and reason for the organization's existence
   C Opportunity for employees to benchmark their own performance
   D All of the above

10 Examples of team building activities are:
   A Staff meeting
   B Myers-Briggs Type Indicator (MBTI)
   C Individual counseling
   D None of the above

11 Outcomes are defined as measurable change over time. Which of the following are outcome measurements?
   A Average age of participants
   B Baseline participant behavior
   C Preprogram/postprogram HbA1c measurements
   D All of the above

12 Quality management is a philosophy that embodies which of the following ways of thinking?
   A Problems in quality are usually employee related
   B Quality costs more
   C Quality is a long-term investment
   D All of the above

See next page for answer key.

Post-Test Answer Key

Management of Diabetes Education Programs 7

1. D
2. D
3. B
4. D
5. D
6. D
7. D
8. C
9. D
10. B
11. C
12. C

A Core Curriculum for Diabetes Education
Diabetes Education and Program Management

Payment for Diabetes Education — 8

Jan Norman, RD, CDE
Washington Department of Health
Diabetes Control Program
Olympia, Washington

Susan L Barlow, RD, CDE
Amylin Pharmaceuticals, Inc.
Indianapolis, Indiana

Introduction

1 Diabetes educators who understand reimbursement policies of the major plans provide a valuable resource to their patients for accessing healthcare services. An important content area from the National Standards for Diabetes Self-Management Education (DSME)[1] concerns teaching individuals with diabetes how to use the healthcare system and understand their entitlement to benefits for diabetes. This is an area that should be taught to individuals once basic management skills have been taught.

2 Private payors cover all types of healthcare problems and persons of all ages. Public payors cover specific populations established by federal or state laws. Understanding the variety of payors and the types of plans improves understanding of reimbursement. Each plan establishes conditions for coverage that include eligibility, medical necessity, authorization, and definition of benefits, coding, payment rates, documentation requirements, and utilization controls.

3 The Centers for Medicare and Medicare Services (CMS), formerly known as the Health Care Financing Administration (HCFA), changed coverage for diabetes education services and supplies as part of the Balanced Budget Act in 1997. The final mandate for coverage of diabetes education services was enacted in early 2001, and all practicing educators should be familiar with the guidelines for reimbursement of diabetes education and supplies.[2,3] Medicare's diabetes education benefit requires the diabetes education provided by Medicare certified providers to meet the National Standards for Diabetes Education.

4 Nearly all states require health insurance policies and managed-care plans to provide coverage for diabetes education and supplies in addition to that provided by CMS (formerly HCFA) to Medicare patients. Commercial payors are subject to the laws in the state in which the policy is sold or delivered. Therefore, it is important for diabetes educators to know the laws in their state so they can teach their patients about these benefits and how to access them.

5 A claim that is submitted is not automatically paid. Documentation and eligibility requirements must be met, and appropriate justification must be provided in the claims submission process. The actual amount reimbursed for diabetes education or supplies is subject to a complex structure of rules and regulations designed to prevent fraud and abuse and to ensure payment only for justifiable claims.

Objectives
Upon completion of this chapter, the learner will be able to
1 Describe the public and private payor mix of healthcare coverage, including who they are, their target population and how their plans are administered.
2 Define the elements that determine coverage, such as eligibility, exclusions, medical necessity, and coding.
3 Explain the 4 different coding methods, when and how they are used, and how they determine payment.
4 Describe the current Medicare regulation for reimbursement for diabetes education and supplies.

5 Summarize the state laws for coverage of diabetes education and supplies.
6 Identify the role of the regulation process in defining coverage policy.
7 Describe the steps in the claims process for reimbursement, identifying the key role of the diabetes educator in each step and the appropriate documentation needed to obtain payment.

The Payor Mix

1 "[The] United States spends more on health-related services than does any other nation. In 1998, it spent more than one trillion dollars on health care, or almost 14% of the gross domestic product."[4] The flow of these healthcare dollars is managed through 4 categories of participants:
   A *Purchasers* (those who purchase health care): individuals, their employers, and/or the government
   B *Consumers* (those who receive health care): policy holders, beneficiaries
   C *Providers* (those who provide health care): individuals (physicians, other healthcare providers) and the entities that employ or contract with them (hospitals, outpatient clinics, physician practices, durable medical equipment suppliers)
   D *Payors* (those who assume the financial risk of health claim losses and/or administering reimbursement for healthcare claims): Medicare, Medicaid, private insurance companies

2 No single nationwide system of health insurance exists to cushion the expenses of health care to consumers. Which payors reimburse for health care varies by the type of service provided and the type of consumers they serve. The percentage of health services paid by payors and consumers are shown in Table 8.1.[5] Consumers may pay as little as 3.3% of hospital care but as much as 32.5% of nursing home care. Payors have a central role in the reimbursement process, assuming much of the financial risk and thus creating many of the rules that govern this process.

3 The distinction between public (government) and private payors is important in understanding the reimbursement industry. The payor mix for the nation as a whole, based on what proportion of the US healthcare dollar is paid by each payor, is shown in Figure 8.1.[5]
   A *Public payors* include federal and state programs that target specific segments of the population. The largest of these programs are Medicare and Medicaid, but there are also a variety of smaller programs.
   B *Private payors* consist mainly of private insurance companies and self-insured employers.
   C The proportion of public and private payors for the population of healthcare purchasers varies by state and locale and is referred to as the *payor mix*.

Public Payors: Federal and State

1 Public payors include federal and state government programs that target specific populations.

Table 8.1. Percentage of Health Services Paid by Payors and Consumers

Service	Payors			Consumers
	Federal Government	State/Local Government	Private Insurance	Out-of-Pocket
Hospital care	49%	11.9%	30.8%	3.3%
Physician services	26.5%	5.4%	50.5%	15.6%
Home health care	44.7%	8.2%	13.7%	20.5%
Nursing home care	40.3%	20.2%	5.4%	32.5%

Source: Centers for Medicare and Medicare Services 1998 estimates.

Figure 8.1. Payor Mix of the US Healthcare Dollar

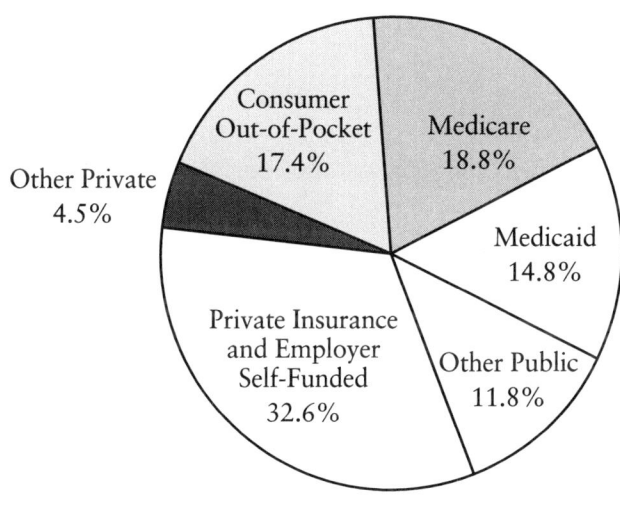

Source: Centers for Medicare and Medicare Services 1998 estimates. "Other public" includes workers' compensation, public health activities, and state/local hospital and school health programs. "Other private" includes in-plant services and charitable funding.

2 The CMS (formerly HCFA) has recently been divided into 3 centers of service:
- Center for Beneficiary Choices (Medicare + Choice, beneficiary information)
- Center for Medicare Management (fee-for-service programs)
- Center for Medicaid and State Operations (all programs administered by states)

A *Medicare* is a federal entitlement program administered by the CMS that provides healthcare coverage for people 65 years and older, people of any age who are permanently disabled, and anyone with end-stage renal disease. Medicare benefits are divided into Part A, Part B, and Part C.

- Part A covers inpatient services of a hospital, skilled nursing facility, home agency, or hospice. Beneficiaries must pay deductibles and coinsurance when seeking covered benefits.
- Part B covers services provided by physicians and other specific providers, outpatient clinics, and labs as well as supplies and equipment. Part B is elective, funded by monthly premiums of approximately $45, and subject to deductibles and coinsurance.
- Part C, or Medicare + Choice, offers Medicare beneficiaries the option of joining a managed-care plan that provides services at least equal to Parts A and B plus other selected preventive benefits. Beneficiaries continue to pay their monthly premium for Medicare Part B but give up their right to seek treatment from fee-for-service providers. Medicare + Choice plans are not available in all areas of the country.

B *Medicaid* is primarily a state-administered program that provides healthcare coverage for specific groups of low-income and needy people: families with children; people who are aged, blind, or disabled; and people with federally assisted income maintenance payments.

C The *Veterans Administration* provides medical care, long-term care, and support services to veterans who served in the active military, have a service-related disability, have served in specific wars, suffer from environmental exposure to contaminants, or are designated as low income. Care is provided free of charge to the extent that it is available. Other veterans receive medical services with a coinsurance payment.

D The *Indian Health Service* provides personal and public health services to American Indians and Alaska Natives in federally recognized tribes. Services are provided free of charge.

E The *Federal Employees Health Benefit Program* provides healthcare coverage for federal workers, retirees, and their dependents through contracts with 400 private health plans operating across the country. The program establishes minimum benefits that each plan must cover, including diabetes education, equipment, and supplies. Group health insurance plans of the federal government are not subject to state coverage mandates.

F The *Bureau of Primary Health Care* offers medical services to underserved and vulnerable people with financial, geographic, or cultural barriers to accessing health care. Care is available on a sliding-scale fee through federally qualified health centers or rural health centers.

G *TRICARE* is a healthcare program that provides coverage for active duty and retired members of military service, their families, and their survivors through the medical facilities of all branches of the service and networks of civilian healthcare professionals. Three choices are offered: TRICARE Prime, TRICARE Extra, and TRICARE Standard (formerly Civilian Health and Medical Program of the Uniformed Services, or CHAMPUS).

Private Payors

1 Commercial (private) payors are for-profit and not-for-profit insurers that sell policies to individuals and groups to cover specific healthcare services and supplies. Included in this private payor category is self-funded employer plans. The payor assumes the financial risk of health claim losses of the individuals insured by the health plan.

A *Individual policies*, or policies covering a single family, can be obtained from insurers or managed-care plans. Consumers pay their premiums direct to the carrier and select their policy from those offered by the insurer. The range of policies offered to individuals can vary by the amount of deductibles, coinsurance requirements, and applicable premiums.

B *Group policies* are far more common, accounting for about three fourths of individuals covered by health insurance. Group policies are incorporated into an employer's total benefit package. Premiums can be paid in full by the employer or shared between the employer and the employee. Smaller employer-sponsored group health plans typically purchase coverage from a selection of policies assembled by insurers or managed-care providers. The premium cost of these plans varies based on annual deductible, coinsurance, or copayment amounts. Larger employer-sponsored plans have the bargaining power to tailor their plan benefits to suit their group needs.

C *Employer self-funded/self-insured plans* were created by Congress through the Employee Retirement Income Security Act (ERISA) and are regulated by the United States Department of Labor. Employers pay the expenses for the covered services of their employees and dependents, dollar-for-dollar, and hire a plan administrator to collect the claims and pay the bills. ERISA plans comprise approximately half of all employer-sponsored health insurance plans. These plans do not have to offer benefits that are required by state mandate laws. Therefore, about half of the insurance plans in a state are exempt from following any state mandate law that requires plans cover diabetes education or supplies.

2 Consumers are often covered by more than one benefit plan (primary and secondary payor coverage). For example, a retired person may have Medicare plus supplemental insurance, or a married couple may each have their own employer coverage and be covered secondarily by the spousal plan. In this instance, one is considered the primary payor and the other is the secondary payor. When claims are filed, the primary payor pays first. The secondary payor considers for reimbursement only the remaining charges after the primary payor reimburses its covered expenses. The insurance industry has rules for determining the primary and secondary plan.

3 Preexisting conditions clauses exclude coverage for a health condition present before a policy takes effect. Federal law limits a preexisting condition exclusion generally to no more than 12 months. People who change from one health plan to another without a discontinuation in coverage of more than 63 days usually are not forced to comply with a preexisting-conditions waiting period in the new plan. This law is especially important for people with diabetes who want to change jobs without losing health benefits, or when the employer changes health plans for employees.

Types of Insurance Plans

1 *Indemnity or fee-for-service plans* indemnify, or reimburse, the insured for medical expenses incurred and typically require the completion and filing of claim forms.

A These health insurance policies generally allow healthcare consumers to receive services from their choice of medical provider, applying a deductible of $100 to $500 per calendar year to initial expenses. After the deductible is satisfied, these plans typically reimburse eligible expenses at 80%.

B Most plans cover a broad list of medical expenditures, including hospital expenses, surgical expenses, physician outpatient office visits, diagnostic X-ray and laboratory services, prescription drug expenses, and many other types of medical expenses including outpatient diabetes care and supplies when prescribed by a healthcare provider. The plans simply reimburse the insured person for the medical expenses incurred.

C Indemnity plans typically have the highest premiums but the fewest restrictions.

2 *Managed-care plans*, which are administered by health maintenance organizations (HMOs), place controls on the provider and the insured person as to what services are provided, under what circumstances the services are provided, and who can provide the service. Managed-care plans emphasize comprehensive (including preventive) care and typically have few exclusions, no deductibles, and nominal copayments.

3 Between these two extremes are a wide variety of plans that offer diverse controls in an attempt to control costs. Some of these plans include provider networks and point-of-service options. Common insurance plans, services offered, and cost controls are shown in Table 8.2.[5]

Table 8.2. Insurance Plans and Benefit Design Considerations

Provider Structure	Services Offered	Cost Controls	
Traditional fee-for-service	Services from any provider	Some screening for fraudulent claims	**INDEMNITY** Higher premiums Fewer restrictions Less cost control
Managed fee-for-service	Services from any provider	Precertification for some procedures	
Provider network (PPO)	Services from any provider but discounts for using a network of preferred providers	Discounts negotiated with providers Precertification for some procedures	
Point-of-service option (POS)	Enrolled in HMO but may use provider outside the network at additional cost	Utilization of services is managed Incentives to use network providers	More cost control Greater restrictions Lower premiums **MANAGED CARE**
Health maintenance organization (HMO)	Restrictions on providers, depending on model (some HMOs are provider-owned)	Utilization of services is managed	

Source: Reprinted with permission from the American Association of Diabetes Educators.[5]

Determinants of Diabetes Education and Supply Coverage

1 Regardless of who the payor is for the diabetes education service, everyone wants to make sure that the payment is legitimate, appropriate for the service rendered, and delivered to a person who is eligible for the service. For these reasons, many safeguards are put in place by third-party payors to ensure that they only pay for or deliver (in the case of HMOs) services that are specified in the insurance policy. Safeguards make certain that payments are for appropriate services.

2 The conditions of coverage control the amount of payment for diabetes services, care, education, or supplies. Payment is subject to conditions that are established by the third-party payor; these conditions define who is eligible for coverage. If these conditions are mandated by legislation or regulation, the payor must meet the requirements for coverage established in the language of the legislation or regulation. If that language is not specific, the payors can define conditions under which they will pay for services or supplies.

  A While the conditions under which payors grant coverage for diabetes education services and supplies vary greatly based on who the payor is, 3 concepts define the conditions under which payment will be made:
  - Where the service can be provided
  - Who may provide the service
  - Whether the service is reasonable and necessary for the patient's condition

  B Each third-party payor can define these criteria differently for the same service, which makes it difficult to gain a thorough understanding of the conditions of coverage. The 3 concepts are applied by CMS to the Medicare benefit for diabetes self-management training in the following ways:
  - Where can the service be provided? Diabetes education services can be provided in hospital outpatient departments, physician offices, durable medical equipment supplier facilities, and end-stage renal disease facilities.
  - Who may provide the service? Training may be provided by a physician, individual, or entity that (1) furnishes other services for which direct Medicare payment may be made; (2) is accredited by an accreditation organization approved by CMS to meet the National Standards for Diabetes Education or the CMS quality standards; and (3) provides documentation to CMS as requested, including diabetes outcome measurements determined by CMS. Although nurses and dietitians may deliver the education, the provider of the service to CMS is the person or entity (eg, a hospital) who gets paid for it.
  - Are the services reasonable and necessary for the patient's condition? CMS defines the conditions under which a patient can receive diabetes education, and this determines what medical condition must be present to receive the benefit.

3 *Eligibility* is one of the first decision points of coverage. The characteristics of the beneficiary (Medicare) or policy holder (private payor plans) determine coverage, such as age (people over 65 are eligible for Medicare), diagnostic category (type 1 diabetes), or type of medical treatment (people taking insulin).

4 *Covered benefits* are the specific types of medical services, procedures, equipment, or supplies that a medical plan will consider for reimbursement. Health plans have detailed stipulations that describe the circumstances under which they will reimburse.
  A Physician office visit: Medicare will pay for face-to-face visits only
  B Laboratory tests: Medicare will cover lab tests to diagnose symptoms but not for screening
  C Glucose monitors: some policies only cover meters for people using insulin
  D Supplies: reagent strips may be limited to specific brands, quantities, and distribution schedules

5 *Exclusions* are specific items listed in the plan benefit book that are excluded from coverage. Typically these include eyeglasses, dental work, cosmetic surgery, and investigational or experimental services. Other exclusions are those services, procedures, or supplies determined by the plan to be not medically necessary for all patients in that plan.

6 Interpretation of *medical necessity* determines the services or supplies that are not specifically excluded or included within a plan. They must be determined as medically necessary on an individual basis, usually by the plan medical director. Often healthcare consumers are provided rights to appeal a denial of coverage based on medical necessity. The procedures for these appeals are also found in the plan benefit manual. However, some states and Congress are examining the issue of patients' rights and considering establishing standardized procedures for disputing denials of coverage along with guarantees for an impartial hearing on the issue of medical necessity.

Coding

1 *Codes* are the language of reimbursement and are used to match services or items described on a claim form to the amount of payment that has been determined appropriate by the payor. *Coding systems* define medical diagnoses, symptoms, conditions, treatments, services, and supplies.[6] Proper coding ensures correct reimbursement for services, equipment, or supplies.

2 There are 4 coding systems that are organized into 2 categories for coding. These systems have been widely accepted by all the major payors.
  A Diagnosis codes are based on the International Classification of Disease (ICD)9 (9th edition) Clinical Modifications (CM)—ICD-9-CM (see Table 8.3). These codes
  • Identify why services, equipment, or supplies are ordered
  • Define specific diagnoses, symptoms, or conditions
  • Categorize diseases and injuries into 17 groups according to established criteria
  • Assign numeric codes with a description
  • Are revised every 10 years by the World Health Organization with annual updates published by CMS
  • Describe diabetes and its complications by codes 250.0 through 250.9. The fifth digit indicates type 1 or type 2 diabetes, and 250.03 describes diabetes mellitus without mention of complication, type 1, and uncontrolled.

Table 8.3. Overview of ICD-9-CM Codes for Diabetes

Basic Codes

250.0	Diabetes mellitus without mention of complication
250.1	Diabetes with ketoacidosis (no mention of coma)
250.2	Diabetes with hyperosmolarity (nonketotic coma)
250.3	Diabetes with other coma (diabetic coma with ketoacidosis, hypoglycemic coma, insulin coma NOS [nonspecified])
250.4	Diabetes with renal manifestations
250.5	Diabetes with ophthalmic manifestations
250.7	Diabetes with peripheral circulatory disorders
250.8	Diabetes with other specified manifestations
250.9	Diabetes with unspecified complication
648.0	Diabetes mellitus complicating pregnancy (conditions classifiable to code 250)
648.8	Abnormal glucose tolerance complicating pregnancy (gestational diabetes)

Fifth Digits

Category 250 requires the use of a fifth digit:

0	Type 2 or unspecified type, not stated as uncontrolled, even if the patient requires insulin
1	Type 1, not stated as uncontrolled
2	Type 2 or unspecified type, uncontrolled, even if the patient requires insulin
3	Type 1, uncontrolled

Examples

For example, inserting the fifth digit with category 250.0 yields:

250.00	Diabetes mellitus without mention of complication, type 2
250.01	Diabetes mellitus without mention of complication, type 1
250.02	Diabetes mellitus without mention of complication, type 2, uncontrolled
250.03	Diabetes mellitus without mention of complication, type 1, uncontrolled

Note: These examples are for illustrative purposes only. For more specific guidance, consult the ICD-9-CM code book.

■ *Procedure codes* are divided into 3 levels: Level I CMS Common Procedure Coding System (HCPCS, pronounced hick-picks) defined by Common Procedural Terminology (CPT) codes; Level II HCPCS for professional services, procedures, and supplies; and Level III state and local HCPCS codes.
  • Level I codes are for physician services and use CPT codes developed by the American Medical Association. The physician's standard CPT evaluation and management (E&M) coding scheme is shown in Table 8.4.[5] Level I codes (1) are 3-digit codes with a fourth digit that represents the edition of the code; (2) include evaluation and management codes (E&M) that describe face-to-face patient encounters to evaluate the patient's condition; (3) describe professional services related to surgery, radiology, lab services, and medicine; and (4) describe a provider's unique service and are essential for assigning payment for the complexity of the service delivered.

Table 8.4. Standard CPT Codes for Physician Evaluation and Management (E&M)

Office visit... which requires at least 2 of the 3 key components:	E&M Code				
	99211	99212	99213	99214	99215
History	NA*	Problem focused	Expanded problem focused	Detailed	Comprehensive
Examination	NA*	Problem focused	Expanded problem focused	Detailed	Comprehensive
Medical decision making	NA*	Straightforward	Low complexity	Moderate complexity	High complexity
Presenting problem(s)	Minimal	Self-limited or minor	Low to moderate severity	Moderate to high severity	Moderate to high severity
Time spent**	5 minutes performing or supervising services	10 minutes face-to-face with patient and/or family	15 minutes face-to-face with patient and/or family	25 minutes face-to-face with patient and/or family	40 minutes face-to-face with patient and/or family
Average reimbursement	$16	$30	$42	$64	$98

* May not require the presence of a physician.
** Time is *not* the criterion for determining the proper level of E&M code.
Source: Reprinted with permission from the American Association of Diabetes Educators.[5]

- Level II procedure codes include most services delivered by nonphysicians as well as diabetes equipment and supplies (HCPCS code A4253 is for blood glucose test or reagent strips for home blood glucose monitor, per 50 strips). Temporary national non-Medicare codes were established in 2000 to describe the services shown in Table 8.5. These codes are to be used by commercial payors.
- Level III state/local HCPCS procedure codes are for unique coverage. Payors developed these codes to handle unique aspects of their benefits.

3 All claims must have an ICD-9 code to indicate the problem, as well as a Level I, II, or III HCPCS code to delineate what service or supply was used to treat the problem.

Table 8.5. Temporary National Non-Medicare Codes

Code Number	Service
S9140	Diabetic management program, follow-up visit to non-MD provider
S9141	Diabetic management program, follow-up visit to MD provider
S9455	Diabetic management program, group session
S9460	Diabetic management program, nurse visit
S9465	Diabetic management program, dietitian visit
S9470	Nutritional counseling, dietitian visit

4 Medicare *diagnostic related groups* (DRGs) were also created by CMS. This coding system groups all of the services needed to treat a specific diagnosis in the hospital under one code connected to a reimbursement amount. Bundling services and supplies to cover a specific reason for a hospitalization is called the *prospective payment system*.

A The hospital completes a CMS 1450 claim form.

B Revenue codes are used to group services by type and location. Revenue code 942 is often used by hospitals to bill for diabetes education as a hospital outpatient service.

C ICD-9 codes are included on the CMS 1450 form to indicate why a service was performed.

D CPT and HCPCS codes can also be used on the CMS 1450 form. Medicare intermediaries process the form and determine the DRG for the specific coverage and the specific reimbursement amount.

Pricing of Payment for Services and Supplies

1 The amount that is reimbursed or paid for a service or supply is determined by the payors financial arrangement with the provider and the financial responsibility of the consumer. The following pricing arrangements define how much the payor will pay for a service, assuming that the coding is correct and the coverage and eligibility requirements have been met.

A Payment for *usual, customary reasonable charges* (UCR) is made based on the UCR charge in that geographic area for the service. Payment then is paid at a certain percentile of the service based on the benefit plan specifications. For example, CPT code 99214 (physician consultation and treatment for diabetes) is paid at 75% of the UCR of $64, or $48. UCR charges are adjusted periodically to account for inflation.

B *Fee schedules* are an alternative to UCR charges and are attached to services, equipment, and supplies at either the national or state level.

- State-established fee schedules can vary from state to state based on the cost of living in that area.
- CMS establishes a floor and ceiling payment for durable medical equipment codes, for example on blood glucose meters. For laboratory services, CMS establishes national limitation amounts, or a fee cap, that is the median of all the individual state fees for a particular test. Fee schedules established by CMS are required to

be adjusted according to the consumer price index. CMS can also adjust fees based on inherent reasonableness. In this case, the amount that CMS allows is adjusted when the allowed fee is either grossly above or below the market value.

C *Percent of charge* means that some payors will pay a fixed percent of a provider's charge as its allowed amount. For example, a provider may charge $12 for an in-office blood test. The payor will pay 75% of that charge, or $9. The patient's payment responsibility may also affect what the payor pays the provider.

D With *capitation* arrangements, services are not reimbursed individually. Providers are paid a monthly fee per member to deliver all of the services that a patient needs or that are defined by the managed-care contract. The capitation rate can be fixed or adjusted for age and sex based on actuarial projections. Providers can accept patients under full capitation (hospitalizations, lab tests, equipment, and supplies) or partial capitation (office visits). A stop-loss limit for providers identifies when the payor will take over the financial risk of the patient up to the maximum benefit in the patient's plan.

E *Maximum benefit* means that payors establish in policies a lifetime maximum dollar amount they will reimburse for an individual policyholder. This protects the payor from catastrophic medical expenses. For example, the maximum benefit could be $1 million. Once this amount is reached, additional claims will be denied. Maximum benefits can also be established for specific services. For example, a $500 maximum allowable benefit for diabetes education services could be included in the benefit plan.

Consumer's Responsibilities

1 Most health plans require patients to share in the cost of their health care through several different ways.

A A *deductible* is usually required in fee-for-service or indemnity plans. Consumers must pay the first expenses each calendar year before reimbursement begins. Usually, the higher the deductible in a policy, the lower the premium is for the health plan. Deductibles are also a part of the Medicare program. For example, with Medicare Part B (outpatient and physician services), the patient is responsible for the first $100 of medical costs before Medicare begins coverage. Medicare Part A requires the patient to pay a deductible of $765 for each hospitalization.

B *Coinsurance requirements* are also a part of fee-for-service or indemnity plans. Once the plan deductible is met, the insurer pays a certain percentage of the allowable charge for the medical service, usually 80%. The patient is responsible for the remaining 20%. If there is no secondary coverage, the healthcare consumer is responsible for the remainder of the charge not covered by their insurer.

C *Copayments* are frequently required in medical plans offered by managed-care plans or HMOs, where a nominal copayment is applied to each office visit, procedure, and prescription that is filled. Under a copayment provision, the patient is usually required to pay a set or fixed dollar amount (eg, $5 or $10) each time a particular medical service is used. The health plan is responsible for paying the provider for the remainder of the charge for medical services or prescriptions.

D Use of provider networks is a characteristic of managed-care plans and HMOs. The two general models of provider networks are the group model HMO and the preferred provider organization (PPO).

- The group model HMO employs physicians and nonphysician healthcare providers to treat patients enrolled in its plan at its own facilities.
- The PPO allows enrollees to choose a physician, nonphysician healthcare practitioner, or hospital from a list of preferred providers to receive full benefits. These preferred providers have a contractual relationship with the insurance carrier for services agreed to be paid at a preferred rate. If the patient goes to a doctor or hospital not on the list, the plan may cover a smaller percentage or none of their costs.

E Some HMOs offer a point-of-service option, whereby patients may opt for a type of indemnity coverage (with a deductible and coinsurance) when they desire medical treatment outside the HMO network.

F Most policies include a consumer's stop-loss limit, which places a cap on the consumer's out-of-pocket expenses, usually at $1000 to $2000 per year. Once the consumer reaches that cap through deductibles and coinsurance, the plan pays the remainder of covered expenses to the limit of coverage specified in the policy.

Utilization Controls

1 *Utilization controls* are determined by the payors to specify when and how often they are willing to reimburse services, equipment, and supplies. The payors interpretation of medical necessity determines the level of usage for which they will pay. These limits may be exceeded if medical necessity is documented appropriately. Utilization controls can be set before the service is provided and identified in the benefit plan. This can include frequency, total number, and timing by which the service or supply is covered. Control can also be applied after the claim has been paid to identify patterns of patient or provider overutilization.

   A *Frequency* means that payors can limit how often they will pay for something. For example, Medicare will only pay for 100 strips every 3 months for people with diabetes who are not using insulin. Providers must document medical necessity to override this limit.

   B The *maximum allowed benefit* in the lifetime of the policy determines the upper limit the plan will pay for specific services or supplies. For example, Medicare limits diabetes education to 10 hours for the initial instruction during the year the patient is eligible. This 10-hour training benefit cannot be used again for the remainder of the time the patient is on Medicare.

   C *Timing* means that plans may only allow access to a service when a certain condition is present or has been met. For example, Medicare will not pay for diabetes education unless the patient meets specific eligibility requirements. Then the service must be used within a certain time period.

Documentation Requirements

1 All plans require documentation that the service for which they are reimbursing is medically necessary and reasonable for the patient's condition.

2 Medicare and most managed-care plans require a written order signed by the patient's primary care provider to document or certify that the referral for services is consistent with the care plan for the patient. Documentation is done through a prescription or physician's order that must be written and kept on file by the person to whom the patient has been referred. Information required by the payor must be included in the physician's order.

A Figure 8.2 is a form that has been created to capture all of the information required by CMS for referral for diabetes education.

B The Medicare certified provider who delivers the education must maintain a record of this information to meet CMS requirements for reimbursement.

3 The patient record must contain documentation that a service was provided. Auditors for payors work on the premise that a service that was not documented was not done. Payors audit patients' charts as a means of postpayment utilization control. The detail of the documentation must match the level of service that was reimbursed.

Site of Service

1 Payors can reimburse different amounts for different sites at which a service is performed. For example, glucose testing payment done at the hospital bedside cannot be billed as a separate service but would be reimbursed under a CPT code when done in a physician's office.

2 Similarly, diabetes education payment under Medicare can only be delivered in the facility of specific certified providers for Medicare. These are physician offices, hospital outpatient departments, end-stage renal disease facilities, and durable medical equipment suppliers with an accreditation certificate from a CMS certifying body. The coding must be correct for the site of the service.

Diabetes Education and Supply Benefits

1 The Balanced Budget Act of 1997 for expanded Medicare diabetes self-management training (DSMT) services was established by the final ruling enacted on February 27, 2001.[2] The program memorandum that implements the rule through Medicare carriers was released June 15, 2001, with implementation by July 17, 2001. The full text of the final rule and carrier program memorandum can be downloaded from the AADE Government Relations Web page at *www.aadenet.org/gov_frame.html*, or through the "What's New" link at *www.hcfa.gov*. The full implementation of this rule will take place over the next 2 years.

A To be eligible for coverage, the Medicare recipient must have one or more of the following medical conditions within a 12-month period before the physician's or qualifying nonphysician practitioner's order for diabetes education. New Medicare beneficiaries and those not previously receiving services for initial training under the G codes or through an American Diabetes Association Recognized Program may receive training. The referring physician or practitioner must document in the patient's record at least one of the following conditions to be eligible for the training:
- New onset diabetes
- Inadequate glycemic control defined by two HbA1c levels over 8.5% for two or more tests at least three months apart
- Changes in treatment regimen from no medication to oral medication, or oral medication to insulin

Figure 8.2. Certificate of Medical Necessity for Diabetes Self-Management Education

Patient Name: _____ SSN: _____

Patient Address: _____

City: _____ State: _____ Zip: _____

Need for Diabetes Education

I certify that diabetes self-management education services are needed under a comprehensive plan for this patient's diabetes care:
❑ To ensure therapy compliance
❑ To provide the necessary skills and knowledge to enable the patient to manage his/her condition

Reason for ordering diabetes self-management education:
❑ Newly diagnosed ❑ Gestational diabetes
❑ Change in condition/treatment regimen _____

Only through a program of diabetes self-management education can the patient acquire the necessary skill and knowledge to comply with the treatment plan. The following plan is ordered:

❑ Group instruction: ❑ Initial _____ ❑ Follow up _____

❑ Individual instruction: ❑ Initial _____ ❑ Follow up _____

Reason for individual instruction: ❑ Language ❑ Impaired hearing/sight ❑ Other _____

Diagnosis

❑ 250.00 type 2   ❑ 250.02 type 2, uncontrolled   ❑ Other _____
❑ 250.01 type 1   ❑ 250.03 type 1, uncontrolled

Is the patient treated with insulin? ❑ Yes ❑ No   Using an insulin pump? ❑ Yes ❑ No

Frequency of Testing
❑ Daily   ❑ 2 times a day   ❑ 3 times a day   ❑ 4 times a day   ❑ Other: _____

Documentation

Variability of blood glucose values (provide range): _____ % of time out of range: _____

Glycosylated hemoglobin A1c _____ %   (normal range) _____

Comorbidities: ❑ Hypertension   ❑ Peripheral vascular disease ❑ Other _____
                ❑ Visual impairment ❑ Dyslipidemia   _____
                ❑ Neuropathy   ❑ ESRD

Complicating/aggravating circumstances: ❑ Hospitalizations: Last date admitted: _____
                                        ❑ Other: _____

Signature must be handsigned – Stamped signature not acceptable

Physician's signature: _____ Date: _____

Physician's name (printed): _____ Phone: _____

Address: _____

City: _____ State: _____ Zip: _____

- High risk of acute complications based on inadequate control that resulted in an emergency room visit or hospitalization
- High risk based on at least one of the following documented complications: lack of feeling in the foot or other foot complications, preproliferative or proliferative retinopathy, or kidney complications with albuminuria or elevated creatinine

B The following conditions must be met for CMS to cover diabetes self-management training:
- A physician or qualified nonphysician practitioner who is treating the patient's diabetes must order it.
- The provider documents a comprehensive care plan that describes the content, number, frequency, and duration of the education service.
- The provider certifies that the education is needed.
- The services must be delivered in a group setting unless (1) the individual has special needs resulting from a hearing, sight, or language problem that would require individual teaching; (2) a group session is not available within the next 2 months; or (3) additional insulin instruction is needed.

C CMS has established the following utilization limits on the diabetes self-management training benefit.
- Initial training of 10 hours must be received within the 12 months the patient was eligible and referred, with payment only for those sessions attended.
- Follow-up training of 2 hours is allowed each calendar year following the completion of the initial training. The provider must order the follow-up training, but the patient does not have to meet the initial eligibility criteria.
- Billing will occur in 30-minute increments.
- One hour of the initial training and all follow-up training may be done individually (without justifying a special need as listed above) to allow for individual assessment.

D The providers of the diabetes self-management training must be certified providers or approved entities for Medicare, have previously received payment under Title XVIII, and accept assignment.
- Approved entities include physician offices, hospital outpatient clinics, end-stage renal disease facilities, durable medical equipment suppliers, and other entities that provide a service or supplies covered by Medicare and are accredited to provide DSMT services.
- Approved individuals for the provision of DSMT include physicians and specific nonphysician practitioners paid under the physician's Medicare fee schedule (eg, physician assistants, nurse practitioners, nurse midwives, clinical psychologists, and clinical social workers).
- CDEs, nurses, dietitians, and pharmacists employed by or under contract to certified providers or approved entities may deliver the training but cannot receive direct payment for the service. The payment will be made to the certified provider who then pays the CDE, nurse, dietitian, or pharmacist.
- All DSMT must be approved by a CMS-approved accreditation organization. At this writing, only the American Diabetes Association is able to approve DSMT programs for Medicare reimbursement through its Education Recognition Program.

- All CMS-approved accreditation organizations must ensure that the providers of DSMT meet quality standards. The quality standards used by the ADA are the National Standards for Diabetes Self-Management Education.[1] Therefore, all DSMT programs must meet the National Standards for Diabetes Self-Management Education as determined by the ADA Education Recognition Program.
- All approved entities must document on a quarterly basis duration of diabetes, medications to control diabetes, height and weight by date, results and date of the last lipid test, results and date of the last HbA1c test, results and date of the last blood pressure measurement, date of the last eye exam, self-monitoring of blood glucose results, educational goals, assessment of educational needs, training goals, 6-month and 1-year follow-up training plans, and documentation of training received.
- All billing must be done using code G0108 for individual teaching and code G0109 for group teaching. Payment will be made following the physician fee schedule. Hospitals use the CMS 1450 form and everyone else uses the CMS 1500 form.

2 Medicare coverage for blood glucose monitors and supplies took effect October 1, 1998. Details about coverage should be referred to the durable medical equipment regional carrier (DMERC) for your state. DMERCs are shown by region in Table 8.6, and the American Association of Diabetes Educators guide to Medicare reimbursement for education and supplies is shown in Table 8.7.

A To establish Medicare medical necessity, all of the following criteria must be met:
- Patient has diabetes and is being treated by a physician
- Meter and supplies are ordered by the physician treating the diabetes
- Patient or caregiver has completed training on the use of the meter and supplies
- Patient or caregiver is capable of using the test results to monitor and improve control
- Meter is designed for home use

B The supplies that will be covered are reagent strips, batteries, control solution, lancet device, and lancets. Cleansing solutions for the skin, urine test strips, insulin, and syringes are not covered supplies.

C Monitors for the visually impaired are covered when the criteria for establishing medical necessity have been met and the physician documents visual impairment severe enough to need this equipment.

D Utilization controls have been placed on the distribution of reagent strips. Medicare limits on test strips, lancets, and lancet devices for blood glucose monitoring are listed in Table 8.8.

E The physician must document how often the patient should test. No more than a 3-month supply can be dispensed at a time, and refills require authorization by the patient or the physician. Quantities that exceed the stated limits require a physician's order stating that the patient is testing more than specified, with proof from a meter printout or logbook to demonstrate the use of the additional strips. This documentation must be present every 6 months to receive the higher quantities.

3 Refer to the American Association of Diabetes Educators Reimbursement Primer[5] for information on Medicaid coverage of diabetes education and supplies, including which states cover insulin, syringes, blood glucose monitors, test strips, self-management training, and other factors.

Table 8.6. Durable Medical Equipment Regional Carriers

Following are the addresses to which patient claims for DME should be sent. Claims should be addressed to the DMERC for the region *in which the patient resides*, even if the equipment and supplies were purchased in another region.

Region	Carrier Address for Claims	States	Web Site
A	Blue Cross Blue Shield of Western New York (eff. 10/1/00) P.O. Box 6800 Wilkes-Barre, PA 18773-6800 Patient claims: 800-842-2052	Connecticut, Delaware, Maine, Massachusetts, New Hampshire, New Jersey, New York, Pennsylvania, Rhode Island, Vermont	Changing, see *www.umd.nycpic.com*
B	AdminaStar Federal Inc. P.O. Box 7031 Indianapolis, IN 46207 Patient claims: 800-270-2313	District of Columbia, Illinois, Indiana, Maryland, Michigan, Minnesota, Ohio, Virginia, West Virginia, Wisconsin	*www.astar-federal.com*
C	Palmetto Government Benefit Administrators (Blue Cross Blue Shield of South Carolina) P.O. Box 10054 Columbia, SC 29202-3254 Patient claims: 800-583-2236	Alabama, Arkansas, Colorado, Florida, Georgia, Kentucky, Louisiana, Mississippi, New Mexico, North Carolina, Oklahoma, Puerto Rico, South Carolina, Tennessee, Texas, Virgin Islands	*www.pgba.com*
D	Connecticut General Life Insurance Co. (CIGNA) P.O. Box 690 Nashville, TN 37202 Patient claims: 800-899-7095	Alaska, American Samoa, Arizona, California, Guam, Hawaii, Idaho, Iowa, Kansas, Missouri, Montana, Nebraska, Nevada, North Dakota, Northern Marianna Islands, Oregon, South Dakota, Utah, Washington, Wyoming	*www.cignamedicare.com*

Source: HCFA web site at: *www.hcfa.gov.* Updated August 2000.

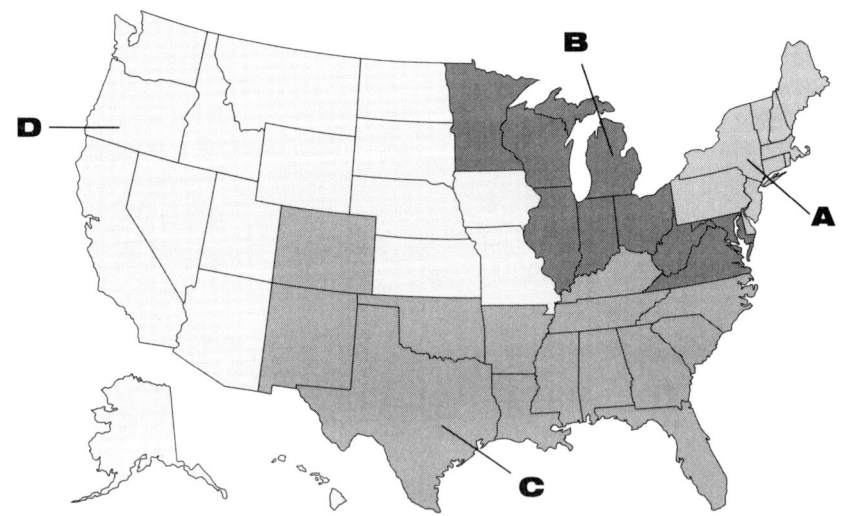

Table 8.7. American Association of Diabetes Educators Guide to Medicare Reimbursement for Diabetes Education and Supplies

Revised February 2001

Services Provided by Individual Practitioners

Type of Provider	Recognition Reimbursement	Whose Provider Number	Coding & Requirements
Physicians	Must have ADA-ERP*	Their own	(G0108) Individual Training $62.74 per patient hour (G0109) Group Training $36.73 per patient hour
Physician assistants	Employer must have ADA-ERP	Their employer's	(G0108) Individual Training $62.74 per patient hour (G0109) Group Training $36.73 per patient hour
All others*	Must have ADA-ERP	Their own	(G0108) Individual Training $62.74 per patient hour (G0109) Group Training $36.73 per patient hour

*Limited by CMS to those who can bill under the Physician Fee Schedule—eg, Nurse Midwives, Nurse Practitioners, Clinical Nurse Specialists, Clinical Psychologists, Clinical Social Workers; or provide some other service or supply to the Medicare program—eg, hospital outpatient departments, ESRD facilities, DME suppliers.

Outpatient Programs Offered by Physician Offices/Clinics

Type of Provider	Recognition Status	Coding & Requirements
Physician office/clinic with outpatient program	Has ADA-ERP	(G0108) Individual Training $62.74 per patient hour (G0109) Group Training $36.73 per patient hour
Physician office/clinic with outpatient program	Does NOT have ADA-ERP	Not eligible for reimbursement until program receives ADA-ERP

Outpatient Programs Offered by Hospital Providers

Type of Provider	Recognition Status	Coding & Requirements
Hospital outpatient program	Has ADA-ERP	(G0108) Individual Training $62.74 per patient hour (G0109) Group Training $36.73 per patient hour
Hospital outpatient program	Does NOT have ADA-ERP	Not eligible for reimbursement until program receives ADA-ERP (any prior eligibility ends 2/27/2001)

Services provided in rural health centers (RHCs) or federally qualified health centers (FQHCs) are bundled under the facility cost payment

*American Diabetes Association Education Recognition Program certification

©1999-2001 American Association of Diabetes Educators. All Rights Reserved.

Table 8.8. Medicare Limits for Diabetes Supplies

Product	Insulin Treated Patients	Non-insulin Treated Patients
Test strips	100 per month	100 every 3 months
Lancets	100 per month	100 every 3 months
Lancet device	1 per 6 months	1 per 6 months

Note: Limits shown may be exceeded with a written order from the primary care provider. Patients may be required to submit testing logs for review.

4 Refer to the American Association of Diabetes Educators Reimbursement Primer[5] for information on state-mandated private payor coverage of diabetes education, equipment, and supplies.

Reimbursement

1 There are several steps to getting your claim reviewed favorably and paid appropriately. Completing these steps prior to the delivery of the service can streamline the payment process.

2 Many payors, including Medicare, require a certificate of medical necessity. This document contains all of the required information for the payor and is signed by the physician. It can also be used as the referral form for those payors who require this certificate.
   A The form in Figure 8.2 can be used as a certificate of medical necessity. It serves to document the criteria by which the patient qualifies for the service, the purpose for the education referral, the kind of instruction needed, the key clinical measures and medical information of interest to the payor, the ICD-9 diagnosis code, identifying information about the patient, and the physician's signature.
   B Gathering this information well before the service is delivered will assist with the assessment of the patient and documentation of outcomes following the delivery of the service.

3 Verifying eligibility and coverage is essential. Before the service is delivered, it is important to verify a patient's eligibility for a service and that the patient is covered for the service that is to be delivered. Verification should be obtained from both the primary and secondary payor.
   A Copy the insurance cards, front and back, for your records. Call the payor's member services department to confirm that the patient is insured and eligible for the service.
   B Confirm that the plan covers the service. This does not guarantee reimbursement, however, because the payor still needs to determine medical necessity. By taking this step, you can advise patients of the extent of their coverage so they can determine if they can meet their financial obligation for the service.

4 Some health plans may require prior authorization or precertification before the service is delivered if it is to be reimbursed. In the case of a managed-care plan, the health plan will specify if prior authorization is to be obtained from the payor or the primary care provider.

   A The responsibility for obtaining the prior authorization could rest with the referring physician, the diabetes educator, or the educator's billing office. When you make the call to the payor, be prepared to answer certain questions about the patient and your services. The health plan customer services representative will either grant, deny, or hold on the decision until further information can be obtained from the referring physician.

   B Once the service is preauthorized, the educator will be given a precertification number to use when submitting claims. The extent of the service will also be defined, including number of visits, group or individual instruction, time limit for the delivery of the service, and approval for follow-up visits. This definition of the service will help you know what to expect the next time you call for prior authorization.

   C It may be necessary to call for prior authorization more than once for the same patient. When additional treatment is necessary, evidence of progress is required by the plan, or if there is a change in the medical condition of the patient, additional precertification may be necessary.

5 The CMS 1500 universal billing form is required by CMS and many third-party payors without additional attached documentation. This form can be found at *www.hcfa.gov/medicare/edi/1500info.htm* and must be submitted electronically to Medicare and Medicaid. The following data must be included on the claim form:
   - Provider's tax identification number or social security number
   - Precertification number, if required
   - Place of service
   - Name and ID number of the referring physician (UPIN) or other indication of documented physician referral
   - Diagnosis code
   - Procedure code (CPT or HCPCS or payor-defined code)

6 Coding, which involves matching the diagnosis and procedure codes to the service being billed, is the most important step to reimbursement. Be sure to use all 5 digits of the ICD-9 codes to define why the service is needed. Then include the procedure code that matches the diagnosis code. Be sure to include codes for all of the diagnoses of the patient, even if you are not treating them all. Make sure your documentation supports the codes you have selected. See the coding section to determine the types of codes that could be used in your program. There is a wide range of codes that could be used as procedure codes (see Table 8.3 for ICD-9 codes for diabetes). A copy of this book can be ordered from Practice Management Information Corporation at *www.medicalbookstore.com*.

7 Claims processing happens when a claim is submitted to a payor. The claim is then evaluated to determine if it meets the payor's requirements for eligibility, coverage, coding, pricing, utilization control, and site of service. From this analysis, the payor determines whether to pay the claim and how much to pay.

A After a claim is submitted, the payor will return a remittance advice that provides the following information:
- Claim number
- Service date
- Procedure code
- Place of service
- Charge
- Allowed amount
- What the payor reimbursed
- Explanatory code for why the claim was not paid in full, if denied

8 Denials and appeals are the final step. Most of the time denials are for small errors that can be identified from the remittance advise. These claims need to be resubmitted on a new claim form. Do not hesitate to call the provider relations department of the health plan for an explanation of a denied or partially paid claim. Use this as an opportunity to educate the payor as to the value of your service.

A If the claim continues to be denied when all of the information is correct, and you know that you have a state law requiring the coverage of this service, contact your state insurance commissioner. Make sure that the patient's insurance is not through a self-funded plan that is not subject to state laws. The insurance commissioner's office can be found at *www.naig.org/consumer/state/members.htm*.

B Each payor has its own appeals process that is identified on the remittance advise. The first step usually involves writing a formal letter stating that you are appealing the claim. Disputes may be sent to external arbitration or reviewed by an internal committee. Self-funded employers will specify the appeals process in their employee handbook. It is recommended that the patient contact his employer's human resources department to discuss the necessity of covering the denied service to maintain the health of a productive employee.

Key Educational Considerations

1 To understand reimbursement, the diabetes educator must know the conditions of coverage for the health plan, which includes eligibility, medical necessity, authorization, definition of benefits, coding, payment rates, required documentation, and utilization controls.

2 Federal healthcare programs provide health benefits for specific populations at no cost or low cost.

3 Medicare's new diabetes education benefit requires all eligible providers of the service to meet the National Standards for Diabetes Self-Management Education. In 2001, the American Diabetes Association is the only accrediting body for CMS that can certify that a program has met the National Standards.

4 Once a claim is filed, there is no guarantee that it will automatically be paid. Documentation is essential to the diabetes education process. It requires specific pieces of information in specific places to comply with regulations governing reimbursement for diabetes education and supplies.

5 Proper coding of a claim is essential to receive proper payment for the service.

6 Employer self-funded plans are exempt from state-mandated laws. Nearly half of all employers have self-funded plans.

7 Persons with diabetes need to be taught their responsibility for reimbursement. They need to understand their plan coverage, criteria for submitting claims, utilization controls, and coinsurance/deductibles.

Self-Review Questions

1 Explain the major differences between public and private payors.
2 What is the difference between group and individual policies, and what is the major advantage of a group policy?
3 Name 3 populations covered by Medicare.
4 Describe the populations covered by the following federal insurance programs: VA, IHS, FEHBP, BPHC, and TRICARE.
5 Describe an employer self-funded plan, what agency regulates these plans, and whether they are subject to any other insurance mandates at the state level.
6 Describe the extremes of health plan administration by addressing the 3 major differences between indemnity and managed care plans.
7 State the main medical service and procedural coding structures, and give examples of where each would be used.
8 Define precertification, medical exclusions, medical necessity, and conditions of coverage, providing examples of each.
9 What are the determinants of eligibility for diabetes education services under Medicare?
10 Summarize the coverage for diabetes services in the state in which you reside.

Learning Assessment: Case Study

TJ is the manager of a hospital-based diabetes education program that has been operating for 5 years. The staff includes an RN, CDE, part-time RD, and a physician advisor. Because the program has not applied for ADA Education Program Recognition, it has lost Medicare reimbursement following the implementation of the new Medicare diabetes education regulation. The current program involves 16 hours of classroom instruction, with an hour of individual assessment by the RN and RD. The program is being covered by the commercial payors in a state where there is a state-mandated law that requires health plans sold in that state to cover diabetes education. With 50% of the current participants attending the diabetes education program on Medicare, TJ's program faces the threat of potential closure due to the loss of half of the program revenue.

Questions for Discussion

1 What is the most important action TJ can take to save this program from closure?
2 How must the program be revised?

3 What billing codes should be used for future Medicare billing?
4 What data should be maintained by the program, and how should the data be gathered?

Discussion

1 This program must meet the National Standards for Diabetes Education and apply to the American Diabetes Association for Education Program Recognition. With an ADA certification, the program can once again bill Medicare.
   A The ADA Education Program Recognition process is now available online at *www.diabetes.org*. By completing this application, the program will demonstrate to CMS that it meets the National Standards for Diabetes Self-Management Education.[1]
   B Meeting these standards will take time, resources, and administrative support from the leadership of the organization.

2 The Medicare regulation places specific limits on program structure and patients' eligibility. This program can only bill Medicare for 10 hours of diabetes education, including no more than 1 hour of individual assessment, unless a group program is not offered within 2 months, the patient has special needs, or the patient needs insulin injection instruction. Therefore, a decision must be made as to how to revise the current program to meet these limitations.
   A You cannot bill various payors differing amounts for the same product. Therefore, a separate program could be designed just for Medicare patients that is 9 hours long, with 1 hour of one-to-one assessment and instruction by the RN and RD prior to the group program. Or the entire program could be revised so that the patients with a commercial third-party payor would receive a 10-hour program. The potential lost revenue from the commercial payors needs to be weighed against the gained revenue from the Medicare patients.
   B Because follow-up is required to meet the National Standards, time should be allotted in the initial diabetes education program to provide follow-up instruction. For example, the 10 hours of instruction could include a half hour of individual instruction before the 9-hour class and a half hour of individual follow-up instruction at 3 months.

3 The new billing codes for Medicare in 2001 are G0108 for individual instruction reimbursed at $62.74 per hour and G0109 for group instruction reimbursed at $36.73 per hour. These rates are subject to deductibles and coinsurance in a fee-for-service plan and copayments in a managed-care plan. Medicare Part B carriers also adjust the local payment rates.

4 The new Medicare regulation requires certified providers delivering the diabetes self-management education to collect and record quarterly several pieces of data. These are in addition to any data the ADA Recognition process requires to meet the National Standards.
   A The Medicare regulation requires the following information:
   • Assessment of educational need
   • Educational goals

- Training goals
- Follow-up plan for 6 months and 1 year
- Duration of diabetes
- Medications
- Height and weight
- Blood pressure and date taken
- Results and date of most recent HbA1c, lipid test, and eye exam
- Self-monitoring of blood glucose frequency and results

■ Some of these data can be collected on the certificate of medical necessity, which functions as the education referral form in Figure 8.2. All data must be documented in the patient's chart. It is highly recommended that diabetes education programs maintain an electronic registry of their patients to store and analyze the data.

References

1 Mensing C, Boucher J, Cypress M, et al. National standards for diabetes self-management education. Diabetes Care. 2001;24:S126-S133.

2 Medicare Program; expanded coverage for outpatient diabetes self-management training and diabetes outcome measures. Federal Register. 2000;63(2511):83129-83154.

3 US Department of Health and Human Services. Program memorandum carriers. Transmittal B-01-40, June 15, 2001. Change request form 1455 available on the Internet at: *www.hcfa.gov/pubforms/transmit/BØ14Ø.pdf*. Accessed May 2001.

4 Hoffman ED Jr, Klees BS, Curtis CA, et al. Brief summaries of Medicare and Medicaid, Title XVIII and Title IX of the Social Security Act as of June 1, 2000. Available on the Internet at: *www.hcfa.gov/pubforms/actuary/ormedmed/*. Accessed May 2001.

5 American Association of Diabetes Educators and Roche Diagnostics Corporation. The American Association of Diabetes Educators Reimbursement Primer. Chicago: American Association of Diabetes Educators and Roche Diagnostics Corporation; 2000 (revised 2001).

6 American Diabetes Association. American Diabetes Association Guide to Diabetes Coding. Alexandria, Va: American Diabetes Association; 1999.

Resources

American Association of Diabetes Educators Legislative Update. E-mailed monthly to subscribers. Register at *www.aadenet.org*. Accessed May 2001.

American Diabetes Association Advocacy E-News Newsletter. E-mailed to subscribers. Register at *www.diabetes.org*. Accessed May 2001.

Learning Assessment: Post-Test Questions

Payment for Diabetes Education 8

1. What is the Centers for Medicare and Medicaid Services, formerly known as the Health Care Financing Administration (HCFA)?
   A A private organization that facilitates Medicare reimbursement
   B The carriers and intermediaries that pay Medicare claims
   C The lobbying organization that influences Medicare legislation
   D A government agency that administers Medicare reimbursement

2. Which of the following populations are covered by Medicare?
   A US citizen, >65 years, or <65 years with end-stage renal disease, or >65 and permanently disabled
   B US citizen, <65 years, or <65 years with end-stage renal disease, or <65 years and permanently disabled
   C US citizen, >65 years, or <65 years with end-stage renal disease, or <65 years and permanently disabled
   D US citizen, retired before age 65 years, <65 years with end-stage renal disease, or 65 years and permanently disabled

3. To be eligible to receive reimbursement for diabetes self-management training, what documentation is required by the approved diabetes education program?
   A Educational goals and training goals
   B Assessment of educational needs
   C 6-month and 1-year follow-up plans
   D All of the above

4. The codes for billing for diabetes education for Medicare patients are
   A G108 and G109
   B CPT codes
   C ICD-9 codes
   D S codes

5. Coding is the key to appropriate filing of a claim and eventual reimbursement because
   A Coding matches services to the correct amount of payment determined by the payor
   B Only 1 code provides payment for an individual service
   C Codes define medical symptoms, diagnoses, symptoms, conditions, treatments, services, and supplies
   D A and C
   E All of the above

6. Utilization controls govern which of the following for specific services covered by an insurer?
   A Frequency and quantity
   B Eligibility and definition of coverage
   C Amount reimbursed and coding
   D Place of service and deductible

7. To receive payment for the delivery of diabetes self-management training services from Medicare, the program provider must
   A Be a certified provider for Medicare
   B Meet the quality standards established by the Centers for Medicare and Medicaid Services
   C Collect specific program outcomes data
   D All of the above

8. Which of the following must be met to ensure coverage?
   A Eligibility
   B Correct coding
   C Deductible, coinsurance, and/or payment
   D All of the above

9. What kind of health plans are not subject to state mandates?
   A Managed-care plans
   B Employer self-funded/self-insured plans
   C Fee-for-service plans
   D Medicaid

10 The amount that is actually paid for a service or supply is determined by
   A Who files the claim
   B The documentation in the provider's chart
   C The payors financial arrangement with the provider and the financial responsibility of the consumer
   D Filing the claim within 90 days of the service

11 The consumer's financial responsibility in a managed-care plan is defined by
   A Deductibles
   B Coinsurance payments
   C Copayments
   D Maximum allowable rates

See next page for answer key.

Post-Test Answer Key

Payment for Diabetes Education

1. D
2. C
3. D
4. A
5. D
6. A
7. D
8. D
9. B
10. C
11. C

A Core Curriculum for Diabetes Education
Diabetes Education and Program Management

Index

Acculturation, 101, 102
Adherence, patient, see Patient compliance
Adjustment disorders, 156, 157, 165-166
Adolescent Coping Orientation for Problem Experiences Scale, 44
Adolescents, 45
Advertising, see Patient education programs
Affective exercises, 7, 11
African Americans
 attitudes toward health professionals, 106
 community outreach, 108
 depression, diabetes and, 149
 diabetes and, 104
 diabetes type 2, 103
 preventive health measures, 107
Aging, diabetes prevalence, 103
Alcohol abuse, see Substance abuse
Alprazolam, 155
Ambulatory care reimbursement, 234, 243
American Association of Diabetes Educators
 financial assistance, information, 47
 health-related behavior (measurable outcomes), 204
 professional values and behaviors, 103
 reimbursement primer, 249
American Diabetes Association
 Education Recognition Program, 6, 186, 189, 197-199, 210-212, 243, 248
 financial assistance, information, 47
 guide to Medicare reimbursement, 243, 249
 National Standards for Diabetes Self-Management Education Programs, 6, 183, 186, 197
American Red Cross, 47
Amitriptyline, 151
Anorexia nervosa, 38, 158
Anthropology, 100
Antianxiety medications, 155
Antidepressant medications, 150-152

eating disorder treatment, 161
 technological and therapeutic advances, 69
Anxiety
 diabetes and, 8, 153-154
 diagnosis and treatment, 154-155
 disorder, clinical, 37-39, 153-155
 disorder, generalized, 154
 Hospital Anxiety and Depression Scale, 36, 37
 hypoglycemia fears, 38, 154
 injection-related, 38, 154
 learning barriers, 8
 pregnancy and, 154
 psychosocial assessment, 26
 symptoms, 153, 154
Appointments (patients with low literacy skills), 131
Asian Americans
 diabetes and, 104
 eating pattern (case study), 111-112
Assessment questionnaires, see Questionnaires
Ativan, see Lorazepam
Attitudes, see Affective exercises; Behavior change; Culture; Health beliefs; Mental states; Patient education programs; Patient empowerment
Attitudinal learning, see Learning
Audiovisuals, 10, 129-130
Audit of Diabetes-Dependent Quality of Life, 41
Autonomy, 29, 31, 67, 71
Behavior
 focus on, 77
 health-related, as measurable outcomes, 204
 intentions, 26, 32-34
 objectives of education programs, 5
 problem-solving skills, 43
Behavior change, 67-96
 behavioral contract, 33-34, 77-78
 compliance perspective, 70-71
 diabetes educators and, 84
 eating problems and, 160
 empowerment perspective, 71-74
 intentions and, 32

motivation and, 69-70
 motivational interviewing, 70
 patient readiness, 8-9, 34-35, 71, 73-74
 protocol for promoting, 70-71
 psychosocial assessment, 27-28
 review (educational exercises), 49-54, 61-64, 84-89, 93-96
 skills development, 79-81
 suggested readings, 92
 transtheoretical model of, 34, 70
Behavioral contract, 33-34, 77-78
Beliefs, see Affective exercises; Behavior change; Culture; Health beliefs; Mental states; Patient education programs; Patient empowerment
Benchmarking, 207
Benzodiazepines, 155
Best practices, 207
Bibliography
 behavior change, empowerment, 92
 culturally competent diabetes education, 114-117
 educational programs, 217
 learning, teaching, patient education principles, 17
 low literacy skills, 139-140
 psychological disorders, 171-172
 psychosocial assessment, 59
 reimbursement for diabetes education, 249
Binge-eating, see Eating disorders
Biofeedback-assisted relaxation training, 157
Bipolar disorders, 152-153
Blame, see Self-blame
Blood pressure (fight-or-flight response), 156
Board games, see Games
Body, and self-image, 39, 160
Budgeting, see Costs
Bulimia nervosa, 38, 158, 159
Bureau of Primary Health Care, 228
Burnout, professional, 83
Business plans, see Patient education programs
BuSpar, see Buspirone
Buspirone, 155

Capitation, 236
Catastrophic medical expenses, see Reimbursement
Center for Epidemiological Studies Depression Scale, 36
Centers for Medicare and Medicaid Services, see US Centers for Medicare and Medicaid Services
CHAMPUS, see TRICARE
Chance orientation, see Locus of control theory
Change, see also Behavior change; Lifestyle; Patient empowerment readiness, 8
readiness, stages, 34-35, 73-74
treatment plans, 74
Children, 43, 44-45
Choice, see Decision-making
Cigarette smoking, see Substance abuse
Civilian Health and Medical Program of the Uniformed Services, see TRICARE
Claims filing, see Insurance
CLAS (National [Health Care] Standards for Culturally and Linguistically Appropriate Services), 99
Clear and Simple: Developing Effective Print Materials for Low Literate Readers, 131
Clinical anxiety disorder, see Anxiety
Clinical depression, see Depression
Clinical practice improvement, 205
Clorazepate, 155
CMS, see US Centers for Medicare and Medicaid Services
CMS (HCFA) 1500 universal billing form, 245
Coding systems, 232-235, 245
Cognitive-behavioral therapy, 150
Cognitive maturity, see Children
Common Procedural Terminology, see CPT
Communication, miscommunication potential, 102
Community outreach, 108
Compliance, see Patient compliance
Complications of diabetes, 3, 35, 161-162

Computers, 11, 82
Confidence, see Self-efficacy
Consumers, see Patients
Continuous quality improvement, 198, 199-201, 212-214
Contracting, see Behavioral contract
Conventional medicine, 101
Coping, see Psychology
Cortisol, 156
Costs, see also Reimbursement
educational program budgeting, 189-190
educational program financial management, 196-197
medical and other expenses, 47
pricing for reimbursement, 235-236
self-care, 28, 30
CPT, 233-235, 238
Cross-cultural education and care, 101-102
Cultural relativism, 103
Culture, 99-120
assumptions about, 106
community outreach, 108
description of, 100
diabetes education programs and, 107-108
diabetes educators as a cultural group, 102, 103
gender roles, attitudes, 110-111
glossary of terms, 100-101
importance, assessment, 47-48
patient psychosocial assessment, 8
review (educational exercises), 108-113, 118-120
standards for services, 99
suggested readings, 114-117
underserved groups, 104
worldview and, 101, 102, 103
Culture, organizational, see Patient education programs
Current Procedural Terminology, 233-235, 238
D-ET, see Diabetes Educator Tool
D-SMART, see Diabetes Self-Management Assessment Report Tool
Data, educational, see Patient education programs
Death, thoughts of, 37, 149

Decision-making, see also Patient empowerment; Self-management
decisional balance, 70
empowerment-based educational approach, 4
enhancement of, 11-12
informed choice, 73
Definitions, see Terminology
Delivery of healthcare, see Healthcare delivery; Reimbursement
Demonstration (teaching technique), 10, 129
Depression, 26, 36-37, 148-152
antidepressant medications, 150-152
case study, 164-165
clinical, symptoms, diagnosis, 37, 148, 150
diabetes and, 148-150
psychotherapy, 150
Depressive disorder, see Depression
Desipramine, 151
D-ET, see Diabetes Educator Tool
Diabetes
anxiety about, 26
coding systems for payments, 232-235
prevalence, demographic characteristics, 103-104
severity, 28, 29, 30
treatment plans, 74
Diabetes complications
compliance-based educational approach, 3
psychological disorders as sequelae, 161-162
self-care and, 35
Diabetes education, see Learning; Patient education; Patient education programs; Patient education team; Self-management; Teaching
Diabetes Educator Tool, 206-207
Diabetes educators, see American Association of Diabetes Educators; Patient education team; Patient relationships; Teaching
Diabetes Empowerment Scale, 32, 33
Diabetes Fear of Injecting and Self-Testing Questionnaire, 38
Diabetes mellitus, type 1

biofeedback-assisted relaxation training, 157
coding systems for payments, 232-235
eating disorders, 38, 158, 159
psychosocial factors (case study), 53-54
self-management benefits, 68
stress and, 156
susceptibility, vulnerability, 28
Diabetes mellitus, type 2
biofeedback-assisted relaxation training, 157
coding systems for payments, 232-235
emotional well-being, 36
myths, 83
patient education, 13-14
psychosocial factors (case studies), 50-53
self-management benefits, 68
sexual dysfunction, 162
stress and, 156
susceptibility, vulnerability, 28
women and, 103
Diabetes Outcomes Intervention Tool, see Diabetes Educator Tool
Diabetes Quality of Life Clinical Trial Questionnaire–Revised, 41
Diabetes Quality of Life Measure, 41
Diabetes self-management, see Self-management
Diabetes Self-Management Assessment Report Tool, 206-207
Diabetes self-management training, see Patient education programs; Self-management
Diabetes Treatment Satisfaction Questionnaire, 41
Diagnostic and Statistical Manual of Mental Disorders, 147
Diagnostic related groups (DRGs), 235
Diet pills, 159
Dieting, 160
Dietitians, see Patient education team
Disabilities, perception of, 28
Discussion (teaching/learning strategies), 9-10

DO-IT, see Diabetes Educator Tool
Drug abuse, see Substance abuse
Drugs, see also Insulin; names of specific drugs
errors due to reading/understanding problems, 131
injection-related anxiety, 38, 154
medication schedule, 34
D-SMART, see *Diabetes Self-Management Assessment Report Tool*
DSM-IV, see *Diagnostic and Statistical Manual of Mental Disorders*
Durable medical equipment, 235, 242
E&M codes, 233-234
Eating disorders, 26, 38-39, 157-161
binge eating, 158
case study, 166
psychotherapy, 160
Eating patterns, see Nutrition
Economic considerations, see Costs; Reimbursement
Education, see Learning; Patient education; Patient education programs; Patient education team; Self-management; Teaching
Educational needs assessment, see Patient needs assessment
Educational outcomes, see Outcomes
Educational programs, see Patient education programs
Educational status, 104, see also Literacy
Educational team, multidisciplinary, see Patient education team
Educational techniques, see Learning; Teaching
Educator-patient relationship, see Patient relationships
Educators, see American Association of Diabetes Educators; Patient education team; Teaching
Effexor, see Venlafaxine
Elavil, see Amitriptyline
Emotional well-being, see Psychology

Employee Retirement Income Security Act, see Employers
Employee health coverage, see Employers
Employees of programs, see Patient education programs
Employers
insurance coverage, 229
payor mix in US, 226, 227
Employment, 47
Empowerment, see Patient empowerment; Self-management
Enculturation, 101
Equipment, see Durable medical equipment; Glucose meters
ERISA (Employee Retirement Income Security Act), see Employers
Erispan, see Fludiazepam
Ethnic groups
assumptions about beliefs, 106
community outreach, 108
culturally competent diabetes education, 114-117
diabetes and, 104
Ethnicity, 100
Ethnocentrism, 101
Ethnographer, 101
Evaluation and management codes, 233-234
Evaluation of educational programs, see Outcomes
Examples (teaching/learning strategies), 11
Exercise
benefits, 68
excessive, and eating disorders, 159
psychosocial assessment, 26
walking, 26, 34
Family
cultural aspects of food preparation, 105
involvement and empowerment, 78
parental involvement in diabetes management, 44-45
patient readiness to learn, 7
powerful-other locus of control, 30, 31
psychosocial assessment, 8, 25, 26
self-care and, 28, 45-46

stress and eating disorders, 159
support and coping, 81
Fate, see Locus of control theory
Fatigue, 37, 38, 149, 153
Federal Employees Health Benefit Program, see US Federal Employees Health Benefit Program
Feedback, see Learning
Fight-or-flight response, 156
Films, see Audiovisual aids
Finances, see Costs
Fludiazepam, 155
Fluoxetine, 151, 161
Food, see Nutrition
Food models, see Audiovisual aids
Foreign-language speakers, 48, 124, 130
Formative evaluation, see Outcomes
Friends, see Social support
Games (teaching/learning strategies), 10-11
Gender roles, attitudes about, 110-111
Glucose control
  compliance-based educational approach, 3
  culturally competent education, 107-108
  eating disorders and, 159
  fight-or-flight response and, 156
  goals, 7
  internal locus of control and, 29
  self-efficacy, intentions, 26
Glucose meters, payment, 235, 241
Glucose monitoring
  behaviors, intentions, 34
  benefits of, 68
  Medicare coverage, 241
  reimbursement for, 232
Glycosylated hemoglobin, see Hemoglobin
Group education, 5, 8
Group support, see Social support
Hallucinogens, see Substance abuse
HCFA, see US Centers for Medicare and Medicaid Services

HCFA (CMS) 1500 universal billing form, 245
HCPCS, 233-235
Health Belief Model, 28, 29
Health beliefs
  assessment, 29, 30
  chance orientation, 29, 30, 31
  cultural and religious influences, 47-48
  educational needs assessment, 7
  educator/professional acculturation, values, 102, 103
  educator/professional burnout, 83
  empowerment counseling model, 72
  importance of, 27, 28-29
  internal orientation, 29, 31
  locus of control, 29-31
  powerful-other orientation, 29, 30
  psychosocial assessment, 25, 26
Healthcare delivery, 48
Health Care Financing Administration, see US Centers for Medicare and Medicaid Services
Health Insurance Portability and Accountability Act, 47
Health literacy, 45, 123
Health maintenance organizations, 230, 231, 236, 237
Health professionals, see Health beliefs; Patient care team; Patient education team
Health-related quality of life, see Quality of life
Health status, see also Diabetes complications
  importance of, 27-28, 35
  psychosocial assessment, 25
Hemoglobin, 68, 151
Herbal medicines, 109-110
Hispanic Americans
  cultural aspects of food preparation, 105
  depression, diabetes and, 149
  diabetes and, 104
  educational exercises, 109-110
HMOs, see Health maintenance organizations
Home health care, payor mix, 227

Hospital Anxiety and Depression Scale, 36
Hospitals, see also Patient education programs
  Medicare reimbursement, 235, 243
  payor mix, 227
HRQL (health-related quality of life), see Quality of life
Humor, 81
Hyperglycemia
  brittle diabetes and psychiatric disorders, 161
  health status assessment, 35
  symptoms and depression, 37
Hypoglycemia
  fears of, 38, 154
  frequent, severe, 159, 161
  health status assessment, 35
Hypomanic episodes, 153
ICD-9-CM, 232-235, 245
IDDM (Insulin-dependent diabetes mellitus), see Diabetes mellitus, type 1
Illiteracy, see Literacy
Imipramine, 151
Immunosuppression, 156
Income and diabetes, 104
Indian Health Service, see US Indian Health Service
Information acquisition (patient learning styles), 8
Informed choice, 73
Injections, see Drugs; Insulin
Insulin
  cultural concerns about, 109-110
  disruption of administration, 161
  dosage adjustment, 34
  injection-related anxiety, 38, 154
  manipulation and eating disorders, 38
  omission and eating disorders, 159
  technological and therapeutic advances, 69
Insulin-dependent diabetes mellitus, see Diabetes mellitus, type 1
Insurance, see also Reimbursement
  claims processing, 245-246
  benefits, coverage, plan types, 47, 228-232

deductibles, coinsurance, copayments, 236
denials and appeals, 246
diabetes education payment, 225
documentation requirements, 237-238
healthcare access and, 48
indemnity, fee-for-service, 229-230
managed care, 230, 236, 237, 238
payor mix in US, 226, 227
prior authorization, precertification, 245
Intentions, see Behavior
Internal orientation, see Locus of control theory
International Classification of Disease, 232-235, 245
Interpersonal therapy, 150, 160
Interviewing, motivational, see Behavior change
Job training, see Employment
Juvenile Diabetes Research Foundation International, 47
Ketoacidosis, diabetic, 159, 161
Knowledge, 7
Kovacs' Issues in Coping With Diabetes Scales for Children and Parents, 43
Laboratory services reimbursement, 235
Lancets, Medicare reimbursement, 244
Language, first (non-English), 48, 124, 130
Laxatives, 159
Leadership, see Patient education programs
Learning, 3-22
adult learner characteristics, 9
affective (attitudinal) exercises, 7, 11
audiovisual aids, 10
continuing (review, updating), 12
demonstration method, 10
discussion method, 9-10
enhancement, techniques, 11-12
feedback, 11
game-playing, 10-11
group, 5, 8
immediate application, 11
lecture method, 9
motivation, 7, 67

one-to-one, 5, 8
pace of, 12
past experiences, active participation, 9, 11-12
patient examples in, 11
patient readiness, 7
printed materials, reading, 10
problem-oriented, 9
psychological barriers, 8
review (educational exercises), 12-14, 20-22
role-playing method, 10
strategies, 9-11
style of, preferences, 7-8
suggested readings, 17
Lifestyle, see also Behavior change; Self-management
changes and diabetes self-care, 69
choices, positive, 81
self-management as living, 73
Lions Club International, 47
Lipid goals, 7
Literacy, 123-144; see also Reading
assessment, 126-128
defining, 123
functional, 123, 126-128
health, 45, 123
importance, assessment, 44-45
levels, United States, 124, 126
low, teaching approaches, 128-133
patient needs assessment, 8
readability formulas, 128
review (educational exercises), 133-138, 142-144
signage and form completion, 130-131
suggested readings, 139-140
Locus-of-control theory, 29-31
Lorazepam, 155
Major depressive episodes, 153
Managed care, 230, 236, 237, 238
Manic episodes, 152
Marketing, see Patient education programs
Meals, see Nutrition
Medicaid, 47, 241, 226-228
Medical Achievement Reading Test, 128
Medical necessity determinations, see Reimbursement
Medical Outcomes Survey, 41

Medical record coding, see Coding systems
Medicare, 47, 190, 197
ADA guide to reimbursement, 243
diabetes education and supplies, 238-241
diabetes education payment, 225, 248-249
documentation requirements, 237-239
DRGs, 235
Parts A, B and C, 227-228
payor mix in US, 226, 227
+ Choice, 228
Medicine, conventional, 100
Men (gender roles, values), 110-111
Mental states, see also Anxiety; Depression; Stress
learning barriers, 8
psychological disorders, 147-176
sequelae of diabetes complications, 161-162
subclinical syndromes, 147, 162-163
suggested readings, 171-172
symptoms of clinical anxiety disorder, 38, 153
Mexican Americans, see Hispanic Americans
Military health care, see TRICARE
Minority groups, see Ethnic groups
Miscommunication, 102
Mixed episodes, 153
Mood disorders, 152-153
Motivation, see Behavior change; Learning
Multidisciplinary educational team, see Patient education team
Muscle tension, 38, 153
Myths, see Health beliefs
National Adult Literacy Survey, 124, 126
National Diabetes Education Outcomes System, 205-207
National Diabetes Education Program, 18
National (Health Care) Standards for Culturally and Linguistically Appropriate Services, 99

National Standards for Diabetes Self-Management Education Programs, see American Diabetes Association
Native Americans
  case study, Navajo woman, 112-113
  diabetes and, 104
  Indian Health Service, 228
Navajo language, 112-113
NDEOS, see National Diabetes Education Outcomes System
Necessity, medical, see Reimbursement
Needs assessment, see Patient needs assessment
Nefazodone, 151, 152
Neuroendocrine system, 149
Newspapers (patient learning styles), 8
Non-English speakers, 48, 124, 130
Noninsulin-dependent diabetes mellitus, see Diabetes mellitus, type 2
Norpramin, see Desipramine
Nortriptyline, 151
Nurses, see Patient care team; Patient education team
Nursing homes, payor mix, 227
Nutrition
  Asian American eating pattern (case study), 111-112
  binge eating, 158, 159
  community food banks, 47
  cultural and religious influences, 47-48
  eating disorders, 26, 38-39, 157-161
  eating habits, health beliefs, 26
  ethnic and cultural constraints, 105
  meal plan use, 34
  normal eating patterns, 159
  patients with low literacy skills, 131
Obsessive-compulsive disorder, 155
Office visit reimbursement, 234, 243
One-to-one education, 5, 8
Organizational culture, see Patient education programs
Outcomes
  behaviors and, 77

data capture, reporting, 205-207
educational program evaluation, 6
formative evaluation, 6
health-related behavior, 204
impact of diabetes education, 3
measurement, 201-205, 217
National Diabetes Education Outcomes System, 205-207
responsibility for (myths), 83
sharing, 208
summative evaluation, 6
Outpatient visits, see Ambulatory care visits
Oxazepam, 155
Pacific Islander Americans, 104
Pamelor, see Nortriptyline
Paroxetine, 151
Patient adherence, see Patient compliance
Patient attitudes, see Affective exercises; Behavior change; Culture; Health beliefs; Mental states; Patient education programs; Patient empowerment
Patient care team
  burnout among professionals, 83
  collaborative perspective, comanagement, 71
  multidisciplinary educational teams and, 6
  powerful-other locus of control, 29, 30, 31
Patient compliance
  -based approach to education, 3, 4
  behavior change and, 70-71
  complex, life-long, prophylactic, 68
  myths of, 83
Patient education, see also Outcomes; Patient empowerment; Patient education programs; Self-management
  adult learner characteristics, 9
  benefits of empowerment, 84
  change readiness, 8-9
  compliance-based approach, 3, 4
  continuing, follow-up, 12
  cultural competence, 99-120

diabetes educators as a cultural group, 102, 103
diabetes self-management education, definition, 208
empowerment and, 4, 84
health-related behavior (measurable outcomes), 204
impact on outcomes, 3
literacy levels and, 8, 125, 128-133
Medicare coverage, 238-241
myths about, and professional burnout, 83
ongoing process, 12
past experiences, active participation, 9, 11-12
payment for, 225-252
philosophy of programs, 4
principles of, 3-22
printed material readability, 128, 132
printed materials, low-literate readers, 131-133
problem orientation of learners, 9
readiness to learn, 7
review (educational exercises), 12-14, 20-22
suggested readings, 17
teaching/learning strategies, 9-11
Patient education programs, see also Outcomes; Patient education; Patient education team; Reimbursement
ADA Education Recognition Program, 186, 189, 197-199, 210-212, 243, 248
advisory committee, 5
annual planning and review process, 198
attitudes of patients toward, 7
benchmarking for best practice, 207
budgeting, 189-190, 196-197
business plans, 183
classrooms, 185
continuing education, follow-up, 12
continuous quality improvement, 198, 199-201
coordinator, 7, 198
course levels, 5
culturally competent, 107-108

curriculum development, 187-188
customers, 191-192, 208-209
data collection, analysis, 198, 199, 200, 201-207, 212-214
design of, 3, 4-6
diabetes self-management education, definition, 208
diabetes self-management training, 238-241
documentation, record keeping, 6
evaluation, 6, 201-207
financial aspects, 5, 182, 196-197, 225-252
goal and treatment priorities, 67, 68
goals and objectives, 4-5
group vs. individual education, 189
individualized plans, 67, 76
knowledge-based organizations, 193, 194
leadership styles, 195
management, leadership, 192-197, 217
managing, 181-220
market analysis, 182, 183-184
marketing, 191-192, 208-209
National Standards for Diabetes Self-Management Education Programs, 6, 183, 186, 197
new program annual plan, 190
office areas, 185
organization and structure, 81-82
organizational culture, characteristics, 192-193
patient-staff ratios, 185-186
payment for, 190, 197, 225-252
people management, 194-195
philosophy of, 4
positioning message, 182
resource and space identification, needs, 184-185
review (educational exercises), 12-14, 20-22, 209-214, 218-220
salaries, 189
services development, 187-189

staff hiring, position descriptions, 186-187, 194
stakeholders, 5
strategic planning, 193-194
team building, 194
visiting other programs, 187
Patient education team
burnout among professionals, 83
coaching, 194-195
coordinator, 7
creating, 185-187
description, 6-7
dietitians, 13, 186
help, consulting, 79
hiring, 186-187, 194
makeup, members, 5, 7
Medicare payment for services, 238-241, 243
meetings, 7
new program annual plan, 190
nurses, 185
organizational culture of programs, 193
patient-staff ratios, 185-186
professional acculturation, values, 102, 103
referrals and, 81-82
team building, 194
Patient empowerment, 67; see also Self-efficacy
behavior change, 71-79
benefits to educators, 84
community outreach, 108
educational approach, 4, 82-83
feelings, 32, 33
readings, 92
review (educational exercises), 84-89, 93-96
twelve steps to, 74-79
Patient health status, see Health status
Patient learning, see Learning; Literacy; Patient education; Patient education programs
Patient needs assessment, 7-9
Patient outcomes, see Outcomes
Patient psychology, see Anxiety; Depression; Mental states; Psychology; Stress
Patient relationships
attitudes toward health professionals, 106-107
behavioral contracts, 33-34, 77-78

contact between visits, 78
culturally competent encounters, 109
culture and diabetes care, 105
emotional content, 83
empowerment and benefits to educators, 84
frequent contacts, 82
frustrating, and empowerment, 82-83
help, consultations for educators, 79
interaction in, 102
listening and rapport, 105
miscommunication potential, 102
rapport, 81
twelve steps to empowerment, 74-79
Patients, see also Health beliefs; Literacy; Patient compliance; Patient education; Patient education programs; Patient empowerment; Patient relationships; Self-efficacy
adult learner characteristics, 9
consumer out-of-pocket health expenses, 227
deductibles, coinsurance, copayments, 236
diabetes education program customers, 191-192
example use in learning, 11
financial considerations, 47
past experiences, active participation, 9, 11-12
quality of life, 26, 40-41
Patients' families, see Family
Paxil, see Paroxetine
Payment, see Reimbursement
Phobia, specific, 154
Physical health, see Health status
Physician assistants, Medicare reimbursement, 243
Physicians
diabetes education program customers, 191-192
diabetes education team, 185
Medicare reimbursement, 243
payor mix, 227
visits, 82
Point-of-service option, 230
Power, of patient, see Patient empowerment; Self-efficacy

Powerful-other orientation, see Locus of control theory
PPOs, see Provider networks
Pregnancy, 154
Primary care, 48
Print materials, see Bibliography; Literacy; Reading
Problem Areas in Diabetes Scale, 42
Problem-solving, 43, 77, 81
Professional acculturation and values, 102, 103
Provider networks, 230, 236, 237
Prozac, see Fluoxetine
Psychoeducational therapy, 160
Psychology, see also Anxiety; Depression; Stress
 bipolar disorders, 152-153
 coping skills, 43-44, 79, 80-81
 disorders as sequelae of diabetes complications, 161-162
 emotional content of patients' problems, 83
 emotional well-being, 26, 35-37
 empowerment counseling model, 72
 goals of psychosocial assessment, 27
 identification of issues, 25
 injection-related fear, 38, 154
 learning barriers, 8
 medical crisis and psychopathology, 161
 psychological disorders, 147-176
 psychosocial assessment, 8, 25-64
 relaxation techniques, 81
 review (educational exercises), 49-54, 61-64, 162-167, 173-176
 self-esteem, 26
 stress, 41-42
 subclinical syndromes, 147
 suggested readings, 59, 171-172
 susceptibility, vulnerability, 28, 29, 30
Psychomotor skills, see Skills

Psychosocial assessment, see Culture; Family; Psychology; Religion; Social support
Psychotherapy, 150, 156-157, 160
Publications, see Bibliography; Literacy; Reading
Quality improvement, see Continuous quality improvement
Quality of life, 26, 40-41
Quality of Well-Being Instrument, 41
Questionnaire on Stress in Patients With Diabetes— Revised, 42
Questionnaires
 behaviors and intentions, 33
 brief, selective psychosocial assessment, 26
 coping skills, 43, 44
 Diabetes Fear of Injecting and Self-Testing Questionnaire, 38
 health belief assessment, 30
 locus-of-control assessment, 31
 quality of life, 41
 self-efficacy, 33
 social support assessment, 46
 stress, 42
Rapid Estimate of Adult Literacy in Medicine, 127-128
Rational emotive therapy, 80
Reading, see also Literacy
 patient learning styles, 8
 print materials, 128, 131-133
 readability, formulas, 128, 132
 teaching/learning strategies, 10
Reading lists, see Bibliography
Reframing, 80
Reimbursement, 225-252; see also Insurance; Medicare
 capitation, 236
 catastrophic expenses, 236
 claims processing, 245-246
 CMS (HCFA) 1500 universal billing form, 245
 coding systems, 232-235, 245
 coverage, eligibility verification, 244
 denials and appeals, 246
 determinants of coverage, 231-232

 diabetes education and supplies, 238-246
 diabetes self-management training, 238-241
 documentation requirements, 237-238
 equipment, 235
 medical necessity determinations, 232, 239, 241, 244
 payor mix in US, 226-227
 pricing for payment, 235-236
 prior authorization, precertification, 245
 private payors, 225, 226, 228-230
 public payors, 225, 226-228
 review exercises, 246-249, 250-252
 suggested readings, 249
 usual, customary, reasonable (UCR), 235
 utilization controls, 237
Relaxation techniques, 81, 157
Religion, 8, 47-48
Retinopathy, diabetic, proliferative, 162
Role-playing (teaching/learning strategies), 10
Salvation Army, 47
Self-blame, 29, 31
Self-care, see Self-management
Self-determination theory, 69, 71
Self-efficacy
 assessing, 32, 33
 behavior change and, 70
 importance of, 31-32
 internal locus of control, 29
 learning enhancement, 11
 optimum self-care and, 67
 psychosocial assessment, 26
 self-esteem and self-care, 26, 36
Self-esteem, see Self-efficacy
Self-image, 39, 160
Self-management, see also Patient education; Patient education programs; Patient empowerment
 attitude change (rules, work, living), 72-73
 behavior and, 27-28, 68-69
 behavior change, review exercises, 84-89, 93-96
 behavior intentions, 32-34
 behavioral contract, 33-34, 77-78

benefits of, 68
collaborative perspective, comanagement, 71
compliance-based approach, 3, 4
complications and, 35
coping skills, 43-44, 80-81
costs of, 28, 30
demanding and pervasive nature of, 27
design of educational programs, 4-6
diabetes self-management education, definition, 208
education, medical necessity certificate, 239, 240, 244
education programs, 181-220
educational processes, 3
emotional toll of, 35-37
empowerment and, 4, 71-79
facilitating, 79-81
family and social support, 45-46
flexibility in, 80
importance of, 25
individualized plans, 67, 76
learning, decision-making enhancement, 11-12
level of, and educational needs, 7
lifestyle changes, 69
locus-of-control theory, 29-31
optimum, through self-efficacy, 67
parental involvement in diabetes management, 44-45
plans for achieving goals, 72
problem-solving skills, 77
psychosocial factors, 49-54, 61-64
relapse prevention, 81
review, educational exercises, 12-14, 20-22
self-determination theory, autonomy, 71
self-esteem and, 36
skills importance, assessment, 42-43
skills training, 73, 79-81
stress management and, 166
treatment plan change, 74
Serax, see Oxazepam
Serotonin reuptake inhibitors, selective, 151, 152, 161
Sertraline, 151
Serzone, see Nefazodone

Sexual dysfunction, 161-162
SF-36 scale, 36
Simulation, see Computers
Site Registration Form, 206-207
Skills, see also Literacy
 coping, 43-44
 coping, and empowerment, 73, 79, 80-81
 evaluation, 28
 immediate application, 11
 importance, assessment, 42-43
 mastery, 11
 practice, rehearsal, 11
 problem-solving, 77, 81
 psychomotor, 7
 psychosocial assessment, 25
Sleeping difficulties, 37, 38, 149, 153
Slides, see Audiovisual aids
Smoking, see Substance abuse
Social support, see also Family
 diabetes self-care and, 45-46
 friends and family in diabetes care, 26
 group education, 5, 8
 group support, 82
 patient empowerment and, 78
 patient psychosocial assessment, 8
 self-care behaviors and, 28
SRF, see Site Registration Form
Staff, see Patient education programs
Stakeholders, see Patient education programs
Standards, National, for Diabetes Self-Management Education Programs, see American Diabetes Association
State laws, reimbursement, 225
 Medicaid, 47, 241, 226-228
State social services, 47
Stimulant abuse, see Substance abuse
Stress, 155-157
 case study, 165-166
 family, and eating disorders, 159
 importance, assessment, 41-42
 learning barriers, 8
 psychosocial assessment, 26
Substance abuse, 39-40
 alcohol binges and eating disorders, 159

Suicide, 37, 149
Summative evaluation, see Outcomes
Supplies, see Reimbursement
Teaching, 3-22; see also Learning; Patient education; Patient education programs; Patient education team
 affective exercises, 11
 audiovisual aids, 10
 demonstration method, 10
 discussion method, 9-10
 educational needs assessment, 7
 empowerment approach incorporated into, 82-83
 feedback, 11
 game-playing, 10-11
 group education, 5, 8
 impact on outcomes, 3
 lecture method, 9
 literacy levels and, 125, 128-133
 one-to-one, 5, 8
 pace of, 12
 patient empowerment, twelve steps, 74-79
 patient examples in, 11
 printed materials, reading, 10
 problem definition, 76
 review (educational exercises), 12-14, 20-22
 role-playing method, 10
 "rolling with resistance" technique, 75, 83
 step-by-step approach, 76-77
 strategies, 9-11
 suggested readings, 17
Team, multidisciplinary, see Patient care team; Patient education team
Techniques in education, see Learning; Teaching
Telephones, 82
Television (patient learning styles), 8
Terminology, definitions, 208
Test of Functional Health Literacy in Adults, 127
Test strips, Medicare reimbursement, 244
Time
 medication schedule, 34
 self-management costs, 28, 30
Tobacco smoking, see Substance abuse

Tofranil, see Imipramine
Traditional medicines, 109-110
Transparencies, see Audiovisuals
Transtheoretical model of behavioral change, see Behavior change
Tranxene, see Clorazepate
TRICARE, 228
Tricyclic antidepressants, see Antidepressant medications
Type 1 diabetes, see Diabetes mellitus, type 1
Type 2 diabetes, see Diabetes mellitus, type 2
US Bureau of Primary Health Care, 228
US Centers for Medicare and Medicaid Services, 225; see also Medicaid; Medicare
CMS (HCFA) 1500 universal billing form, 245
US Civilian Health and Medical Program of the Uniformed Services, see TRICARE
US Federal Employees Health Benefit Program, 228
US Health Care Financing Administration, see US Centers for Medicare and Medicaid Services
US Indian Health Service, 228
US Veterans Administration, 228
Utilization controls, 237
Venlafaxine, 151, 152
Veterans Administration, see US Veterans Administration
Videotapes, see Audiovisual aids
Vision impairment, 47, 162
Vulnerability, see Psychology
Ways of Coping Checklist, 44
Weight, see also Eating disorders
 anxiety about, 159
 eating disorders, 39
 goals, 7
Weight loss
 depression symptoms, 37, 149
 motivational interviewing, 70
Women
 cultural aspects of food preparation, 105
 diabetes type 2, 103
 eating disorders, 38, 160
Worldview, see Culture
Xanax, see Alprazolam
Zoloft, see Sertraline
Zung Depression Scale, 36